BROILER BREEDER PRODUCTION

BY

STEVEN LEESON, Ph.D.
Professor of Animal Nutrition

Department of Animal & Poultry Science
University of Guelph
Guelph, Ontario, Canada
N1G 2W1

AND

JOHN D. SUMMER, Ph.D.
Professor Emeritus

Department of Animal & Poultry Science
University of Guelph
Guelph, Ontario, Canada
N1G 2W1

PUBLISHED BY
Context Products Ltd
53 Mill Street
Packington
Leicestershire
LE65 1WN, England

Digitally reprinted in 2013 from:

Broiler Breeder Production
University Books
P.O. Box 1326
Guelph, Ontario
Canada N1H 6N8

British Library Cataloguing in Publication Data
Broiler Breeder Production
I. Leeson, S., II. Summers, J.D.
ISBN 978-1-899043-39-2

Disclaimer

Every reasonable effort has been made to ensure that the material in this book is true, correct, complete and appropriate at the time of writing. Nevertheless, the publishers and authors do not accept responsibility for any omission or error, or for any injury, damage, loss or financial consequences arising from the use of the book.

PREFACE

Our aim in writing this book has been to assemble all the current information available on the biology, production, housing and management of broiler breeders. Management of broiler breeders has become a very specialised task, and to our knowledge there is no previous attempt at capturing all relevant information in a single text. The book is written with the commercial industry in mind because we are aware of the difficult tasks facing breeder managers and technicians in realising the genetic potential of today's breeding stock. Our experience with breeders tells us that although the information given in this book is current at the time of printing, the reader must be aware of ever changing needs and goals of the industry that have an affect on their input in breeder management. Realising this continual evolution of breeding stock management, highlights the importance of understanding the basic principles of management, and that the actual implementation of these techniques may need to be modified over time. Likewise breeders are managed successfully under a wide range of environmental conditions and feeding and disease challenge situations, and this again emphasises the need for flexibility in management techniques. While hopefully we have provided a basis for understanding the range of factors that can influence breeder performance, we also realise that you cannot manage breeders by sitting in an office. Management essentially involves looking at and understanding the birds' reaction to your production systems - there is no substitute for continual appraisal of breeder condition and behaviour, and it is this management input which invariably makes the difference between average and exceptional consistent breeder performance. Use this book as a reference, but don't forget to look at the birds.

We are once again indebted to Wendy Bauer for her major contribution in layout and production of the final manuscript. Cover design, graphic artwork and layout are expertly provided by Ford Papple Assoc., Guelph and our thanks to Martin Schwalbe for photography. Our thanks to Linda Caston, Diane Spratt, and Dr. Dick Julian for their invaluable assistance in proof reading, and lastly a special thanks to the corporate sponsors who sponsored the original publication of this book.

Steven Leeson and John Summers, Guelph
January 2000

TABLE OF CONTENTS

WARNING

Throughout this book we have mentioned various feed additives, vaccines, disinfectants and other pharmacological or chemical treatments. Not all of these products are registered in all countries, and so their legal use must be established prior to farm application. While we have mentioned numerous commercial products, we do not endorse or recommend these, and reliase that effective alternatives may be available. With any pharmacological product, vaccine or biological, it is essential to get local recommendations from qualified personnel, and to always administer products strictly according to manufacturers' label recommendations.

Steven Leeson and John Summers

Guelph, January 2000

CHAPTER 1.	INDUSTRY DEVELOPMENT, GENETICS AND BREEDING PROGRAMS
	PAGE NO.

1.1 INTRODUCTION

Current breeding strategies mean that we no longer have to worry about genetic selection of our commercial broiler breeders. Even at the grandparent level, virtually all selection for heritable traits has been accomplished by the primary breeding company. For grandparents and parent stock, we have only to select birds based on their phenotype for such traits as skeletal integrity, morbidity etc. In large part, such selection is a consequence of birds reacting to adverse environmental factors, where fitness relates to birds performing well under "commercial conditions". The breeding of broiler chickens ultimately comes down to gradual multiplication of the generations necessary to meet the ever increasing demands for broiler meat production. Each generation results in multiplication of bird numbers by factors of about 50 or 100 depending on whether one or both sexes are needed. Within a few generations, pure bred stock measured in just hundreds of birds quickly evolve into commercial broilers measured in hundreds of millions.

Virtually all the genetic selection work is accomplished by the primary breeders working with various pure-line families, and so the job of the commercial grandparent and parent breeders is essentially to expand numbers of offspring from these intensely selected birds. However this multiplication is an important and critical step in the breeding process. The management of broiler grandparent lines is a very specialized industry, and the task is given only to companies that have a history of success in breeder management and that have been carefully screened by the primary breeders. Management problems at the grandparent level have a devastating effect on the ability of a breeding company to maintain its market share of commercial broilers. Inability to meet market demand or production of inferior parent breeding stock or broiler chicks takes considerable time and effort to rectify. Problems at the grandparent breeder level often lead to regional loss in the commercial broiler market for at least 2-4 years.

As will be discussed in the following sections, the selection of broiler breeding stock involves a fine balance between optimizing growth while maintaining a competitive level of reproduction. Unfortunately, these two characteristics move in opposite directions, and consequently the broiler geneticists must develop an index that balances out all the factors of importance to most of their customers. Within a truly integrated broiler meat company, growth-type traits should be of prime concern in selecting commercial strains, while for independent broiler hatching egg or chick producers, there is always a concern about reproductive traits such as egg numbers, fertility and hatchability. Poultry breeding companies sometimes take specialization to extremes, in concentrating on particular niche market needs, or even supplying just one sex to be used within a commercial breeding program. The breeding and multiplication of broiler stocks is being conducted by fewer and larger companies each year, and this seems to parallel the natural evolution of the chicken meat industry. Fears are often raised about the shrinking genetic base that is a consequence of such specialization and amalgamation. However, it must be remembered that most of our so-called poultry breeds were developed within the last 100 years. Breeding strategies were essentially for differentiation of plumage color and body conformation, and so these strains do not have long histories on an evolutionary time scale, and it is doubtful that they possess dormant genes of potential commercial significance. Certainly the primary breeders seem to have little interest in conserving such stock, and presumably the current genetic base is of sufficiently diverse background as to enable selection for new traits should they become necessary at some future time. Coupled with this inherent genetic diversity is the potential of genetic engineering to accomplish specific goals for biodiversity.

1.2 HISTORICAL PERSPECTIVE

Consideration of poultry as a source of meat, rather than just for egg production, started in the early 1900's. The term "broiler" seems to have originated in the eastern USA describing a very young (10-12 week old) bird which was most often prepared by splitting the bird longitudinally and "broiling" over an open fire. As early as 1900 there are reports of flocks of 5000 broilers grown to 12 weeks of age for this specific market. Similar early reports indicate marketing of 700 2 lb broilers from 1000 chicks placed with a market value of 654/lb - at least growth rate and liveability have improved. Production was typically in small wooden houses, with windows, measuring just 2.5 x 3 meters housing 50-60 birds, and early photographs show rows of at least 100 of these buildings. At this time there was little specialized selection for growth rate, and even as late as 1940 there is often mention of White Leghorn males being suitable for broiler production.

BREEDS

A number of different breeds were initially used for producing meat strains suitable for the fledgling broiler industry. Initially there was emphasis on crossbreeding of several strains with focus on such traits as autocolor sexing as well as growth and meat yield.

Barred Rock: Because of its popularity at Cornell University and the University of Guelph, this breed was promoted as a meat producing bird in the early 1900's. Apart from having only moderate growth potential compared to some other breeds, a subsequent disadvantage was the dark pin feathers associated with its feather color.

White Plymouth Rock: Developed in the New England States in the 1870's, this breed was to become the choice for female lines within most breeding programs. Its main advantage was white plumage, and while initially most birds were slow feathering, this characteristic was quickly changed to the fast feathering allele.

New Hampshire: Also used on the female side of early broiler breeding programs, the New Hampshire had reasonable growth characteristics and good egg production and hatchability. As with the Barred Rock, its red/brown plumage prevented the breed from being used exclusively in the female lines of commercial programs.

White Cornish: With white feathers and yellow skin the White Cornish offered great potential for establishing white feathered broilers in the 1920's - 30's. With relatively short legs and a heavyily muscled broad breast, the breed quickly became established as a major contributor to the male lines within the breeding programs. Because of relatively poor egg production, the Cornish was little used in female lines of the 3 or 4 way crosses that were to become the most popular breeding systems.

Light Sussex: More popular in Europe, the Light Sussex was somewhat comparable to the New Hampshire in the USA, in providing a breed that could be reasonably well used in either male or female lines.

Over time, the White Cornish male crossed with the White Plymouth Rock female became the basis for most broiler breeding programs. In addition to being white feathered, the cross gave an excellent balance of growth, conformation and livability together with a reasonably good level of reproduction.

The modern broiler industry started in the Delmarva region of the USA in the mid 1930's. Inducements into this new industry were a general decline in the traditional shell fishing and fruit growing industries of this region, together with the fact that there was a large local market that could easily be served with supply of fresh product. The move from egg to meat production was also hastened due to the fact that Leghorn birds were experiencing high mortality from what was later to be known as Marek's disease. At this time, the broiler strains seemed more resistant to the disease, a fact likely associated with the much shorter life-cycle of the new fast growing birds. New Hampshire also quickly developed a new broiler industry, although this New England region was soon to become more important as the location of many influential primary breeding companies. The willingness of primary breeders to locate in this area was greatly helped by an active and effective pullorum testing program. While the North Eastern USA was quickly becoming a leader in broiler production, Georgia was one of the first to apply sharecropping systems to broiler production. As farms became larger with 10,000+ birds, the local feed dealer became the major source of credit. There was a move to also supply chicks on credit, and so there was a natural development of tying chick and feed sales together, and this became the basis for contract production and integration within the industry.

During World War II, the Delmarva region accounted for almost 50% of the chicken meat production in the USA, with much of this contracted to the government. At the end of the war, the government cancelled these contracts, and this placed considerable pressure on an industry that was grossly overproducing for local needs. Competition quickly resulted in the development of even larger farms.

Improvements in nutrition, housing and disease control helped the broiler producers to realize the continually improving genetic potential of the bird. The early years of the broiler industry coincided with the discovery of many trace nutrients, such as some critical B vitamins, and because the chicken was such as easy animal to work with, a wealth of information developed on the nutrient needs of the young bird. Dr. H.M. Scott, at Connecticut was an advocate of higher energy diets for meat birds, and corn became the cereal of choice in broiler diets. Together with soybean meal, corn provided the basis for diets fed to the majority of broilers grown world-wide.

As bird numbers increased, processing became a limitation and innovators such as Gordon-Johnson in New England met the demand by developing automated equipment. Subsequent major growth in the industry has occurred in response to needs for further processing and here Harland Sanders with Kentucky Fried chicken in the 1960's and McDonalds Corp., with their Chicken McNugget in the 1980's typified the general thrust of the expanding industry. Today we continue to see yearly improvements in genetic potential of the bird, although it is obvious that this phenomenal trend cannot continue indefinitely. Table 1.1 indicates the changing pattern of broiler performance throughout its brief history.

A corollary of this improved genetic potential has been the consolidation of primary breeding companies. At the present time (1999) there are only seven companies world-wide that are major international suppliers of broiler breeding stock.

TABLE 1.1 Growth characteristics of mixed-sex broilers grown to typical "market weights"

Time period	Age (days)	Live wt (kg)	Live wt gain (g/day)	Feed: Gain	Mortality (%)
1920's	120	1.0	8	5.0	20
1930's	100	1.2	12	4.6	15
1940's	85	1.4	17	4.0	10
1950's	75	1.5	20	3.2	8
1960's	70	1.6	23	2.5	8
1970's	60	1.9	32	2.2	5
1980's	50	2.2	44	2.0	5
1990's	50	2.6	51	1.9	4

1.3 GENETIC SELECTION

The primary breeding companies carry out intense selection on very valuable birds maintained within small family groups. The numbers of birds owned by primary breeders are exceptionally small in comparison to the numbers that will eventually be generated as offspring through 3 or 4 generations of multiplication. In fact, most large scale commercial broiler farms will house as many birds as are handled by a primary breeder.

In developing or maintaining a strain of broilers, geneticists must consider a balance of characteristics related to growth vs reproduction (Table 1.2).

The various traits (characteristics) outlined in Table 1.2 are influenced by the genetic make-up of the bird. Unfortunately phenotypic traits are only partially influenced by inherited genetic material, the other major factor being the bird's "environment".

TABLE 1.2 Characteristics most often considered in selecting pure-line breeders

Growth related	Reproduction
Growth rate	Egg number
Weight-for-age	Egg size
Feed efficiency	Hatchability of fertile eggs
Meat (breast) yield	Fertility
Carcass yield and body conformation	Libido
Livability	Mature weight and age
Skeletal integrity	Liveability
Feathering - cover, rate and color	Aggressiveness (±)
Adaptation to heat distress	Adaptation to heat distress

In this context, environment means non-genetic influences such as nutrition, environmental temperature, stocking density, egg size, incubation conditions etc. The balance of variation between individual birds caused by genetics relative to total variance is termed heritability.

$$\text{Heritability (H)} = \frac{\text{genetic variance}}{\text{observed variance}}$$

The heritability for growth characteristics (Table 1.2) is quite high, being in the order of 0.4-0.6 (or 40-60%). This means that fairly rapid progress can be made by simply selecting as breeders, the heaviest birds in a flock. Reproductive traits (Table 1.2) on the other hand have much lower heritabilities of 0.05-0.20, meaning that the selection of a hen based on its own egg production record is a very slow process for improving overall egg production in her progeny.

There is a common misconception that a heritability of 0.5, for growth rate for example, means that we can increase the growth potential of a bird by 0.5 (50%) each generation. In reality, the response to selection for each generation is defined as H^2x selection differential. The selection differential is the difference between the selected individuals and the average of the flock. For example some male birds are selected because they are 200g heavier than the flock average. Heritability for growth is 0.5, and so selection response will be 0.5^2x200 = 50g. Due to genetic selection, the next generation can be expected to be 50g heavier than the mean of the two parent lines. The male only provides 50% of the genetic material to his offspring, and so this effect is further diluted by the selection response that can be applied on the female line. The bottom line is that the 25-50g increase each year in weight-for-age that we have seen is our broilers over the last 15-20 years is rather a remarkable achievement by the primary breeders. This situation is even more impressive when consideration is also being given to so many different traits (Table 1.2) in a breeding program.

Within the male lines of a breeding program, the growth related characteristics receive major emphasis. Traditionally growth rate or more specifically body weight at a specific age has been the major criterion for selection. During early development of broiler strains, it was fairly easy to make rapid progress with this trait. Over time however the geneticist is confronted with metabolic problems associated with fast growth rate, and also reproduction starts to decline. There is little doubt that metabolic disorders such as ascites, SDS and skeletal abnormalities are a function of growth rate per se rather than the bird having to carry a heavy weight at any specific age. These traits will have some genetic basis, and primary breeders now have to consider these potential problems as being negatively correlated with growth rate. Metabolic disorders are best observed in very fast growing birds, and this poses a special problem for geneticists who will want to select certain birds for subsequent breeding. Successful reproduction in heavy meat birds is achieved through body weight control that is usually achieved through feed restriction. In genetic selection programs, birds must be grown under commercial broiler-type conditions to about 42-49d and the heaviest birds are selected. These selected birds must then be managed as potential breeder candidates through the remainder of the growing period and as adult breeders. This usually means exceptionally heavy feed restriction, because, the broiler weight at 49d is little different from "desired" mature weight at 22-24 weeks. This type of fast early growth rate is now even more essential when geneticists attempt to select birds with metabolic problems, because they are best identified using pelleted diets of high nutrient density.

Modern broiler breeding programs now also place major emphasis on carcass conformation and meat yield, as well as feed efficiency. Breast conformation has traditionally been determined through measurement of breast angle. While this is still an important attribute influencing breast conformation that may influence breast blisters, breast meat yield is now of greater importance and can really only be ascertained from carcass dissection. It is very difficult and expensive to determine breast muscle size on a live bird, and this trait is a general example of a selection problem that is best solved through sib or progeny testing. Sib testing involves observations on brothers or sisters while progeny testing involves measuring traits of the offspring from the potential breeder. Although such testing is very expensive and time consuming, the changes in bird type in response to such selection are now obvious in the so-called "yield" broilers available today.

Currently most breeding companies also undertake measurements of feed efficiency in the pedigree birds. As shown in Table 1.1, feed efficiency of broilers has improved dramatically during the time period that birds have been heavily selected for growth rate. In large part, this improvement in efficiency has been due to an ever decreasing age for a specific weight, and this translates into less feed being used for maintenance and more being directed towards growth. However, feed efficiency per se has a heritability of around 0.25 and so there should be fairly rapid progress in selecting directly for this trait. Birds of the same weight at a comparable age, may have different feed efficiencies. Differences in efficiency, independent of weight-for-age, may be caused by differential digestibility or metabolizability of nutrients, differences in carcass composition (more fat leads to reduced feed efficiency) or more heat loss due to poorer feathering or more activity. Measurement of feed efficiency is very difficult to achieve. Birds to be selected can be held in small individual pens, and feed intake measured over a 10-14d period. Birds can also be maintained in cages for these tests. While caged broilers often grow more slowly than floor-reared birds, the genetic selection process essentially involves finding birds that are above average for any trait, so even in cages, relative growth or feed efficiency can be ascertained.

As previously discussed, a pedigree breeding program must retain a balance between growth and reproductive traits. There is a negative correlation between growth rate and reproductive traits such as egg numbers and fertility. To some extent, we can correct this problem by not allowing breeders to reach their genetic potential for growth by using techniques such as physical feed restriction. As roosters get heavier there is greater semen yield. Generally however this semen contains more dead or abnormal sperm that have a lower metabolic rate, and so are less motile. Heavier males also have reduced libido. In hens, there is a positive relationship between body size and Erratic Ovulation and Defective Egg Syndrome (EODES). Erratic ovulation leads to multiple ovulations, meaning that 2 or more ova are released from the ovary at one time. Two ova in the oviduct can lead to double yolked eggs or slab-sided eggs, both of which will fail to hatch if fertile. With multiple ovulation, some ova can completely miss the opening of the oviduct, and end up in the body cavity leading to peritonitis. Heavy breeders also have a higher incidence of shell defects, such as "rough-ends", extra calcification, loss of pigmentation etc. all of which cause loss in hatchability. The female lines of the pedigree program must therefore be carefully selected so as to minimize these problems of reproduction. Egg size is also an important characteristic, because this influences chick size and subsequent growth rate of the commercial broiler. During incubation, egg size influences rate of moisture loss, because of the associated relationship to egg surface area. Consistency of egg size is therefore also very important in commercial breeders. Most of these egg characteristics are correlated with mature body size of the hen. This means that it is very difficult to convince a small-bodied bird to lay an egg of optimum size, while for very heavy birds it is often difficult to temper egg size during the latter part of the production cycle.

Table 1.2 mentions liveability as an important characteristic of both broilers and adult breeders, and there is a genetic basis for resistance to some diseases. Inherent genetic resistance to disease, together with isolation, eradication and vaccination/medication programs form the basis of broiler health management. Heritability of resistance to certain diseases is quite high, for example, with Marek's disease the value is around 0.5-0.6. However heritability of general liveability in young birds (0-6 wks) is quite low at around 0.01. Selection for disease resistance is again difficult to implement, because it necessarily involves sib or progeny testing and challenging these birds with pathogens. Such testing must obviously be carried out under strict isolation.

In mammals, the male dictates the sex of its offspring. In birds however the situation is reversed and it is the hen's genetic make-up that dictates sex of the embryo. The sex chromosomes are usually described as the Z and W chromosomes, with males being homogametic (ZZ) and females heterogametic (ZW). For females, this is sometimes written as Z- rather than ZW. The difference in the sex chromosomes can be used to advantage in order to identify the sex of the bird or to manipulate some other traits. Having feathers of different color in the male and female was a popular system of "autosexing" in traditional crossbred birds. An example of the technique utilizes the genes for gold vs silver feathering. Silver (S) is dominant to gold (s). This means that a bird will be silver if it carries the silver gene on one or both of the chromosome pairs. With two dominant silver genes, the bird is said to be homozygous silver (SS). If the bird carries a silver gene on one chromosome and a gold on the other, it is heterozygous (Ss), but still appears silver because silver is dominant (or gold is recessive). When these genes are on the sex chromosome, we can use the dominant/ recessive characteristics to differentiate sex of the offspring. For example, a cross between a gold feathered male and a silver female, will result in the following:

Parent	<u>Male</u> ss(Gold)	x	<u>Female</u> S-(Silver)
Offspring	Ss(Silver)		s- (Gold)

For the parent male to have gold feathering, means it must have two recessive gold genes. The female has only "one" sex chromosome, and this must carry the dominant silver gene, because phenotypically she is silver feathered. The male offspring must carry the gene pair, and this will always be Ss, with the silver color being dominant. The female offspring will be gold because these are the only genes held by the male parent. The offspring can therefore be color sexed at day of age. A number of other feather colors and characteristics can also be used to color sex chicks. While a few modern primary breeders have developed color-sexed broiler lines, this system has not been used extensively in commercial production.

An alternative system of sexing relies on genes for rate of feathering, rather than feather color, although the basic genetic principles are very similar. Rate of development of feathers is quite variable in birds, and within an unselected population there can be up to 4 weeks variation in the age at which birds progress through various feather molts. Most birds undergo 4-6 molts, involving the feather down, chick feathers, 1-3 generations of juvenile feathers and finally the adult plumage. The rate of feather development is influenced by a sex-linked recessive gene and while the gene affects the growth rate of all feathers, the most noticeable differences are in the wing and tail regions. Slow feathering (K) is dominant to fast feathering (k). Slow feathering birds can therefore be KK or Kk in males or K-in females. Chicks from these parents characteristically have wing coverts which are as long or longer than the primaries. Rapid feathering male, (kk) or female (k-) chicks on the other hand have primary wing feathers that are longer than the coverts. With an appropriate cross therefore, we can produce male and female chicks with different feathering characteristics, and this trait can be used to sex chicks. As shown with the previous example, using color sexing, the color of the male and female chicks is exactly opposite to that of their corresponding male and female parents. The same situation applies with rate of feathering. We are interested in producing fast feathering female chicks and slow feathering male chicks. This means that we will have to cross a fast feathering male breeder with a slow feathering hen.

Parent	<u>Male</u> kk(fast feathering)	x	<u>Female</u> K-(slow feathering)
Offspring	Kk(slow feathering)		k-(fast feathering)

Each generation effectively "reverses" the phenotypic characteristic of the sex-linked traits, and so at each generation back through the breeding program, traits such as rate of feathering have to be changed from the male to the female side of the program. For example, in the above mating, the slow feathering female parent would herself be produced from a grand-parent line that involved a slow feathering male and fast feathering female. At the great-grandparent level, the feathering characteristics are again reversed. Alternatively the various lines have to be homozygous for either fast or slow feathering, and lines are vent-sexed up to this final cross.

A number of primary breeding companies also produce dwarf lines of broiler breeders. Birds carrying only the dwarf (dw) gene are up to 30% smaller in size than regular sized birds (Dw). The dwarf gene (dw) is recessive to Dw, and so the size effect can be corrected with an appropriate mating system:

Parent	<u>Male</u> DwDw (regular)	X	<u>Female</u> dw- (dwarf)
Offspring	Dwdw, (regular male)		Dw- (regular female)

The advantage in using the dwarf female parent is that because she is about 25% smaller in body size, her feed intake is proportionally less. Birds carrying the dwarf gene also seem to be somewhat more resistant to heat stress, a situation possibly related to the fact that these dwarfs are hypothyrotic. Because the Dw gene is dominant to the dw dwarf gene, the male broiler offspring (Dwdw) are regular size. In practice however, the Dw gene is not 100% dominant to the dw gene, and so male broiler offspring are about 97% the size of the regular broiler. The grandparent lines for the dwarf mating can be alternated so as to produce dwarf or regular size breeder hens. If the primary breeder wishes to produce dwarf parent females, then a dwarf male grandparent is used. However if there is need to produce regular sized female parents, then the dwarf grandparent males can quickly be replaced with regular (DwDw) grandparent males. Therefore by simply substituting the male grandparent at various times, the characteristics (needed for different markets) of the female parent breeder can be easily manipulated, using a single flock of grandparent hens.

As previously discussed the primary breeder has to maintain a balance between all of the traits of economic significance. In most situations breeding programs involve steady progress in selection for a variety of characteristics. Periodically new genes have to be introduced within lines, and this is a very difficult task to accomplish because concurrently there can be no loss of other established important traits. A good example of this, was the introduction of the sex linked gene for rate of feathering. If the lines being used do not carry the gene, then it had to be introduced by adding new birds into the population. If these new birds are different from the established line for any trait, then that trait will change correspondingly over time. The geneticist therefore has to introduce new genetic material over a number of generations so as not to compromise traits of economic importance.

The success of various strains of broiler are to some extent a reflection of the balance of traits achieved by the geneticist. Some strains are known to excel in certain traits, but perhaps have weakness in other areas, whereas another strain may not excel in any one trait but rather have an excellent balance of all characteristics of economic importance. The relative value of different traits is usually changing, in keeping with changes in the breeder, broiler and meat industries. For example carcass meat yield, and especially breast meat yield is now a very important economic trait, whereas it was rarely considered in breeding programs 10 years ago. To some extent the geneticists have to be able to predict future market trends, because in most pure line breeding programs selection occurs some 4-5 years in advance of their offspring appearing as commercial broilers. Carte (1986) provided an interesting comparison of traits that may be considered in a breeding program (Table 1.3).

These data suggest that, all other factors remaining the same, then a +0.18 kg increase in live weight at a specific market age will reduce overall costs by 14/ kg broiler live weight produced. Increasing carcass yield by 1% has the same economic benefit etc. Of particular interest are the relatively large changes that have to occur at the breeder level in order to bring about the same economic return. For example, obtaining an extra 29 hatching eggs from every breeder is equivalent (economically) to reducing feed efficiency in all broilers by 0.05 units. An alternative way of expressing this comparison is to suggest that an integrated operation could give up 29 hatching eggs per breeder if the result was -0.05 units improvement in feed efficiency of commercial broilers. In reality the integrator could give up say 15-20 eggs because there would be no economic advantage to reducing output by 29 eggs, because this equals -0.05 units F:G (Table 1.3). However these types of calculations are necessary in order to determine the relative economic worth of various strains, and for selection of traits within a strain.

TABLE 1.3 Relative economic values within an integrated broiler operation, where costs are equivalent to about 14/kg live weight

A. Broiler traits:	+0.18 kg live weight -0.05 feed:gain +1% carcass yield -1.2% condemnation -2.2% liveability
B. Broiler breeder traits:	+29 hatching eggs +16% hatchability all eggs set -1.2kg feed/dozen eggs -164/dozen hatching eggs -14 kg breeder feed
	Carte (1986)

Because most broiler growth traits are more highly heritable than are the reproductive traits, then it is tempting to place more emphasis on these, because progress can be made more quickly. Unfortunately not all customers of the primary breeders are integrated companies, and not all integrated companies are truly integrated in their organization of profit centres. Consequently the reproductive characteristics remain very important in a breeding program, and to date there has been no really successful broiler strain that has poor reproductive characteristics.

1.4 COMMERCIAL BREEDING PROGRAMS

Most commercial broiler chickens are produced by a so-called "4-way cross". This essentially means that the broilers are derived from four different grandparent lines. Figure 1.1 shows a schematic representation of such a program, and the numbers involved indicate flock sizes necessary to generate 500,000,000 commercial broilers annually.

It is very unusual for primary breeding companies to sell great-grandparent stock, and so for most integrated companies the breeding program will start at the grandparent or even parent level depending upon the size of the operation. At each generation there is multiplication of numbers by approximately 50 because only one sex is retained for the program.

Figure 1.1 Commercial breeding programs to produce 500 million broilers

	Male Lines				Female Lines		
Pure lines or Great Grandparents	A♂ x A♀		B♂ x B♀		C♂ x C♀		D♂ x D♀
Grandparents (GP's)	AA♂		BB♀		CC♂		DD♀
	5,000		20,000		16,000		100,000
(Selection)	↓		↓		↓		↓
	2,000	X	15,000		8,000	X	80,000
Parents (PS)		AB♂ 400,000		X		CD♀ 4,000,000	
Commercial Broilers				ABCD♂,♀ 500,000,000			

The pure lines, or great grandparents will essentially come from birds not retained by the primary breeder. For example, in the pure line A male (Fig 1.1), the primary breeder will be selecting the top 5-6% of birds (based on traits considered important by the geneticists) for reproducing the next generation of this line. Of the remaining pureline birds, some 40-60% could be used for production of great-grandparent chicks. In general, males from within male lines will be selected more heavily than females within this line, or from males within the female line (D, Fig 1.1). The great-grandparents are therefore very close in genetic make-up to the pure lines, and for this reason breeding companies rarely allow these birds outside of their immediate control. However where customers require large numbers of parent breeders, it becomes more logical to consider the purchase of grandparents or great-grandparents if allowed. The choice of entry into the breeding system depends largely on the numbers of birds involved. For example in Figure 1.1, it would be impractical for a single customer to purchase 4 million PS ♀'s and 400,000 PS ♂'s needed to generate 500 million broilers annually. With this scale of operation, it is more logical to purchase about 100,000 of the various GP ♂ and ♀ chicks. These numbers could be reduced by a factor of about 50, if great grandparents (GGP's) were purchased for the initial part of the program.

In the example shown in Figure 1.1, it requires about 4 million PS ♀'s and 400,000 PS ♂'s to produce the 500 million broiler chickens. At this level there is very little selection carried out. Obviously deformed or runted birds will be culled, which together with normal mortality will only account for about 3-4% of chicks placed depending upon local disease challenge. At the grandparent level however, some breeding companies suggest an intensive selection, especially in the males. In males from the male line (A, Figure 1.1) only about 40% of chicks placed will be selected as breeder candidates. For males of the female line (D, Figure 1.1) selection is slightly less intense, but still only 50% of males will be moved to the breeding pens. For males the main selection criteria will be growth rate, general body conformation and leg/foot condition. Other breeding companies recommend no such selection of their GP's, their position being that genetic selection per se has been carried out at the GGP level, and the GP customer should only have to deal with culling based on "environmental" variance within a flock.

As one progresses back through the breeding program, then obviously the economic value of the stock increases. Figure 1.2 shows average industry costs for day-old chicks at various levels in the breeding program.

Figure 1.2 Day-old chick costs of grandparent and parent breeders ($US)

	Male line		Female line		Total investment for 500 million broiler chickens
Grandparents (GP's)	AA♂ $30	BB♀ $30	CC♂ $22	DD♀ $18	$2.9m
	↓		↓		or
Parent (PS)	AB♂ $3.50		CD♀ $2.30		$10.6m
					or
Commercial Broiler	500,000,000 $0.25				$125m

Male line grandparent chicks are valued at about $30 each, and these are the most expensive birds in the breeding program. However relatively few of the chicks are needed relative to the female line chicks, and the major capital expense becomes the D-line female chicks of the female line. In order to produce 500 million broiler chicks, the capital cost of grandparent breeding stock is around \$2.9m (Figure 1.2). At the parent level, the male chicks are again the most expensive at \$3.50 each, but again the numbers of female chicks required make them the most expensive overall. For production of the same 500 million broiler chicks, day-old chick cost of parent breeders is around \$10m. The 500 million day-old broiler chicks themselves will be valued at around \$125 m.

In practice the breeding program is usually complicated by the need to sustain continuous production of parent breeder chicks and commercial broiler chicks. Under exceptional circumstances when there are seasonal fluctuations in demand for breeder or broiler chicks, then scheduling is made even more difficult. For continuous uninterrupted production, flocks must be scheduled at regular intervals. With the example shown in Figure 1.1, there would need to be 5-6 flocks, of each line, delivered annually. For the D-line female, this means, for example, 6 flocks each of about 17,000 birds received at 8 week intervals. Obviously corresponding numbers of chicks in the other 3 lines must also be received at the same time. Figure 1.3 shows a schematic representation of such scheduling of D-line females.

In this example we have assumed purchase of 100,000 birds annually, delivered as 6 flocks of 16-17,000 birds each. This means deliveries every 2 months, and each shipment will need 3 grower houses. With a 1 month clean-out of the grower house, there is a need for 9 houses in total, since each group of 3 houses is used for each 4th delivery of chicks. Assuming a 20 week growing cycle and a 10 month breeder cycle, then there needs to be 18 breeder houses to accommodate the mature birds. For the breeder houses, a 2 month clean-out is scheduled to allow for any unforseen delays or problems. Obviously appropriate facilities are required for growing the roosters. If this is a grand-parent facility, then corresponding facilities are required for the other male line breeders, with deliveries arriving at the same times. As with any scheduling exercise, there are pros and cons to having a shorter or longer time between each delivery of day-old chicks. The more frequent the intake of new flocks, the greater the potential of continuous production of eggs and chicks. In the example shown in Figure 1.3, there is only one breeder house empty for clean-out at any one time and there is always production of eggs from different ages of breeder flock. With larger breeder flocks, there will be problems with major effects due to clean-out and turn around, and more variable size of egg and chick produced because of more distinct differences in breeder flock age. Whatever system is used, the hatchery has to be prepared to always handle eggs from breeders of various ages.

Figure 1.3 Scheduling of breeder flocks for placement of 100,000 birds annually. Deliveries of 16-17,000 birds each 2 months, with about 6,000 birds per house. Bird numbers dictate need for 9 growing houses and 18 breeder houses.

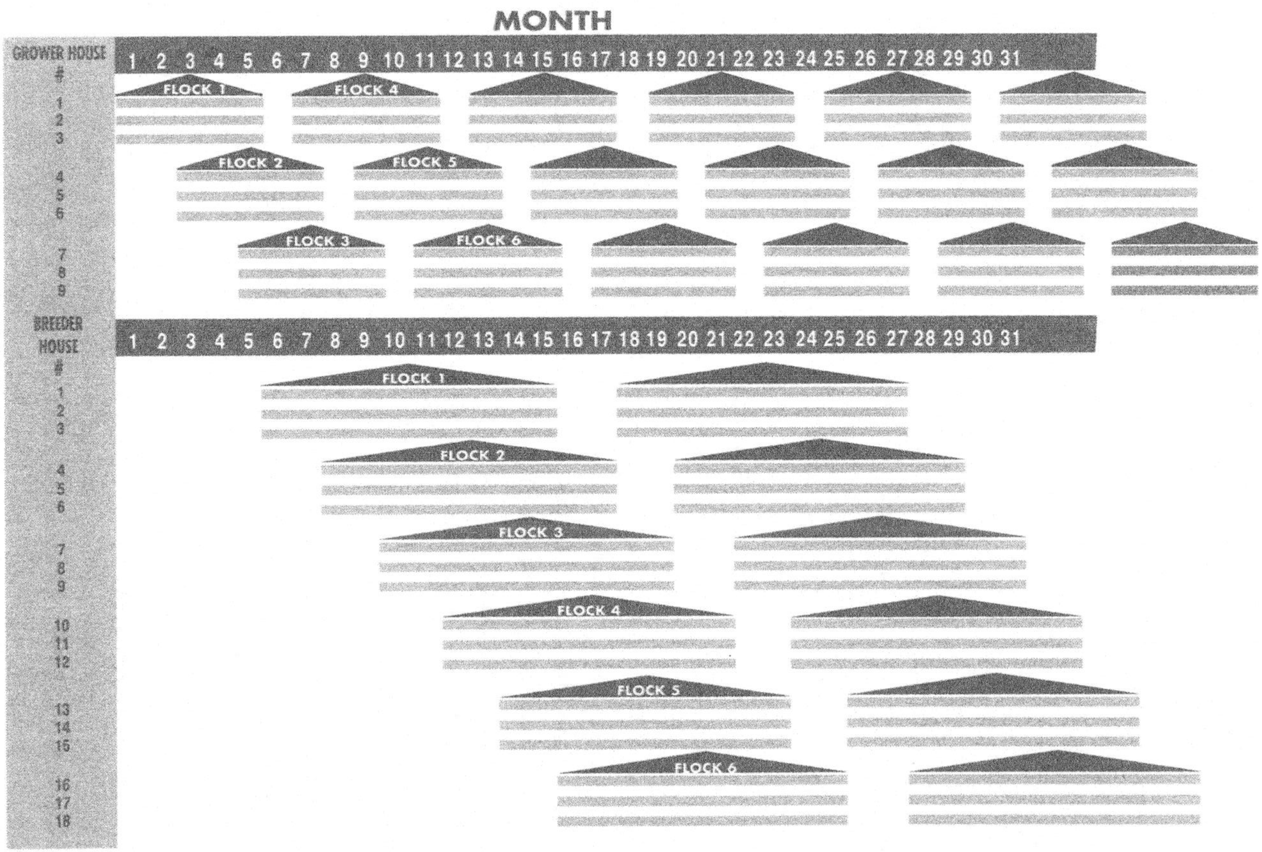

As previously indicated in Figure 1.1, at the pure-line and grandparent level there is selection of the heaviest and fittest male breeders. In part, this selection is for superior growth rate of male offspring, which will eventually result in better growth of male broilers. The same concept could be applied to commercial breeding programs, but this is a very rare occurrence.

It must also be remembered that not all pureline and grandparent day-old male chicks are used as breeders. Selection of only 30-50% of the male birds is based on physical characteristics, and body weight. Because growth rate is quite highly heritable (0.4 - 0.5) then selecting heavier males is expected to have a positive effect on the growth of their offspring. This concept is often applied in commercial turkey breeding programs, but is rarely used with commercial broiler breeders. In selecting the heaviest 25% of a flock of male breeders (PS) at 3 weeks Van Wambeke *et al.* (1979) showed a consistent improvement in growth rate and feed efficiency of their offspring compared to broilers sired by the remainder of the breeder flock. The improved growth rate averaged 1.7%, while feed efficiency was improved by .004 units. If each selected male is ultimately mated to 12 hens each producing 140, 2kg broilers, then a 1.7% improvement in growth equates to an extra 57kg liveweight generated from the superior males. This extra liveweight is also realized on 26kg less feed assuming a feed:gain of 2.0.If broiler liveweight is $1/kg and feed price is 204/kg, then the advantage of the superior males to an integrated broiler company is (57x1.0) + (26x0.2) = $62.2. Selecting the top 25% males, effectively means that 3 males will be discarded, for each superior male selected at 3-4 weeks. If male chick price is $4.00, then there is a "loss" of $12.00 for the discarded males (that could be marketed as broilers). Assuming a $12 loss due to selection, then the advantage to the system becomes about $50 per male placed in the breeder house.

BIBLIOGRAPHY

Cahaner, A. and P.B. Siegel, 1986. Evaluation of industry breeding programs for meat-type chickens and turkeys in Proc 3rd Wld. Congr. Genetics Appl. Livestock Prod.

Carte, I.F., 1986. Genetic economics of chicken meat production in Proc. 3rd Wld Congr. Genetics Appl. Livestock Prod. Vol. 10 pp 228-235.

Hunton, P., 1990. Industrial breeding and selection in Poultry Breeding and Genetics, Ed. Crawford, Publ. Elsevier

Marks, H.L., 1995. Genetics of growth and development in Poultry Production, Ed. Hunton, Publ. Elsevier.

Siegel, P.B. and E.A. Dunnington, 1987. Selection for growth in chickens. Critical Reviews Poult. Biol. 1:1-24.

Van Wambeke, F., R. Moormans and G. De Groote, 1979. Early body weight selection of broiler breeder males in relation to reproductive and growth performance of their offspring. Br. Poult. Sci. 20:565-570.

CHAPTER 2. REPRODUCTION	
	PAGE NO.

Managing the reproductive processes of the hen and rooster is the basis of broiler breeder production. An understanding of the basic reproductive physiology of both sexes is important in applying management principles involving feeding, lighting and health management. Following is an overview of reproductive processes in both sexes which are to some extent subject to manipulation by the breeder manager.

2.1 STRUCTURE OF THE OVARY AND OVIDUCT

The mature hen has only one ovary and oviduct even though left and right reproductive systems are evident during very early incubation. Unlike the situation with testes in the male, the right ovary and oviduct regress during mid-incubation, and are non-functional in all "normal" hens.

The left ovary is found deep in the body cavity lying in close proximity to the left kidney. During incubation as many as 20,000 eggs develop, of which about 2,000 are visible to the naked eye. There should be minimal development of these oocytes in the growing pullet, and consequently the ovary should be fairly difficult to find during necropsy. During maturation, a hierarchy of ovum will develop so as to supply a sequence of eggs for daily ovulation. In the mature hen the ovary should weigh around 35g, being composed of 3-4 large "maturing" follicles, and a series of 8-12 follicles of ever diminishing size. The follicles consist of concentric layers of "yolk" that are continually being deposited. If fat soluble dyes of different color are given to the hen daily, then daily concentric deposits are clearly visible if the follicle is bisected. The greatest mass of the follicle, which comprises about 50% fat and 50% protein per unit of dry matter, is deposited in the last 3-4d prior to the follicle being ovulated.

If follicles fail to ovulate, then they start to regress which can involve gradual re-absorption or rupture and loss of contents into the body cavity which itself can contribute to peritonitis. Such regression of the follicle is most commonly caused by molting or under feeding. The oviduct is not attached to the ovary, and so when follicles are released they must "fall" into the funnel shaped opening of the oviduct called the infundibulum. Follicles that fail to reach the oviduct are lost into the body cavity which most commonly occurs with multiple ovulations (see Chapter 2, Section 2.4) which unfortunately is a more common occurrence in broiler breeders rather than Leghorn hens. The infundibulum also contains sperm storage glands (see Chapter 2, Section 2.6). Albumen is formed in the next region of the oviduct known as the magnum while the shell membranes are deposited in the mid isthmus region. The egg spends the majority of its time in the shell gland, where over 15-18 hours the shell material is gradually deposited. The shell pigments are finally deposited during the last 2-3h before egg laying.

2.2 OVULATION

Ideally, breeders will lay eggs on a consistent cycle with a minimum of non-laying days. At peak production, we routinely see flocks laying at 85-87%, and periodically individual flocks reach 90% production for 10-14d. This sustained high rate of production means that birds are ovulating close to a 24h cycle. The release of the follicle from the ovary is controlled by hormones produced within the pituitary and the follicles themselves, and both are under control of the lighting schedule (see Chapter 3). As the largest, or so-called F1 follicle, in the ovary "matures", its production of hormones changes resulting in greater output of progesterone. This change itself is controlled by output of luteinising hormone from the brain, which is controlled by the light/dark cycle. The release of luteinising hormone from the brain only occurs during a 6-8h period each day, and this is influenced by the pattern of light:dark each day. It is the failure to release luteinising hormone in this "window" that results in a non-egg laying day, or a pause in the clutch sequence.

2.3 CLUTCH LENGTH AND PATTERNS OF OVULATION/ OVIPOSITION

Like most birds, the broiler breeder hen produces her eggs in the form of clutches, which are eggs produced on consecutive days. With the selection for high sustained peak egg numbers of today's breeder strains, we now have quite extensive clutch sizes. Clutches of eggs are separated by 1 or 2 days of non-ovulation, and so the length of the clutch in relation to the non-egg days, dictates the maximum possible rate of production (Figure 2.1).

Figure 2.1 Egg production relative to clutch length

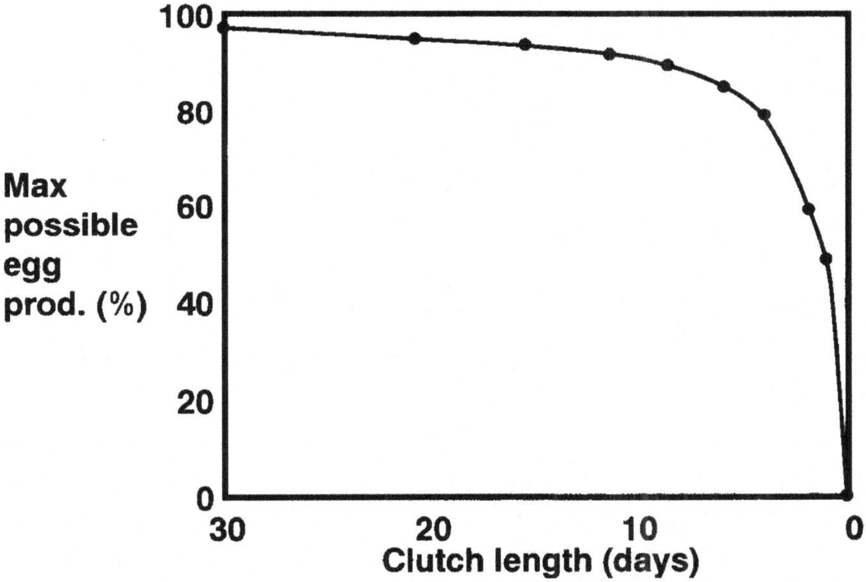

In this example, the longest clutch length shown is 30 days. This large clutch size results in 96.7% egg production, because 30 eggs are produced each 31d assuming a single non-ovulatory day between clutches. For breeders at 85% production, the mean clutch length of the flock will be between 7-8 eggs. With breeders in cages, we sometimes see sustained clutches of 30-40 eggs, and clutches of 15-20 eggs are quite common. This means that a considerable number of birds must have very erratic and/or short clutch sizes. As breeders get older, the clutch size declines naturally, and this is the reason for the observed decline in flock production over time.

Long sustained clutches are only possible when successive ovipositions (egg laying) lag each other by only a short time. Table 2.1 shows the type of pattern that can be expected for birds laying clutches of 9 (90% production), 5 (83% production) or 3 (75% production) eggs in a sequence.

TABLE 2.1 Time of day of egg laying in relation to clutch length assuming lights on 5:00 - 22:00 h

Successive days	9 egg clutch	5 egg clutch	3 egg clutch
1	6:00	6:30	7:00
2	7:00	8:30	11:00
3	8:00	10:30	15:00
4	9:00	12:30	None
5	10:00	14:30	7:00
6	11:00	None	11:00
7	12:00	6:30	15:00
8	13:00	8:30	None
9	14:00	10:30	7:00
10	None	12:30	11:00
11	6:00	14:30	15:00
12	7:00	None	None

Birds will obviously not lay with such precise timing each day but these types of patterns will appear at the different levels of production. The cumulative lag for the clutch is about 8h as shown in Table 2.1, meaning that the first and last egg in the clutch is separated by about 8h. After accumulating a lag of 8h, the "window" of time for release of luteinizing hormone does not correspond to development of the F1 follicle or the light program, and so there is a one day pause. Release of the follicle is restricted to the time of about 5:00→14:00h, assuming "lights-on" at 5:00h. Following the pause (one day in Table 2.1), the F1 follicle is again ovulated early in the cycle, such that the clutch of eggs is repeated, in sequence.

The time of egg laying as shown in Table 2.1 influences a number of management situations, and especially egg collection. With "lights-on" occurring early in the morning it is obvious that the higher the egg production (or the younger the flock usually), the greater the number of eggs that will be laid before 12 noon. It is this longer clutch length of younger birds that dictates the usual management practice of needing at least one conventional type nest per 4 breeder hens. The first egg of a longer clutch is usually laid earlier in the day (Table 2.1). For young flocks at peak-production, this can cause some problems of conflict between the desire of the bird to nest versus the urge to feed. With lights on at 5 a.m., there will (should) be active feeding for the first 30-40 minutes, followed by continuous but less active feeding, until clean-up some 2-4h later. For some birds the desire to feed is greater than the desire to seek out a nest, and consequently eggs are dropped along the feeder line. This should only be a problem for first eggs within a long clutch that are laid early in the day, but does undoubtedly contribute to floor egg production. If there are more than 1% eggs found on the slats around the hen feeders, then this is a good indication that initial feeding time is too late in relation to the time of "lights-on".

The position of the egg in a clutch also affects its physical characteristics, and also possibly the chances of producing a viable chick. Eggs laid early in the day tend to be larger, while eggs laid later (end of clutch) tend to have more shell material (Table 2.2).

TABLE 2.2 Egg and shell weight as affected by time of lay

Time of lay (h)	Egg wt. (g)	Shell wt. (g)	Shell wt. (as % egg wt.)
7:00-9:00	65.2	5.93	9.1
9:00-11:00	63.5	5.73	9.0
11:00-13:00	63.3	5.76	9.1
13:00-15:00	64.0	5.99	9.4
15:00-17:00	64.7	6.12	9.5
17:00-19:00	62.9	6.08	9.7

Adapted from Brake (1985)

While large eggs are helpful in maximizing chick size, and especially with young breeders, there is an indication that first eggs within a clutch have a slightly higher rate of embryo mortality. This may be due to longer retention time of the "first" egg within the oviduct (+2h) where "pre-incubation" causes higher embryo mortality. Robinson *et al.* (1991) recorded 78.7 vs 83.2% ($P<.05$) hatchability for first vs subsequent eggs within a clutch. Because this is a characteristic of only the first egg in a clutch, it indicates the incentive to attain as long a clutch sequence as possible because this mathematically reduces the proportion of this type of egg. High rates of egg production are often associated with good hatchability and vice versa, and clutch length may play some role in this relationship. It is theoretically possible to select for increased egg production by selecting hens that have shown long clutch length *ie.* short time between successive ovipositions. This is best achieved by selecting hens under conditions of continuous lighting, so as to potentially extend the length of the normal clutch seen within a regular light program. This experimental situation works well with Leghorn birds. However with broiler breeders, because of the need to impose a restricted feeding program, the birds entrain to the daily routine of feeding, and so this counteracts the potential "freedom" for ovulation under constant light. The breeders essentially cue to the feeding time as a replacement to the normal light/dark cycle. While only of academic interest to geneticists and physiologists, the experiments do show the powerful effects that daily routines such as limited feeding have on the bird's cycle of reproductive processes.

The decline in egg production after peak is more rapid in broiler breeders compared to Leghorn birds, and this is often referred to commercially as "lack of persistence". In part, this decline in egg numbers is due to reduction in clutch length, with a greater proportion of non-egg laying days occurring. Additionally, however, there is an indication of a slower rate of recruitment of small follicles into the hierarchy of larger follicles that make up the potential clutch. There is also an increase in follicular regression together with more eggs ending up in the body cavity and also a greater incidence of soft-shelled or improperly shelled eggs which obviously reduce production of settable eggs. As discussed in the following section, nutrition and feeding management can have a major effect on such erratic or abnormal patterns of ovulation and egg formation.

2.4 EFFECT OF FEEDING LEVEL ON OVULATION

Unfortunately the broiler breeder sometimes exhibits the very undesirable characteristic of multiple ovulation. Instead of releasing just one follicle per day, she can release 2 and sometimes 3 or 4 follicles per day. This trait of multiple ovulation is usually in response to overfeeding, and especially when there is an excess of energy. Multiple ovulation therefore, often precedes or accompanies obesity in breeder hens. When more than one follicle is released, there can be double or even triple yolked eggs produced, although more commonly the extra follicles end up in the body cavity. The practical consequences of multiple ovulation are either the production of unsettable double yolked eggs, or an erratic pattern of egg laying, because of so many lost follicles. For example, with two follicles released at one time, the production rate can be no greater than 50%. When broiler breeders are overfed, they develop more large follicles and in extreme cases there may be two or three replicate hierarchies present in birds fed close to ad-libitum. Even overfeeding adult birds as little as 10%, can lead to increase in multiple ovulations. Apart from there being a net loss of settable eggs, any normal eggs that are produced often appear at unusual times of the day because of erratic times of ovulation. An early warning sign of overfeeding, apart from the obvious associated increase in body weight, is increase in egg laying between 15:00-6:00h. These eggs often appear as floor eggs if nests are closed at night.

Multiple ovulation can also cause more shell defects. Slab-sided eggs are a consequence of two eggs being formed simultaneously and physically contacting each other in the upper regions of the shell gland. With erratic timing of eggs entering the shell gland, shell calcification may be incomplete or missing on some eggs. Unfortunately erratic ovulation most often results in shell-less eggs, and these are rarely seen by the breeder manager, because most are eaten by the hens or roosters. Once hens become obese, they also have fewer sperm in the sperm storage glands, and so this situation coupled with reduced mating activity leads to lower rates of fertilization. Undoubtedly the worse cases of multiple ovulation occur in young breeders that are overweight at sexual maturity. Although heavy birds at maturity must be fed more than standard, because of their greater maintenance need, there is a fine line between giving extra feed for maintenance vs inducing multiple ovulations. All commercial breeding companies provide recommended body weights for their birds at maturity, and this is usually around 2.2kg at 22 weeks. While birds that are slightly heavy *eg*. +0.1kg often excel in many management situations and especially those involving hot weather, weights much in excess of these standards can quickly lead to multiple ovulation and subsequent failure to realize peak egg numbers. Likewise, after peak egg production, failure to practice a gradual withdrawal of feed commensurate with reduced needs also leads to multiple and erratic ovulation. In this later scenario, erratic ovulation coupled with obesity leads to sudden and dramatic decline in post-peak egg numbers. Fatness, independent of body weight, does not seem to be a factor in multiple ovulations, and because of this, it is suggested that birds being too heavy at first egg (rather than simply being overly fat) is the main trigger for the problem. Having accurate, precise records of mature body weight and variance of such weight is therefore an important diagnostic tool under these circumstances. For example Hocking (1996) recorded a mean early production ovulation rate of almost 1.9 follicles/day for pullets that had been fed free-choice during rearing. Pullets restricted to commercial standards had a mean rate of 1.2 follicles/day while birds on an intermediate level of restriction ovulated 1.4 follicles/day. These data demonstrate that even our regular pullets show some multiple ovulations, but that this will be dramatically increased if pullets are overweight at maturity.

2.5 BROODINESS AND MOLTING

Broodiness involves the natural instinct of the hen to stop ovulating and to incubate her eggs. This involves behavioral changes together with major interruption of feeding and drinking. Characteristically, hens resist being moved from the nest exhibiting raised neck feathers and clucking when approached. Fortunately broodiness is a trait of moderately high heritability, and so over time the characteristic has been selected against in breeding programs. While Leghorn birds rarely show broodiness, it is sometimes seen in broiler breeders in moderately warm climates and especially in male line grandparents. As levels of luteinising hormone decline, so levels of prolactin increase, and in the turkey at least, there is a direct relationship between levels of prolactin and duration of broodiness. Since birds rarely exhibit broodiness in cages, then it is obvious that environment must play a major role in stimulating this behavior in hens. Broody hens seek out a nest site that is isolated, dark, warm, moist and, ideally, already has a number of eggs present. Providing such environments in a commercial breeder house is therefore simply poor management. Broodiness can be stopped by moving the hens to a new environment, and especially one that has a different floor material. However, even under the best broody management systems, it will take some 15-21d for resumption of egg production, and during this time of rehabilitation, it is time consuming to feed birds according to their changing nutrient needs. The best broody management is prevention by timely collection of nest and floor eggs and to exclude "ideal" nesting sites on the litter.

Of more concern to breeder managers is molting because this also implies loss of egg numbers. Molting involves the orderly loss of feathers from the body and this occurs naturally to some extent in most birds in a flock over time. However extensive molt is usually an indication of reduced ovary function. Under natural molting, the feathers are first lost from the head and neck region, and then the breast and back and finally the wings and tail feathers are lost under extreme conditions. The wing feathers will be lost in order from #1 to #10, with #1 being the primary closest to the body, adjacent to the secondaries. The orderly loss of primaries can therefore be used to assess the stage of molting of a bird. However even birds ovulating quite regularly at 50-60 weeks of age may show some loss of the first few primary feathers, and these are usually evident on the litter.

So called "neck molt" is a common occurrence in some flocks of breeders, and when a high incidence occurs, such flocks invariably fail to show high or sustained peak production. Neck molt is most frequently caused by simply underfeeding birds during the period approaching peak production. This situation most commonly occurs with flocks (or individual hens) that are slightly overweight, and where the manager makes a conscious effort to try and limit feed increases so as to correct the body weight situation. Neck molt is therefore often associated with "stall-out" in weight gain. Natural molting very rarely occurs with flocks that are accidentally overfed.

There has been some interest in induced molting of breeders over the years, although generally this has not been accepted by the industry. Molting and a subsequent second cycle of lay can be induced by feed withdrawal programs as used for commercial egg layers. There seems to be a good correlation between pre- and post-molt breeder performance, and so it seems advisable only to consider molting flocks that have performed well up to 64 weeks of age. Heavy breeders seem less responsive to feed changes than do commercial layers, and so it may be necessary to combine programs such as high mineral (*eg*. zinc) together with feed restriction. Undoubtedly the best second cycle performance is seen when there is a major change in daylength, (down to 6-8h initially) and so this makes effective molting programs very difficult in open-sided buildings. The feathers lost by breeders can cause serious problems with management of the slatted floor area. Extensive feather loss causes blockage of slatted floors, with a resultant build-up of manure. In extreme cases such feather/manure accumulation has to be removed by hand.

Another problem with molting is male management. There have been reports of molting roosters together with the hens. With separate male feeding systems, however, a very limited feed supply (20-30g immediately after the feed withdrawal period) means greater than usual competition at the feeders. For both hens and roosters, the longer the period of molt or non-production, the better the second cycle and 6-8 weeks seems ideal. During a second cycle, peak production of 75% is possible, although the major management concern is sustaining post-peak production and limiting the increase in egg size.

A situation that is often overlooked in discussion on molting of breeders, is loss of yearly genetic progress of both breeders and broilers. Essentially molting involves using "last year's model" compared to the most current genetics available. For breeders themselves, this may be less difficult to quantitate because progress in selection for reproductive traits is relatively slow. However for the broiler offspring we expect at least +25g in weight-for-age as yearly progress. Broiler offspring from molted flocks will therefore have less genetic potential for growth. Table 2.3 shows a calculation of such an effect to an integrator with 100,000 breeders.

TABLE 2.3 Comparison of breeder performance and broiler production from breeders involving single cycle vs molting

	Conventional flock replacement	Molting
Jan 1st Year 1	100,000 breeders each producing 150 broilers @ 2.200kg = 33 m kg	100,000 breeders each producing 150 broilers @ 2.200kg = 33 m kg
Nov 1st - Dec 31st Year 1	Clean-out	Molting
Jan 1st Year 2	100,000 breeder replacements	100,000 molted breeders[1]
Aug 1st Year 2 (end of 2nd cycle for molted flock after only 28 weeks production)	120 broilers @ 2.225kg = 26.7m kg	100 broilers @ 2.200kg = 22m kg
Total broiler production	59.7m kg	55.0m kg

[1]Assuming no mortality

In this example, we start out with 100,000 breeders, and in one case these are replaced with new pullets after a conventional 40 week cycle. The alternative flock is molted and used for a second (28 week) cycle. For ease of comparison, we have assumed an eight week molt period vs an eight week turn-around for clean-out and stocking of the new flock and start of their egg production. The molted flock will not peak as high, and so in this calculation we have assumed 100 chicks/breeder compared to 120 chicks/breeder in 28 weeks for the new flock. Because of genetic selection, the new breeders produce broilers with genetic potential +25g compared to the previous year (2.225 vs 2.200kg broiler weight). This calculation perhaps biases against the molted flock, because they will have slightly better growth rate in broilers as a consequence of a larger egg size. However in this simulation, because of reduced egg numbers and growth potential, the integrator is producing some 4.7mkg less broiler meat from 100,000 breeders due to molting. Coupled with the management challenges of molting, these data shows the limitations of this procedure.

2.6 FEMALE FERTILITY

If sperm are present in the sperm storage glands, and the hen ovulates normally, then the egg is usually fertilized. As a generalization therefore, true fertility problems are most likely a reflection of problems with the rooster (see Chapter 2, Section 2.8) rather than with the hen. Most hens are capable of laying fertile eggs for 7d following natural mating or artificial insemination, although individual fertilized eggs may be produced for as long as 28d following a single mating. It seems as though there is individual (genetic) bird variance in duration of fertility following mating, because birds observed with such long duration following a single insemination retain their ranking regardless of age. Studies have also shown that hens with long duration fertility have more sperm storage glands containing ≥20 spermatozoa, leading to the speculation of genetic differences in the way that hens nourish and nurture sperm within these glands.

As previously discussed, there seems to be a correlation between fertility and the number of sperm penetrating the germinal disc. After a single insemination of hens with a given number of sperm, then as expected, fertility declines over time. However this decline in fertility is correlated with a dramatic decline in the number of sperm penetrating the germinal disc. Bramwell *et al.* (1996) indicate that the decline in fertility usually seen with older hens is associated with a decline in the number of sperm penetrating the germinal disc following a standard insemination procedure. Interestingly, fertility of hens was improved when they were mated to older roosters (64 vs 39 weeks age) and again this improved fertility was correlated with more sperm penetration. This data unfortunately is contrary to industry practice of spiking new males into a flock at around 40 weeks of age. The need for spiking is probably related to ability or willingness of males to mate successfully, rather than to the fertilizing capacity of those males *per se* that are maintaining fertility of the flock. Ideally, it would be advantageous to spike with "older" rather than young males, but this obviously poses management problems of maintaining groups of older mature males. If this is desired, then housing under blue lights does seem to have a calming effect on such large groups of males penned without hens. However, under natural mating a decline in fertility is expected, and so the hen effect seems to be most dominant and/or that factors other than sperm penetration *per se* are responsible for loss in fertility over time. Table 2.4 shows the relationship between fertility in a flock of commercial breeders and mean sperm penetration determined by egg breakout. These data suggest that sperm receptors on the surface of the germinal disc may decrease in numbers or in efficacy with age of the hen. At any age, it is generally recognized that infertility is associated with a relatively small percentage of hens. From a study involving a large number of trap-nested hens with natural mating, about 4% of the hens were found to produce

40% of the unfertilized eggs. If these hens were inseminated, fertility was almost normal, suggesting that periods of infertility for individual hens are likely caused by hens not being sexually responsive to males and/or preferential mating of selected hens by the males. It is further realized that body condition of individual hens will also affect fertility, since there is a correlation of around -0.3 between body weight and fertility.

TABLE 2.4 Relationship between commercial breeder flock fertility and sperm penetration of the germinal disc

Flock age (wks)	Fertility (%)	Sperm penetration holes
27	-	113
30	86	112
33	92	108
36	93	127
45	95	117
56	84	60

Adapted from Bramwell *et al.* (1996)

However there is little indication of change in fertility for hens that are within ±10% of mean body weight-for-age as specified by the primary breeder. Loss of fertility with overweight hens most likely relates to physical changes in the oviduct caused by obesity or simply loss in mating activity and/or successful matings.

McDaniel *et al.* (1995) indicate that fertility in heat stressed hens (≃30° vs 21°C) is associated with reduction in the number of sperm penetrating the previtelline layer. However the usual reduction in fertility seen during heat stress is not due solely to problems with the hen because if normal hens are inseminated with sperm from normal or heat stressed roosters, then the later sperm result in reduced previtelline sperm penetration and fertility.

Parthenogenesis, or the spontaneous development of unfertilized eggs is a very rare occurrence in chickens. The female pronuclei spontaneously develops, and so there is a chance of incorrectly diagnosing an infertile egg as being fertile. The chick rarely completes full development, and on those occasions when the chick hatches they are invariably males, suggesting that the WW sex chromosome combination is lethal.

2.7 MALE REPRODUCTIVE SYSTEM

With natural mating, the function of the male is to produce viable sperm in the testes and then to efficiently transport these to the cloaca of the hen during mating. Unlike the situation in most mammals, the testes of the rooster are deep within the body cavity and so function at the normal body temperature of close to 41°C. The testes are found close to the kidneys. The testes are quite small prior to maturity, being only 1-2g each, although similar to the situation with the ovary in the hen, there is a dramatic increase in size starting at around 18 weeks, and the mature testes are 15-20g and easily visible. There is a direct relationship between sperm production and testes size, and the latter to some extent is positively correlated with body size. Daily sperm production is about 100 million per gram of testes weight. Sperm production is fairly constant regardless of mating or collection frequency. Therefore, with higher frequency of mating, there will be fewer sperm per ejaculate. If ejaculation does not occur over a 2-3d period, then any sperm stored in the vas deferens are reabsorbed. During mating, or collection during artificial insemination, the semen is directed from the vas deferens to the engorged phallic folds on the cloaca. Such engorgement is caused by lymphatic fluid. The semen is usually white and opaque, but can be clear and watery which is often a sign of reduced sperm concentration. The hormone testosterone is produced by the testes under regulation of gonadotrophins, and similar to the female system, overall control of the breeding cycle is ultimately dictated by the photoperiod. Comb size is a sensitive indicator of testosterone level, and so can be used to evaluate stage of maturity in developing roosters. Collection of 4-5 semen samples over a 7-10d period is sufficient to predict a rooster's potential life-time fertility.

2.8 MALE FERTILITY

Male fertility is best assessed by manual collection of semen and subsequent evaluation as detailed in Chapter 2, Section 2.9 involving artificial insemination. It is generally considered that most problems of male fertility relate to mating behavior although nutrition and/or obesity can also be problematic. For roosters at ideal weight and condition, and fed adequate quantities of appropriate diets, frequency of successful mating is the major correlate with successful fertilization of the egg. Modern breeder males exhibit less courting behavior than was observed some 15-20 years ago, or compared to Leghorn strains today. There is some evidence for a negative relationship between courting behavior and general male aggressiveness, and this is especially relevant to so called "high-yield" roosters. Without the normal courtship behavior, the male merely mounts the hen from behind, maintaining his stance by holding on to the comb or neck region of the hen. Unfortunately, these matings rarely involve coupling of the cloacas and so the process is totally ineffective. Roosters have been observed to make as many as 20 such "matings" per day. It is thought that such active "mating" is part of the males establishing dominance in the flock, and particularly in relation to other males. The number of males producing sperm in a flock is often much lower than expected based on visual observation and bird condition. Some estimates suggest that fertility will be accomplished by no more than 60% of males in a flock. Unfortunately it is not always possible to physically select such males, because roosters at both ends of the social scale may be ineffective - the smaller males because of failure to secure hens, and the large dominant males because of ineffective (but active) mating technique. The "average" males in the flock are likely the most effective in maintaining fertility. Males can produce semen as early as 12 weeks of age, depending upon body size and lighting program. However sperm from such roosters is rarely viable, and effective maturity does not develop until birds are around a minimum of 18 weeks of age.

Diet composition and feeding level can have a dramatic and absolute effect on fertility. Both over or underfeeding will lead to loss of semen production (see Chapter 5). There is very good evidence for optimum semen production from roosters fed diet protein/amino acid levels much less than routinely used for hens. Such separate male diets can be as low as 9-10% crude protein. However, low protein diets are less commonly used today because of the inconvenience of handling small quantities of such specialized feed, and the fact that such lower protein diets are often more expensive. However, fertility will be improved by up to 2-3% by using such lower protein diets (see Chapter 5) and so the cost:benefit relationship of such feeding management has to be established for individual breeder operations. Obesity in males is negatively associated with semen production and more importantly with mating activity. Such obesity is most commonly caused by general overfeeding, or more specifically, can relate to there being excess of either protein or energy in the diet. Feeding high protein (>16% CP equivalent) most frequently causes extra muscle growth (especially in high yield males) and this itself causes problems with weight control, although such development is often accompanied by greater fat accretion. If roosters are underfed, males will quickly decline in semen production unless they seek an alternative source of nutrients such as eggs or female feed.

With introduction of high breast yield strains, there has been increased concern about male aggression and its negative impact on mating behavior and fertility. To some extent the problem can be reduced by placing less males in the breeder house, and this certainly has been a trend in recent years. Mating ratios of 1:12 are now more common than 1:8 or 1:10, as used 5-10 years ago. There is also anecdotal evidence for less aggression in roosters given larger quantities of less nutrient dense feed. Experimentally, male aggression can be reduced by feeding very high levels of the amino acid tryptophan. While 0.2% is a normal level of tryptophan in breeder diets, levels as high as 0.75% have been shown to have a calming effect on males (and also hens exhibiting hysteria for whatever reason). Tryptophan acts as a precursor of brain neurotransmitters (serotonin) which can influence behavior. Tryptophan seems to have most effect in reducing the major period of aggression during morning feeding. Unfortunately tryptophan is very expensive at this time and such treatment is currently uneconomical.

2.9 ARTIFICIAL INSEMINATION AND SEMEN EVALUATION

Artificial insemination is sometimes used commercially with caged dwarf breeders and less frequently with regular caged breeders. However the primary breeders now use AI routinely in maintaining pure line breeding stock. The potential advantages to AI are greater use of superior males and better fertility, while the associated cage environment usually means reduced feed intake and cleaner eggs. The disadvantages to AI under large scale commercial production are maintaining efficiency and interest of insemination crews, while cages *per se* have distinct limitations for heavy breeders related to foot pad condition and ease of feed allocation.

Semen collection: It is not really known why the normal manual manipulation of the rooster produces semen because the process in no way mimics natural mating. It is often difficult to produce semen from an individual rooster at the first attempt because they seem to benefit from a "training" session. This means it is difficult to occasionally "milk" roosters in a naturally mated flock in order to assess general sperm production and motility. Collection involves holding the male, breast down, usually on a table or the knee of the collector, who is usually sitting. The bird is held by another operator or alternatively held in some type of mechanical leg clamp. The abdomen is then firmly massaged with one hand while the other hand is drawn across the back and over the tail feathers. Depending upon variation between males, the phallus will enlarge after 3-6 such massages, and at this time, the collector quickly places their hands around the cloaca. The thumb and forefinger of each hand are held diametrically opposite the top and bottom of the cloaca. The fingers above the cloaca squeeze gently down and into the vent region, while below the vent, the pressure is applied upwards and away from the bird's body. The semen is then aspirated from the surface of the phallus directly into a sealed tube. At this time semen should appear on the end of the phallus. The procedure of manipulating the cloacal region can be conducted a second time to produce a second stream of semen. Semen should be routinely examined for concentration, motility and viability. Apart from identifying inferior roosters, such observations are the basis for semen dilution used to increase the mating ratio from around 1:10 under natural mating, up to 1:20 with diluted semen.

Sperm number: It is essential to know sperm concentrations in order to rank individual males and/or to calculate appropriate levels of dilution. The hemocytometer is the only direct method of determining sperm number. However, this is a very tedious and tiring procedure that is used only to "calibrate" other indirect measures. Such indirect methods are packed cell volume, colorimetry and turbidity that all need a correction or conversion system for application. Depending upon the degree of precision needed, published standard curves can be used to give approximations of the relationship between hemocytometer determined sperm per ml vs absorbence in a spectrophotometer, % packed cell volume etc. For more accurate assessment, individual machines must be calibrated (yearly) with a range of diluted semen samples of known sperm concentration.

Sperm viability: The number of dead and abnormal sperm in a sample should be less than 10%. Sperm viability is determined by simple microscopic examination combined with a nigrosin-eosin stain. Live viable sperm do not take up the pink-colored eosin stain, and so remain white, on the blue (nigrosin) background. Dead sperm take up the eosin, and appear pink. When viewed under the microscope at 80-100x magnification, a field of view is measured for live vs dead sperm. At the same time, live abnormal sperm can be counted because these will also likely be incapable of fertilization. Normal avian sperm are "worm-like" in appearance with a thin symmetrical shaped body culminating in a short (15-20% length) thin tail. These normal sperm are gently curved. Most abnormal sperm are characterized by severe bending in the head, mid or tail region.

Sperm motility: Motility, which is a measure of potential viability and fertilizing capacity, is most easily determined by subjectively scoring sperm movement when observed at about 50x magnification. Any subjective scale can be used, with 0-5 being most common and representing no motion, (0) through to fully active sperm, (5) over the whole field of view. All sperm become motionless over time, and so standardization of time of viewing after collection is very important. An objective measure of motility can be obtained using a specialized flow cell connected to a spectrophotometer. Sperm will "swim" against a flow, and in so doing, live sperm align themselves against this flow. Because sperm are "long and thin", having them all aligned in one direction affects light transmittance across the flow. The more % live sperm in a sample, the lower the light transmittance. Sperm motility and metabolism can also be determined by a colorimetric procedure. A sample of sperm and dye (tetrazolium) are incubated for about 10 minutes, during which time sperm are able to produce chemicals that influence color. Color change can be estimated by eye, or with a spectrophotometer following centrifugation, and this method is often used to "rank" roosters. More recently there has been interest in evaluating sperm and/or roosters according to their ability to penetrate the previtelline membrane extracted from a shelled egg. The previtelline membrane is carefully removed from around the yolk and cut into 0.5x0.5 cm squares and incubated with about 10^7 sperm for 10 minutes at 40°C. Under a microscope, sperm penetration holes are distinctively visible, and the number of holes are directly correlated with sperm motility/metabolism and overall male fertility. In the region of the germinal disc, there may be as many as 40-60 holes/mm^2 while in other regions there are often only 5-10 holes/mm^2.

Semen dilution: Semen can be diluted so as to provide coverage for around 20 hens. The degree of dilution will depend upon the initial concentration of sperm which itself varies between roosters and for individual roosters over time. Most diluents contain sodium glutamate, glucose, fructose and specialized buffers so as to maintain pH at around 7.0 and osmotic pressure at 400 mOsm $kg^{-1}H_2O$. The glutamate seems especially important if semen is to be held more than 4-6h prior to insemination. Unfortunately semen cannot be frozen-thawed for adequate routine commercial fertility. The following is an example of calculations used to dilute semen:

a) Add about 5-6ml semen to 1ml of diluent at ambient temperature.
b) Determine sperm concentration and semen volume in order to calculate total sperm number
c) Divide total sperm number by dose of sperm per insemination to derive total volume of diluted semen

   eg: 5 ml semen plus 1 ml extender found to have $8x10^9$ sperm/ml = $48x10^9$ total sperm

   Insemination dose to be $200x10^6$ as a 0.1 ml dose

   $$\therefore \frac{48x10^9}{200x10^6/0.1\ ml} = 24\ ml$$

The semen already represents 6 ml of this volume and so it must be mixed with (24-6) = 18ml diluent.

Inseminating hens: During artificial insemination, the handling and manipulation of the hen is somewhat similar to that previously described for semen collection from roosters. The operation is either a one or two person procedure depending upon equipment available to constrain the hen. Gentle pressure is applied with both hands concurrently from below the cloaca and above the tail region. The insemination tube is then inserted into the everted cloaca to a depth of about 3cm, and then pressure released from the abdomen and tail region. Within a few hours the sperm storage glands will contain their normal complement of sperm. Most data confirm that fertility is maximized with weekly inseminations of about 150 million sperm (Table 2.5).

TABLE 2.5 Influence of sperm number per insemination on fertility and hatchability

Sperm number ($x10^6$)	Fertility (%)	Hatch of fertile (%)	Early dead (%)
25	42a	87a	11.5a
50	70b	91ab	5.2b
100	87c	93b	1.9b
200	94d	94b	2.5b

Adapted from Eslick and McDaniel (1992)

The data from Eslick and McDaniel (1992) confirm many reports of the relationship between sperm number per insemination and fertility. Also of interest in this study, is the negative effect on hatch of fertile, due to early dead embryos, from having a minimal number of sperm in the oviduct. While only one sperm ultimately fertilizes the egg, the number penetrating the vitelline membrane is much greater and may be correlated with early embryo viability. The number of sperm per insemination, or the number of sperm transferred during natural mating, may therefore be of consequence to both fertility and hatchability of such fertile eggs.

Timing of insemination also influences fertility. Data from McDaniel and Sexton (1980) suggest reduced fertility from hens inseminated in the morning (Table 2.6). These same authors conclude that this effect of time is related to occurrence of insemination relative to time of oviposition (Table 2.7).

An egg in the upper oviduct at time of insemination seems to dramatically reduce fertility. Late afternoon or early evening inseminations therefore seem ideal. However such timing does not always correspond to the most efficient work load at the farm, and handling breeders during the time of early shell calcification (late afternoon) can lead to more body checked eggs which themselves rarely hatch due to reduced porosity of the shell.

TABLE 2.6 Fertility of breeder hens as affected by time of artificial insemination

Time of insemination	Experiment 1	Experiment 2
2400h	91.5a	97.9a
0300h	85.1b	95.8ab
0600h	82.7b	92.1bc
0900h	84.8b	87.0c
1200h	91.4a	88.5c
1500h	91.1a	89.9c
1800h	93.1a	91.0bc
2100h	95.3a	97.3a

Adapted from McDaniel and Sexton (1980)

TABLE 2.7 Fertility of breeder hens inseminated at various times relative to occurrence of oviposition

Time of oviposition occurring after time of insemination (hrs)	% Fertility
1	62.9d
2	74.7c
3	84.9bc
4	95.2ab
5	91.3ab
6	96.8a
7	96.1ab
8	97.2a

Adapted from McDaniel and Sexton (1980)

2.10 COMMERCIAL USE OF ARTIFICIAL INSEMINATION

World-wide it has been estimated that only about 0.5% of commercial breeders are maintained in cages and bred by artificial insemination. Many of these commercial flocks involve dwarf breeders, and the majority of these are found in Western Europe. Following are potential advantages and disadvantages of commercial breeding using artificial insemination:

Advantages:

- ✓ Cleaner eggs
- ✓ Better fertility
- ✓ Reduced feed intake
- ✓ Fewer males
- ✓ Greater use of selected males
- ✓ Culling of non-layers
- ✓ Increased bird number/sq m floor area
- ✓ Can use dwarf effectively

Disadvantages:

- ✗ High capital cost
- ✗ High labor cost
- ✗ Training/motivation of inseminators
- ✗ Problems with feed allocation following mortality
- ✗ Footpad lesions

There is little doubt that the dwarf hen is best suited to the cage environment. Dwarfs are eating closer to ad-libitum intake than are regular hens, and so feed allocation becomes less critical for these smaller birds. A major problem with cage systems for breeders is feed allocation, which is usually accomplished with a mechanical hopper system that provides a predetermined depth of feed in front of each cage. The depth is obviously calibrated to provide a given quantity of feed per cage. Alternatively breeders can be fed by an auger system that delivers a weighed quantity to a given row or back-to-back row of cages. However whatever system is used, the feed allocation will be for the cage group which is usually 3 or 4 hens. For example with 3 hens per cage, then at peak egg numbers, the allocation may be 450g per cage group. If one bird dies, then the allocation for the 2 remaining hens is increased by 50%. The only solution is to continually move birds so as to maintain the regular stocking density. However this practice itself imposes continued change in social dominance in these small groups, and this often leads to loss of production. Also because breeders should be fed according to their level of production, then variable performance within a cage group leads to overfeeding of the less productive birds. Obviously the same situation occurs in floor-housed birds, but the overall effect is quite minimal because of the large group size involved.

Footpad lesions are another problem with caged hens, and especially regular sized breeders. After being in cages for 15-20 weeks, many birds start to develop foot pad lesions. It is difficult to control such lesions with nutritional modification, and so severity of the problem relates to cage design, and especially floor design and floor material. Hens with poor foot pad condition quickly decline in egg production. A distinct advantage of caged breeder hens is reduced feed needs caused by less feed needed for maintenance. This saving is estimated at about 15-20% depending upon environmental temperature.

Because it is difficult to inseminate non-laying hens, artificial insemination is not usually started until flocks are at about 25% production. Two weeks prior to this, roosters should be collected twice per week to ensure adequate semen production. Hens are usually inseminated twice the first week, and then at weekly intervals with about 0.05ml of fresh or diluted semen, containing around 150-200 million sperm. Roosters can be collected 2-3 times each week depending upon the need for semen. Each collection will be 0.2-0.5ml, with an average of about 0.35ml. If semen is used undiluted, then each 0.35ml collection will yield sufficient semen for about 7 inseminations, and so if roosters are collected 3 times per week, this represents about a 1:20 "mating" ratio.

Depending upon cage design, the hens do not have to be removed from the cage, but rather their legs brought outside and the vent exposed. With the aid of mechanical leg clamps, the operation can be conducted by one person. Alternatively two people are required, and such a crew should be able to inseminate up to 3200 hens each day - inseminating 5 days per week, means that a 2 person crew should be able to routinely inseminate a flock of about 15,000 breeders. As previously outlined, a major challenge with this work is job motivation, and it is advantageous to utilize crews of 3 people with the 3rd person rotating on to the job of semen collection from the roosters. Inseminating is best done in the afternoon (Table 2.6) and ideally fresh undiluted semen should be used within 1-2h. For diluted semen, the time of insemination can be up to 6 h later.

Both hens and roosters can be culled for poor performance starting after about 30 weeks of age. Roosters giving poor quality semen before this time should probably be culled because there is seldom improvement in reproduction of males over time. Culling of females will be on the basis of appearance of the cloaca coupled with other problems such as molting, obesity, footpad lesions etc.

Reddy (1994) suggests that commercial broiler chick cost will be increased by about 4.04 with artificial insemination vs natural mating. Most of this cost relates to initial capital cost of cages together with the increased labor cost of inseminating. Labor cost for AI alone is about 2.04 per chick (3 people working 5 days per week per 15,000 hens). Charged against this cost is the reduced feed intake, estimated at 15% as discussed previously. For a hen normally eating 45kg, this represents about 6.75kg less feed @ 204/kg = $1.35/hen or roughly 1.04 per chick. The saving in feed cost should therefore recover about 50% of the inseminating costs. Ultimately the use of AI often revolves around the potential to maintain high levels of fertility from dedicated and motivated insemination crews.

2.11 EGG BREAKOUT

Whatever system of breeding and male/female management is used, the success of the reproductive process is established by egg breakout at the farm and/or hatchery. Egg breakout is used to assess fertility prior to incubation and also early dead germs during the first 5-7d of incubation.

For fresh eggs, the shell is carefully broken and the yolk rolled within the shell or on the palm of the hand until the germinal disc is clearly present. The fertile egg has a clearly visible raised disc (doughnut) which is white or of less intense color than the surrounding yolk. For the unfertilized egg, the germinal disc is evident but lacks texture (Fig 2.2, Fig 8.21).

Figure 2.2 Schematic representation of unfertilized and fertilized germinal disc.

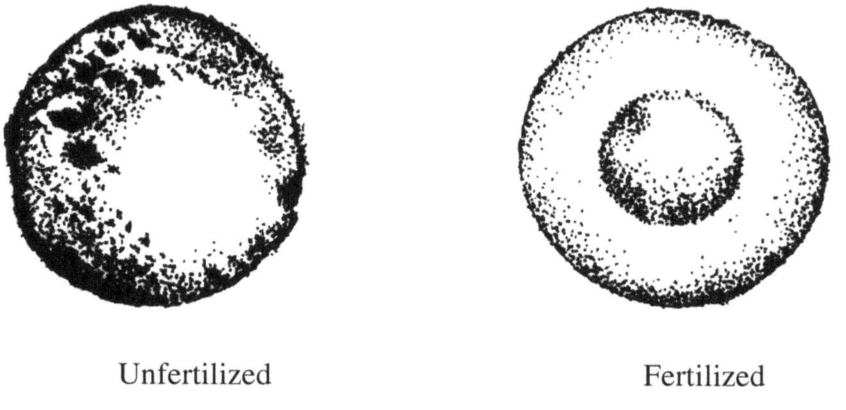

True fertility is calculated as the number of fertile eggs observed expressed as a percentage of all eggs examined. For any breeder flock, at least 60 eggs should be examined.

Eggs can also be examined after 5-10d incubation to determine fertile/infertile numbers as well as occurrence of early dead germs (Table 2.8). Eggs are carefully broken, and the germinal disc/embryo examined within the broken shell or again on the palm of the hand. Infertile eggs retain the original yolk color, and are little different in appearance compared to fresh eggs. The germinal disc is still quite distinct and small. With embryos dying very young, the germinal disc will be larger in diameter and there will not be a distinct raised disc *per se*. The yolk is often paler in color and sometimes has a mottled appearance. When candling at 7d, the total number of viable embryos, expressed as a percentage of all eggs examined, is often referred to as candling fertility. Eggs can be examined after chicks have been taken from the hatch trays to determine general age of embryo mortality. The most common classification is as early, mid and late dead germs which refer to 1-7, 8-14 and 15-21d respectively.

TABLE 2.8 Pattern of embryo mortality related to breeder age

			Expected occurrence (%)		
Description	**Days incubation**	**Embryo identification**	**27 wks**	**45 wks**	**64 wks**
Infertile	0	Germinal disc	10	7	15
Early dead (1-7d)	1 3 5 7	Primitive streak Embryo on left side Appearance elbow/ knee joints Comb evident	4	2	4
Mid-dead (8-14d)	11 13	Tail feathers Feather down	0.7	0.5	0.5
Late dead (15-21d)	16 18 20	Feathers Head under right wing Yolk sac absorbed	2.5	2.0	3.5

It is more difficult to differentiate infertile from very early dead embryos after the eggs have been incubated for 21d. Determining age of embryo mortality is important for problem solving and identifying, for example, any contribution of poor breeder management or nutrition. As a generalization, assuming that no disease situation is involved, then early dead germs are related to improper pre-incubation egg handling and/or egg storage conditions. On the other hand, mid-dead germs (7-14d) are rarely seen under normal conditions, although we can create a very high incidence by feeding diets inadequate in certain vitamins. Mid-dead germs are therefore a clue to inadequate diet formulation or vitamin antagonists being problematic. Late dead germs are more likely caused by incubation conditions, and rarely relate to breeder management or nutrition.

BIBLIOGRAPHY

Brake, J., 1985. Relationship of egg weight, specific gravity and shell weight to time of oviposition and feeding in broiler breeders. Poult. Sci. 64:2037-2040.

Bramwell, R.K., C.D. McDaniel, J.L. Wilson, and B. Howarth, 1996. Age effect of male and female broiler breeders on sperm penetration of the perivitelline layer overlying the germinal disc. Poult. Sci. 75:755-762.

Eslick, M.L. and G.R. McDaniel, 1992. Interrelationships between fertility and hatchability of eggs from broiler breeder hens. J. Appl. Poultry Res. 1:156-159.

Hocking, P.M., 1996. Role of body weight and food intake after photostimulation on ovarian function at first egg in broiler breeder females. Br. Poult. Sci. 37:841-851.

McDaniel, C.D., R.K. Bramwell, J.L. Wilson and B. Howarth, 1995. Fertility of male and female broiler breeders following exposure to elevated ambient temperatures. Poult. Sci. 74:1029-1038.

McDaniel, G.R., and T.J. Sexton, 1980. Effect of time of day of artificial insemination interval on the fertility of broiler breeder hens. Poult. Sci. 59:2544-2549.

Reddy, R.P., 1994. Artificial insemination of broilers:Economic and Management implications in Proc 1st Int. Symp. AI in Poultry. College Park MD, June 1994.

Robinson, F.E., R.T. Hardin, N.A. Robinson and B.J. Williams, 1991. Influence of egg sequence position on fertility, embryo viability and embryo weight of broiler breeders. Poult. Sci. 70:760-765.

SUGGESTED READING

Etches, R.J., 1996. Reproduction in Poultry Publ. CAB Int.,UK.

Bakst, M.R., and G.J. Wishart, 1994. Editors. Proceedings First International Symposium on the Artificial Insemination of Poultry. Publ. Poultry Science Assoc., Savoy, Illinois, U.S.A.

CHAPTER 3. LIGHTING		
		PAGE NO.

Most birds are seasonal breeders and their reproductive cycle is controlled by changes in day length. Through its effect on the hypothalamus, light is responsible for the control over gonadotrophin releasing hormone production by the pituitary, and this is ultimately responsible for control of ovulation in the hen and spermatogenesis in the rooster. Both hens and roosters can, and do, reproduce in the absence of light or the absence of any meaningful change in the daily light:dark cycle. For example, hens kept in complete darkness will eventually mature and ovulate, and commercial breeders are sometimes kept in equatorial regions on farms without any electricity. Light and lighting programs are therefore not essential for reproduction in broiler breeders. Unfortunately, few farms have the luxury of a constant 12h light:12h dark natural photoperiod, and few houses are completely lightproof. Consequently, for most commercial flocks we must manipulate the lighting program so as to initially dictate age at sexual maturity and subsequently sustain egg production and fertility for a predetermined cycle.

3.1 BASIC PRINCIPLES OF LIGHT STIMULATION

Birds differentiate night from day because of the effect of light stimulating the hypothalamus in the brain. Light energy is converted into neural transmissions which ultimately guide the pituitary in releasing the all important gonadotrophin releasing hormones. However, birds are really not "stimulated" by the entire period of light, but rather by two important parts of this period. Birds are sensitive to the time of initial "lights-on" and subsequently during a period 11-13h later. This latter period is called the photosensitive phase, and essentially dictates whether or not the bird perceives the day as being "long" or "short". A short day is not stimulatory, whereas a long day initiates or maintains the cascade of hormonal releases that control ovulation or spermatogenesis. Therefore if birds perceive light during the photosensitive phase which occurs 11-13h after initiation of natural dawn or "lights on", then the ovary or testes can be functional. This pattern of dawn/dusk or lights-on/lights-off sets the circadian rhythm of the bird, which is essentially an inherent biological clock. In commercial situations, we often control and manipulate the time of the photoperiod, and so timing of the photosensitive phase is relative and not fixed according to our time clocks. For example, Table 3.1 shows the relationship of different photoperiods to the photosensitive phase of the bird, and ultimately whether or not such photoperiods are stimulatory for reproduction.

TABLE 3.1 Examples of photoperiods as they relate to the photosensitive time for breeders

Time of day		Day length	Photosensitive period	Stimulatory
Lights on	Lights off			
6:00h	14:00h	8h	17-19:00h	No
6:00h	16:00h	10h	17-19:00h	No
6:00h	18:00h	12h	17-19:00h	Yes
8:00h	18:00h	10h	19-21:00h	No
8:00h	21:00h	13h	19-21:00h	Yes
5:00h	19:00h	14h	16-18:00h	Yes

If lights are on during the photosensitive period, then the light is stimulatory for reproduction. Although it is normal to have continuous light from the time of artificial dawn to dusk, it is not essential. Following the initial stimulation at dawn, the day can be interrupted by periods of darkness. This is the basis of biomittent programs used with adult Leghorns in black-out houses, where the period of "lights-on" is in fact 17 cycles of 45 minutes dark:15 minutes light, rather than 17h continuous light. Both programs are equally effective in sustaining ovary function. This concept has not been tried with breeders, and perhaps this is too extreme a situation for optimum mating activity, but it seems worthwhile to pursue this concept so as to save both feed and electricity. Work with Japanese quail has shown that there is a 2-3 fold change in pituitary hormones in the plasma of birds within 24h of the initial stimulation to long daylength. Even though egg or semen production does not usually occur until some 14-21d following this stimulation, the first major change in photoperiod for the immature pullet does initiate an irreversible change in the endocrine system of the bird. For practical purposes the minimum stimulatory day length is around 12 hours, and there is little benefit to going much beyond 16-17h total light. Usually, the longer the initial stimulus, the greater the change in hormone balance, and the greater the synchronization of maturity in the flock. Therefore if pullets and roosters are at ideal weight, condition and age, then a large initial stimulus seems ideal. However if birds are underweight or in poor condition at a specific age, then early photostimulation should be delayed. If early photostimulation is essential due to the need to transport birds to breeder facilities then the initial light stimulation should be somewhat less and increased more slowly commensurate with bird development.

The light:dark cycle is really a change in light intensity, where darkness is non-stimulatory to the hypothalamus. Change in light intensity can be important to the bird, especially in moving pullets from black-out growing houses to open-sided breeder houses. Under these conditions, the birds are often exposed to changes in intensity during both "light" and "dark" phases of the photoperiod. The important consideration is to ensure that the intensity of the light period is always at least 10x greater than the intensity of the dark period. This is usually easy to achieve with open-sided houses because natural lighting is 5-10x the intensity of the brightest available artificial light, and so even with intense moonlight, the differentiation between dark and light is easily achieved. Complete darkness is rarely achieved in black-out housing, and in fact is not necessary, again assuming that the intensity of the daylight is >10x that of the nighttime intensity. Assuming that the basic principal of 10x intensity in light:dark phase is achieved, then absolute intensity has little effect on reproduction. However, immature pullets should never be subjected to a decline in light intensity when moved from grower to breeder facilities. Egg production is reduced with intensities much less than 5 lux during the light period, and this situation is perhaps related to the fact that it is difficult to always achieve <0.5 lux in the dark period.

Over time, breeders become photorefractory to light, meaning that the endocrine system becomes less active, and output of gonadotrophins from the pituitary decline. In large part this is the reason for the decline in egg production over time. There are some reports of better persistency of lay when older birds are given extra light stimulation later in the breeding cycle eg. +1h at 45 weeks.

The majority of broiler breeders are kept in open-sided buildings, and so the pattern of natural daylength:night time influences both the rate and persistency of egg and sperm production. The pattern of light:dark has two major influences on breeders, namely the age at sexual maturity and secondly, the duration of the breeding season. It is generally agreed that immature birds should not be exposed to an increase in day length while after maturity hens and roosters must not be exposed to a step-down in day length. The aim of any lighting program is to achieve these two basic principles by either using controlled environment (black-out) houses, or by using supplements of artificial light so as to achieve control over the light:dark cycle.

3.2 PERFORMANCE UNDER NATURAL LIGHTING

The natural patterns of light:darkness vary depending upon latitude. At the equator, the photoperiod is constant at 12h light:12h dark year round, and so this provides a simple base for manipulation. With increase in latitude, north or south, then the pattern of light:dark fluctuates throughout the year. At 10° latitude, day length varies by only about 1 hour comparing the longest vs shortest day. However, at 20°, 30° and 40° latitude the differences are about 2,4 and 6h respectively. The higher the latitude, then the greater the potential advantage of using some type of artificial lighting program especially for control over sexual maturity. For example in the N. hemisphere at 30° latitude, January hatched breeders can be expected to mature much earlier than June hatched breeders exposed to natural lighting, because the January hatched chicks will be grown on an increasing light program until the time of expected maturity. Similarly, the June hatched birds will mature later than expected. Such variance in maturity makes it very difficult for the manager to plan the time of move to the breeder house and also schedule feed allocation in relation to impending maturity. A question often asked under these conditions is whether or not all breeder hens should be at the same body weight at maturity, regardless of their age? The answer is likely "yes", but realising such consistent weights for birds of different mature ages is quite difficult to achieve in practice. Of the two scenarios described, the maturity of the January hatched breeders is most problematic, because their earlier maturity is accompanied by much smaller egg size, especially in the first 6-8 weeks of production.

A few years ago we published data on the performance of 900,000 commercial breeders in Mexico maintained at around 20° latitude where there was no light control and natural fluctuation in light was 11-13 h/day (Lopez and Leeson, 1992). After 18 weeks, pullets were moved to the breeder houses and given 14h light/d and then 16 h/d at 22 weeks. Egg production through peak production as affected by month of the year is shown in Fig. 3.1.

A very clear pattern emerges for maturity throughout the year even though daylength during rearing is different by a maximum of only 2h throughout the year. When the latter part of the growing program coincides with increasing day length, then earlier maturity relative to the standard is seen. The extreme is seen with November hatched breeder chicks that mature in May - these birds are subjected to increase in natural day length after about 8 weeks of age, and so they mature much earlier than expected. The other extreme is seen for May hatched breeder chicks, where growing pullets are subjected to decreasing day length for most of the late rearing period, and consequently these pullets mature later than expected (Fig 3.1). Table 3.2 summarizes the major characteristics of these flocks relative to month of hatch.

Figure 3.1 Effect of month of hatch on egg production

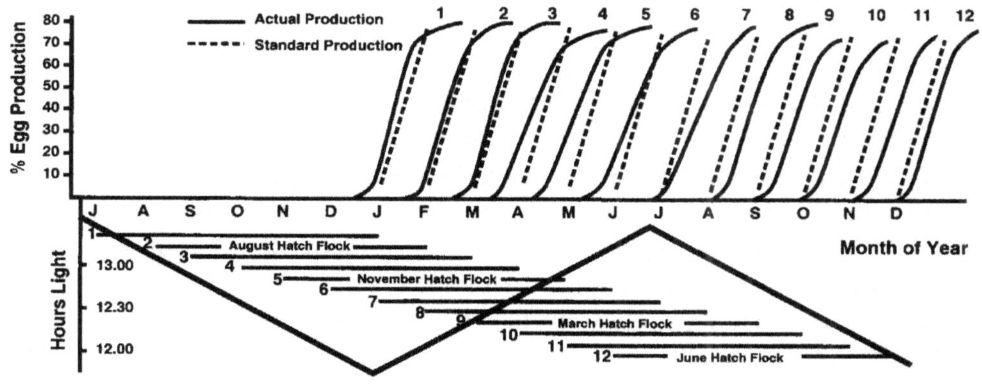

TABLE 3.2 Breeder performance at 20o latitude for pullets reared under natural lighting (Lopez and Leeson, 1992)				
Month of hatch	**Age at 5% production (d)**	**% Peak egg production**	**Age at peak (wks)**	**Weeks >75% egg production**
July	171	81	32	9
August	172	80	32	9
September	172	80	31	9
October	164	77	34	7
November	161	80	33	8
December	165	78	33	8
January	175	80	34	6
February	183	79	33	9
March	182	78	37	6
April	181	76	33	6
May	183	79	34	6
June	182	81	34	7

Age at 5% egg production varies by 22d throughout the year. There was relatively little effect on peak egg production and persistency of production, but in large part, this was due to the manager's prior knowledge of this seasonal fluctuation in performance, and birds were managed differently for summer vs winter hatched breeder flocks. The farm managers were therefore able to predict seasonal changes in maturity, and slow down or speed up growth where appropriate, so as to achieve a standard "mature" weight at first egg.

As latitude increases and as egg production potential of modern breeders increases, then this management technique is more difficult to implement and consequently there is loss in egg production. Knowledge of variation in maturity related to seasonal changes in day length (latitude effect) gives the breeder manager an advantage in growing the young pullet and rooster. However, it is obvious that any management system that reduces such variation in sexual maturity will be a major advantage. This ideal can be achieved with black-out housing or by providing a constant daylength during rearing of birds in open-sided buildings. Control of maturity with black-out housing is quite simple, and this is one of the major advantages of this costly system of management. After 3-5d of age, birds can be maintained at constant 7-10h light/day through to maturity, and consequently seasonal effects are totally eliminated. The situation with open-sided buildings is more complex, but still manageable and the opinion that "lighting programs cannot be applied in open-sided buildings" is merely a reflection of the philosophy of ill-informed breeder managers. With open-sided pullet growing facilities, the lighting program has to be flexible, commensurate with seasonal changes in day length. The goal is to have constant daylength, at least from 10-20 weeks of age, and not to expose birds to step-up daylength at any time prior to 21 weeks or whatever age that first light stimulation is usually given. Table 3.3 shows 3 scenarios for breeder flocks hatched in January, April, or June, again at 20° latitude.

3.3 PROGRAMS FOR GROWING PULLETS

It is generally considered that the pullet's response to light becomes important only as these birds approach maturity. While the most dramatic effects of change in day length and/or light intensity are seen after 16-18 weeks of age, there is little doubt that lighting programs for younger birds can influence their development and subsequent reproduction. Dunn *et al.* (1990) light stimulated dwarf breeder pullets at various times throughout rearing, starting as early as 21d of age. Feeding conventional diets, there was an increase in ovarian weight 14d following stimulation at 15 weeks of age, although no response was seen with younger pullets. However, if the diet was modified to contain 10% corn oil, (diet ME 2770→3350 kcal/kg) then ovarian response was seen in 7 and 11 week old pullets. Interestingly the 500g pullets light-stimulated at 7 weeks, and fed corn oil, showed higher plasma luteinizing hormone levels than did

TABLE 3.3 Lighting programs for January, April and June hatched chicks grown in open-sided buildings at 20^0 latitude

	J	F	M	A	M	J	J	A	S	O	N	D
Hours Light	10.45	11.0	11.30	12.15	12.45	12.45	12.30	12.00	11.30	11.35	10.30	10.15
	Hatch ——— Flock #1 ———➤ Mature											
				Hatch ——— Flock #2 ———➤ Mature								
						Hatch ——— Flock #3 ———➤ Mature						

Flock #1 With +2h light up to 20 weeks, January hatched pullets and roosters will mature very early. This can be corrected by imposing a constant daylength of 12h 45 min after 3-4d. This means 1 h 45 min artificial light in February, 30 minutes artificial light in April.

Flock #2 April hatched birds are exposed to increasing day length up to 12 weeks of age (end June), then a decrease in daylength. This flock is the only one that could successfully be grown on natural daylength. However for consistent age at maturity compared to other flocks, provide 12 h 45 min total light during July and August.

Flock #3 With continuous step-down light up to maturity, June hatched birds will mature very late. While this is less problematic than too early maturity (Flock #1) more consistent age at maturity can be achieved by giving 12 h 30 minute total light during August, September and October.

control fed birds weighing 1380g and light-stimulated at 19 weeks. These authors conclude that the increase in body fat and/or increase in plasma lipids enhances the neuroendocrine pathway, making the younger pullet responsive to light stimulation. Essential fatty acids, such as linoleic found in corn oil, may also have a direct effect on the release of luteinizing hormone from the pituitary. Interestingly, these same researchers indicated that birds on a restricted feeding schedule had higher baseline luteinizing hormone levels than did corresponding ad-libitum fed birds, and suggest that this general effect could contribute to the improved reproductive performance seen with restricted-fed compared to ad-libitum fed pullets.

While it seems as though body composition may influence the very young pullet's response to light, of more commercial significance is the effect of light stimulation closer to anticipated sexual maturity. Robinson *et al.* (1996) observed breeder pullet maturity when light stimulation, changing from 8L:16D up to 14L:10D was initiated at 120-160d of age (Table 3.4). Birds mature earlier corresponding to earlier light stimulation although the relationship is not linear. Very early stimulation (120-130d) does not seem to greatly advance the age at maturity, although later stimulation at 160d seems to have a definite delaying effect on onset of production. However early light stimulation (120-130d) did have a detrimental effect on production of chicks over the breeding cycle (Table 3.4). Other researchers have generally confirmed this work, where light stimulation as early as 15-17 weeks of age causes reduced peak egg numbers and/or very poor persistency of lay after peak.

TABLE 3.4 Effect of light stimulating pullets at 120-160d of age

	120 d	130 d	140 d	150 d	160 d
Age at maturity(d)	173	171	175	176	182
Stimulation to maturity (d)	53	41	35	26	22
Weight of 1st egg (g)	44.1	43.5	45.5	44.8	45.4
#Chicks	119b	117b	133a	130a	127a

Adapted from Robinson *et al.* (1996)

Understanding the effect of light stimulating birds at various ages is always complicated by birds often being of different body weight. There is a correlation between mature weight and age at maturity, with genetically heavier strains maturing later. However most commercial strains of breeder pullet are similar in mature weight, and so this fact is of little practical significance. Of more practical importance, is the decision to light stimulate flocks that do not achieve normal weight-for-age. Lien and Yuan (1994) recently indicated performance of pullets that were either 2kg or 1.8kg at 20 weeks of age when light stimulation was planned. Because the 1.8kg birds were below standard, a group of these pullets were grown to 22 weeks, when they were 2.0kg, and then lighted (Table 3.5). These data confirm that underweight pullets should not be light stimulated until the standard weight (around 2.0kg) is achieved, regardless of age. In practice, this means light stimulating pullets only if they achieve a minimum threshold of both weight and age.

Undoubtedly the greatest control over sexual development is achieved with use of black-out growing houses, where a simple constant day length is used throughout rearing. There are economic advantages to using very short days, such as 8h, because birds are less active, and need less feed for maintenance.

TABLE 3.5 Effect of light stimulation of pullets at 2kg or 1.8kg body weight

	Standard weight birds at 20 wks	Underweight birds at 20 wks	Standard weight birds at 22 wks
Lighting age	20 wks	20 wks	22 wks
Body wt at lighting	2.0kg	1.8kg	2.0kg
Age 1st egg (d)	164	172	173
Age 50% production (d)	179	184	188
Eggs to 45 wks	101b	87a	94b

Adapted from Lien and Yuan (1994)

Managers often overfeed such pullets when first using black-out facilities because standards used for open-sided buildings are initially used. Because of reduced maintenance needs, pullets in black-out vs open-sided buildings will be about 5% heavier when given the same feed allocations. This faster growth potential causes earlier maturity. Obviously the situation is corrected by adjustment to the feed allocation.

3.4 PROGRAMS FOR ROOSTERS

If roosters are grown together with the pullets, then usually the lighting program will be dictated by the needs of the females. With separate sex growing, however, there is the potential to consider male lighting programs.

Males seem to perform optimally as breeders when grown on 6-8h light/day. With longer constant photoperiods, maturity is slightly delayed and testes size is somewhat reduced. When very long photoperiods are used during rearing (16-20h), then there is a linear decline in subsequent sperm production. Males normally mature earlier than females given comparable lighting programs. Commercially males are also light-stimulated ahead of the hens because they are often moved to the breeder houses 7-10d earlier, so as to allow them to become accustomed to the male feeding system.

If males are kept separate from hens in situations where artificial insemination is used, then 10-12h light is adequate for sustained semen production. If males are to be maintained in all-male flocks after maturity, they should be held on 8-10h light. Blue lights can also be used with these all male flocks destined for spiking into other breeder flocks, since this environment has a very calming effect on what otherwise can involve very unstable group dynamics.

3.5 COMMERCIAL LIGHTING PROGRAMS

For reasons not fully understood at this time, it seems as though the breeder hen performs best when she has attained a certain age and body weight/ condition prior to light stimulation. A useful rule of thumb with broiler breeders is to ensure hens are at least 2.1kg and 20 weeks of age before light stimulation. This means that a flock at 2.3kg at 19 weeks will not be light stimulated, and likewise 2.0kg birds at 20 weeks will also be held back. Too early a light stimulation without regard for weight and age will lead to small early egg size and poor persistency of egg production after peak.

In essence this means that pullets must always be at least 20 weeks of age before light stimulation, but even at this age they must also be at least 2.1kg in body weight. The effectiveness of early light stimulation can be "lost" if the bird does not have an appropriate body weight and condition. For example, a program of +2 hours at 19 weeks for a 1.9kg bird will likely have little effect on sexual development. The sexual development of such pullets is dictated by the subsequent smaller increases, either natural or artificial, that are given after this time in the breeder house. As previously mentioned, these smaller increases are much less effective in synchronizing the onset of egg production. This concept is of particular significance to high yield birds where there is usually a need to maximize early egg size in order to optimize chick size and subsequent meat yield.

Controlling the lighting program in black-out houses is fairly simple because the manager has total control over daylength. Both pullets and cockerels will be grown on continuous light for 2-3 days, and then daylength reduced to 8-12h of constant light, up to 20 weeks of age. The shorter the daylength, the greater the saving in feed cost, because birds are less active and spend more time in darkness. However, it should be emphasized that the capital costs of black-out housing will never be recovered by savings in feed cost alone. The major economic benefit to black-out housing will be control over sexual development and thus more consistent breeder performance. Another advantage of a short day length is the potential for a greater light stimulation at maturity. On the other hand, the disadvantage of short daylengths of 8-10h, is that there is greater potential for accidental light leakage through the ventilation system. If leakage is of sufficient intensity, it can effectively add to, or subtract from, the light period depending upon the season. Such leakage can detract from any advantage of black-out housing. Less severe light leakage can also be problematic if the leakage creates an intensity which is ≥10x the intensity of the true black-out period. As previously discussed, birds respond to ≥10x changes in intensity as though they are different light periods, and so effectively the bird is subjected to three different light phases - namely light, dark and brown-out due to excessive light leakage. These three "different" light-dark phases will interfere with the normal ovulation process. Growing houses do not have to be 100% black-out. Achieving such control is often expensive, and invariably affects the ventilation system. Brown-out is acceptable, as long as the brown-out realized is not greater than 10x the intensity of any true black-out period occurring on moonless nights after sundown.

With open-sided buildings, the control over sexual development is a little more complicated, but still possible with the use of a simple timeclock. In order to remove seasonal increases or decreases throughout the growing period, it will be necessary to establish the pattern of natural daylength and then supplement this with periods of artificial light (Table 3.3).

In order to initiate and synchronize sexual maturity, it is ideal to give an initial significant increase in daylength of at least 1 hour and preferably 2 hours or more. If birds are grown in black-out houses, then the initial stimulation can be quite large at +3 or 4h, depending upon daylength used during growout. For birds housed in open-sided houses, the daylength at "maturity" will be dictated by the season of the year. For pullets and roosters grown under naturally increasing daylength, (*eg.* winter hatched in the N. Hemisphere), it is hoped that growing pullets will have received extra light so as to counteract the natural increase in daylength. This means a relatively long daylength used during rearing, and so under these conditions, there is less scope for a large increase in daylength needed to induce maturity. Under these conditions, +1h is often adequate to stimulate maturity. Following this initial light stimulation, there needs to be subsequent weekly or biweekly increases necessary to sustain the maturation process. The maximum day length used will, to some extent be dictated by the growing conditions. With open-sided grow-out, involving long daylengths up to maturity, it may be necessary to eventually provide 16-17h light in the breeder house in order to establish a meaningful stimulation. With shorter daylengths used for birds grown under black-out conditions, it is only necessary to increase to a maximum of 14-15h in black-out breeder houses. The shorter daylengths obviously save on electrical costs, and there is an indication of better persistency of production with 14-15h vs 16-17h under these controlled conditions. Many managers will also limit maximum daylength because it may be beneficial to stimulate post-peak birds with +1h light, in order to try and correct any management or disease-induced declines in egg production (or birds becoming photorefractory as discussed at the end of Section 3.1).

If males are grown with females, then their light program is usually dictated by maturity and conditions of the pullets. Where males are grown separately, it is critical to light stimulate the birds at the same time as the hens, such that both sexes are at comparable stages of maturity when mixed in the breeder house. Having males maturing much earlier than the hens, often leads to excessive aggression while the converse situation can lead to psychological castration in such timid immature males and consequently there is loss of life time fertility. Day length has little effect on egg size, fertility or hatchability. Age at first light stimulation can, however, affect egg size, because too early a light increase invariably results in life time loss of egg size for a particular flock. On the other hand, delaying the age of light stimulation usually results in an increase in life time egg size.

Breeders can perform quite well at intensities as low as 10 lux, assuming there is good control over the dark phase. Most breeders are going to be subjected to much higher intensities, usually around 200-400 lux in controlled environment houses, while birds in open-sided breeder houses may be at 800-1200 lux. One of the most important considerations is not to subject birds to a reduction in light intensity when they are moved from growing to breeder facilities. This sometimes happens when pullets are grown in open-sided houses and the birds moved to controlled-environment breeder houses. Pullets can sometimes be subjected to 10x reduction in intensity and this contributes to delayed sexual maturity, and is often associated with obesity.

Examples of lighting programs are summarized in Table 3.6, which encompasses various combinations of black-out vs open-sided growing and breeder facilities.

TABLE 3.6. Lighting program according to housing type

Black-out growing Black-out breeding	Black-out growing Open-sided breeding	Open-sided growing Black-out breeding	Open-sided growing Open-sided breeding
0-3d, 24 hrs @ 30-40 lux	0-3d, 24 hrs @ 30-40 lux	0-3d, 24 hrs	0-3d, 24 hrs
3-21d, 18 hrs @ 30-40 lux	3-21d, 18 hrs @ 30-40 lux	3-21d 18 hrs	3-21d, 18 hrs
21-140d, 8-10 hrs @ 10-30 lux	21-140d, 8 hrs @ 10-30 lux	21-140d daylength corresponding to natural maximum in this period	21-140d daylength corresponding to natural maximum in this period
140-147d, 12 hrs @ >30 lux	140-147d, 14 hrs minimum or natural daylength	140-147d + 1-2 hrs depending on season	140-147d + 1-2 hrs depending on season
Weekly, + 1 hr to 14-15 hrs	Weekly, + 30 minutes to 17 hrs max	Weekly + 30 minutes to 17 hrs max	If natural daylength ≤ 14 hrs, give + 1 hr weekly to max. 17 hrs. If natural daylength ≥ 15 hrs, give + 30 minutes weekly to max. 17 hrs.

There are many variations of lighting programs used commercially, and many of these can be applied successfully. Table 3.6 gives examples of the concepts that need to be applied with any program, however, poor breeder performance will always result from an ill-designed or implemented light program, while a good lighting program is merely part of an overall management strategy. The breeder hen is flexible in her response to a range of well designed lighting programs but is always adversely influenced by ill-designed or "unnatural" photoperiods.

In discussing lighting programs for breeders, the number of hours in the light:dark cycle is invariably assumed to be 24h. With black-out housing there is potential to consider non-24h, or so called ahemeral cycles. For example a 14h light:14h dark cycle is ahemeral, and the 28h day so created, repeats itself six times in a conventional week. The advantages of ahemeral cycles are improved shell quality, improved feed efficiency and increased egg size and such programs have been used with commercial Leghorns. Improved shell quality may be advantageous with older breeders, although there is perhaps less interest in increasing egg size at this time. Little work has in fact been carried out with ahemeral cycles for breeders, although there is an indication of improved fertility. Shanawany (1993) suggests 2-5% improvement in fertility and 5-6% improvement in hatch of fertile with 28 h ahemeral cycles. Better fertility is explained on the basis of longer clutch length and the fact that the first eggs laid within a clutch usually show slightly less fertility. Better hatch of fertile is discussed on the basis of the egg spending an extra 4h in the oviduct (hence stronger shell) and that this results in a preincubation of the embryo which is subsequently better able to withstand transportation and storage. Unfortunately ahemeral cycles are not conducive to timing of management, because the "working day" for the flock quickly gets out of synchronization with the conventional working day.

The practical problems of using ahemeral light programs is somewhat less problematic with mechanized feeding and egg collection, yet it still imposes some unsocial hours on the labor force. It has been suggested that this latter problem can be resolved by using a light:dim ahemeral cycle rather than a light:dark cycle, such that workers could service the flock in the dim period if necessary. Under such conditions it seems necessary to use light intensities of at least 30:1 in the light:dim phases of the cycle.

BIBLIOGRAPHY

Lopez, G. and S. Leeson, 1992. Manage broiler breeder pullets to reduce seasonal variations. Poultry Digest, Sept. 1992, p.31-35.

Dunn, I.C., P.J. Sharp and P.M. Hocking, 1990. Effects of interaction between photostimulation, dietary restriction and dietary maize oil dilution on plasma LH and ovarian and oviduct weights in broiler breeder females during rearing. Br. Poult. Sci. 31:415-427.

Robinson, F.E., T. Wautier, and R.T. Hardin, 1996. Effects of age at photostimulation on reproductive efficiency and carcass characteristics. Can. J. Anim. Sci. 76:275-282.

Lien, R.J., and T. Yuan, 1994. Effect of delayed light stimulation on egg production of broiler breeder pullets of low body weight. J. Appl. Poult. Res. 3:40-48.

Shanawany, M. M. 1993. Ahemeral lighting and reproductive efficiency in breeding flocks. Wld. Poult. Sci. J., 49:213-220.

SUGGESTED READING

Lewis, P.D. and T.R. Morris. 1998. Responses of domestic poultry to various light sources. Wld. Poultry Sci. J. 54: 7-25.

CHAPTER 4. HEALTH MANAGEMENT

PAGE NO.

Health management and biosecurity are perhaps the most critical aspect of modern breeder production. Disease outbreaks are especially catastrophic with breeders because of disruption in egg supply to the hatchery. Today it is becoming more difficult to achieve adequate isolation of breeder farms so as to ensure a comfortable degree of protection against flock infection. However even with isolation and optimum biosecurity procedures, it is impossible to ensure absolute protection for a flock of breeders. Health management today revolves around appropriate use of vaccines, biosecurity, and where appropriate, careful use of feed and water additives. We are now acutely aware of the importance of priming and maintaining optimum immune response in the bird, a situation that starts with the day old breeder and continues through to the end of the breeder cycle. Health management involves not only studying the immune function of the breeders themselves, but also the effect that these programs have on the immunity and health status of the embryo and young broiler chick.

Actual disease challenge obviously varies from country to country and even for different geographical locations within a country. Health management programs should obviously be tailored to combat local potential disease challenge. However breeder managers must be continually updated on new potential diseases and be prepared to modify the protective programs for their flocks. In this chapter, we have given only a brief description of potential diseases, because these are more adequately described elsewhere (Calnek *et al.,* 1997). Although we have briefly outlined the most important diseases and have detailed a number of currently important global disease situations facing the broiler breeder industry, the main aim of this chapter is to review principles involved in developing health management programs.

4.1 IMMUNE RESPONSE

The body protects itself against foreign material, such as bacteria and viruses, through the action of its immune system. Understanding the function of the immune system is important in breeder management, because this is the basis of our extensive vaccination programs.

Invading viruses and bacteria trigger the action of lymphocytes (white blood cells) and/or macrophages (scavengers) in the body. The lymphocytes are produced and programmed by the bursa (B-cells) and the thymus (T-cells). The bursa reaches maximum size and activity about 2 weeks after hatching, and there is little new development after 8-12 weeks of age. Early destruction of the bursa, through natural IBD infection for example, is therefore a major problem to the health status of the pullet and adult breeder. The B-cells migrate to the spleen and lymph nodes where there is antigenic (foreign protein) stimulation of antibodies - this activity is often referred to as humoral immunity. The thymus, found in the neck of the bird, produces T-cells under control of hormone production. These T-cells are produced up to sexual maturity, and work in cooperation with the scavenging macrophages to kill invading bacteria, viruses etc. This action is referred to as cell mediated immunity.

Humoral immunity (bursa) is the main defense against bacteria, while cell mediated immunity is critical for protection against viruses. The B-cells may be induced to divide and specialize, and it is such sensitized B-cells that release antibodies into the blood, with a life span of 3-5 days. Some B-cells have a memory system, and this enables a much greater activation the second time that an antigen is recognized - again, this action is important in developing the immune response through vaccination. The T-cells from the thymus, on the other hand, respond to antigens by producing so called effector cells and also memory cells. The effector cells act directly on the viral cell and release chemicals known as lymphokines which help to confine the antigen (virus) to the immediate site of infection.

The various lymphocytes will therefore be produced in response to natural infection or to vaccination. A vaccine will contain an attenuated (weakened) live virus, or a killed or inactivated virus. Memory cells are then able to respond very quickly and precisely if the bird is subsequently exposed to a natural infection. Vaccination therefore "sensitizes" the immune system. Unfortunately the vaccination response takes some days to develop, and this is of little use to the day old chick that is very susceptible to natural infection prior to vaccines becoming effective. For this reason, we rely heavily on the adult breeder hen to pass on some "immunity" to the chick, via the egg. This short-lived immunity is often referred to as passive or maternal immunity, compared to active immunity, which will develop following the chick's own vaccination program. These maternal antibodies are often called IgG and IgA. The IgG circulates in the blood of the breeder hen and can be deposited in the yolk and these will subsequently be "absorbed" by the embryo during incubation. The IgG act as do regular antibodies, but they have a finite life and cannot themselves reproduce in any way. The IgA antibodies on the other hand remain in the hens epithelial tissue, such as the uterus, and so these antibodies can be secreted with the albumen. The IgA antibodies confer less protection than do the IgG, yet they are active in the chicks intestine and respiratory tract and are useful in protection against Newcastle and Infectious Bronchitis virus infection.

The success of passive immunity depends upon adequate vaccination and antibody titer of the breeder hen. Within reason, the higher the titer (measure of circulating antibodies) in the hen, the greater the transfer to the chick. For Newcastle, Infectious Bursal Disease, Infectious Bronchitis and Reovirus, there is about a 50% transfer of titer from the breeder hen to the chick. If the breeder hen's titer is low then at least 10% of chicks usually fail to exhibit any measurable titer to the virus. Even in breeders with high titers, 5-6% of chicks may show low or no titer, especially with Reovirus. The most important factor in protecting all chicks seems to be uniformity of titers in the breeder hens. As will be discussed in the following sections, high uniform titers in breeders are usually obtained with vaccination programs that involve initial administration of a live virus (primer) followed by a killed virus at some older age. If the immune system is not adequately primed then there are fewer memory cells, and so the response to the secondary killed virus is much less.

To some extent the effectiveness of vaccination programs is influenced by the nutritional status of the bird. If breeders are fed nutritionally inadequate diets, then immune response is likely to be adversely affected. This situation has often raised concerns about the effect of skip-a-day feeding on vaccination response. Where possible, vaccination should be in the late afternoon of the feed day. There is also some recent evidence to suggest that results of vaccination (*eg.* ELISA response) are better for hens fed higher than normal levels of vitamin E. Optimum results in breeders and broiler offspring are seen with 10x the normal level of dietary vitamin E (up to 300 IU/kg). Unfortunately vitamin E is very expensive, and so the economics of such a management procedure must be carefully considered for specific local situations.

4.2 VACCINATION PROGRAMS

Vaccines are used to stimulate the bird=s own immune system without causing overt signs of disease. They are most commonly used to protect birds against infection by viruses, although more recently there has been development of vaccines for protection against selected bacteria (often called bacterins rather than vaccines) and also for coccidiosis. When an exact dose of attenuated (weakened) or killed virus is given to the bird, it will produce antibodies as directed by the thymus and/or bursa depending upon the age of the bird. This controlled priming dose means that antibodies will be produced more quickly and in greater quantities if the bird is subsequently infected with the natural, more virulent, virus.

Live vs inactivated vaccines: There are essentially two types of vaccine available to the poultry industry, namely live or killed. The live viruses are attenuated in some way, and to be effective, must grow and replicate in the bird's own tissue. As the virus is live, it can be sprayed onto the birds, because the virus will establish itself in the mucosa of the eye or respiratory tract etc. Killed or inactivated viruses must be injected, either intramuscularly or sub-cutaneously. The main characteristics of live vs dead vaccines are summarized in Table 4.1.

The main advantages of a live vaccine are that they can be administered very quickly by spray or via the drinking water. They are relatively inexpensive and give almost immediate immunity. Killed vaccines on the other hand are much longer lasting, are easy to transport and handle, and pose no disease threat.

In practice, a life cycle vaccination program usually involves a combination of live and killed virus vaccines. The live vaccines can be used to give an initial priming reaction, and then this is followed at later ages with inactivated vaccines. Killed vaccines must always be injected because they cannot replicate in the bird's body. These killed vaccines are usually mixed with an adjuvant, such as oil, which helps the vaccine to be released much more slowly into the bloodstream. Live vaccines can be administered in a number of different ways (Table 4.2.).

Breeder pullets and cockerels are likely going to be vaccinated almost every week up to transfer to the breeder house. The exact vaccination program will depend entirely upon the natural infections endemic in a given area. All vaccines are stressful to the bird, and so the number of different vaccines used, and their frequency of use should be kept to a minimum commensurate with achieving optimum protection.

Table 4.3 outlines a potential vaccinating schedule for pullets.

TABLE 4.1 Comparison of live vs killed vaccines

Parameter	Live Vaccine	Killed Vaccine
Bird reaction	Greater	Generally less, and local
Cycling	Present	Absent
Effective time period	Short	Long-lasting
Application method	Complex	Simple
Effective coverage	Some misses	Uniform exposure
Disease potential	Yes	No
Storage needs	Yes, refrigeration	No, long shelf life
Multivalents	Potential for interference	No interference
Cost	Less	More
Application time	Short	Long
Labor needs, cost	Low	High
Time for immunity to develop	Days	3-6 weeks
Quantity vaccine	Less - live virus replicates	Large quantity needed
Immunity	Local and cell mediated	Blood antibodies only

TABLE 4.2 Vaccination techniques for attenuated live virus-based products

Virus	Vaccination method
Marek's	Injection
Infectious Laryngotracheitis	Eye drop
Infectious Bronchitis	Drinking water or spray
Newcastle Disease	Drinking water or spray
Infectious Bursal	Drinking water
Fowl Pox	Wing web
Avian Encephalomalacia	Wing web

TABLE 4.3. Potential vaccination schedule

Vaccine	Age	Method	Type
Infectious Bronchitis, Newcastle	1 d 3 wks 16 wks Repeat each 30-60d, if necessary	Spray Water Water	LA LA LA
Infectious Bursal Disease	1 d 3 wks 16 wks	Subcutaneous Water Subcutaneous	LA LA Killed
Marek's	1 d or 18d incubation	Subcutaneous Egg injection	LA LA
Avian Encephalomalacia	10 wks	Wing-web	LA
Infectious Laryngotracheitis	6 wks	Eye drop	LA
Fowl Pox	1 d	Wing Web	LA
Tenosynovitis	1 d 6 wks	Subcutaneous Subcutaneous or Wing Web	LA LA
Fowl Cholera	8,12,16 wks	Subcutaneous	KB
Infectious Coryza	8,12 wks	Subcutaneous	KB
Coccidiosis	1 d	Water or gel puck	LA
LA = Live attenuated; KB = Killed bacterin			

4.3 VACCINATION METHODS

a) Subcutaneous or Intramuscular Injection: All dead vaccines and some live vaccines can be given by injection. The advantage of this system is that all birds are equally covered, but obviously at the expense of greater time and labor. Marek's vaccine is almost universally given as an injection into either the 18d embryo or the day old chick at the hatchery (see later section on Marek's). With older birds, vaccination should not occur in the morning of a skip-a-day program because the physical handling of the birds can cause regurgitation of feed.

b) Drinking water: Administering live vaccines via the drinking water has become a common practice for IB, ND and IBD. In order to ensure complete coverage of the flock, it is essential to turn-off or raise waterers for 1-3h prior to vaccinating. In warm weather (30°C), 1h water deprivation is adequate, while at a more moderate temperature (22°C), 3h may be necessary. The idea of water deprivation is to ensure that birds are interested in water, but not necessarily excessively thirsty. If dehydration occurs prior to water vaccinating, then uneven vaccine uptake can occur because 50-60% of the dominant birds in the flock may drink all the water/vaccine that is subsequently delivered.

Because the vaccine is live, it must be handled carefully in terms of ensuring no temperature shock, or presence of foreign organic material. Many poultry farms chlorinate the drinking water in order to kill such natural viruses. Chlorine and other disinfectants will also kill the virus in the vaccine and so this must be removed from the system. Ideally, the chlorinator should be switched off for 48h prior to water vaccination. In order to further protect the vaccine, skim milk powder is usually added to the vaccine-water mixture to "buffer" any adverse action of residual chlorine (up to 1 ppm) or other water contaminants. If water is heavily contaminated with viruses or bacteria and the removal of chlorine for 48h will cause other problems for the birds, then it is advisable to import water for vaccinating and give the vaccine in separate drinkers. Waterers must also be thoroughly cleaned before vaccine is given. The vaccine should be carefully mixed with water and skim milk powder. It is usual to administer the vaccine in about 30% of the water that would normally be consumed by the birds. To this water is added skim milk powder at about 1 kg/400 litres. The vaccine pellet is carefully dissolved in a small quantity of water then added to the water/milk powder solution in a holding tank. The stock solution is then pumped into the water system. Vaccines should not be administered via medicators. Following is a guideline for normal water intake of breeder pullets at 20° and 30°C, together with suggested quantities of water/vaccine and skim milk powder per 10,000 birds (Table 4.4).

As vaccine is pumped through the water system, the end of the line furthest from the pump should be opened until the milky fluid is detected. The birds should be "walked" 2-3 times, especially along the outside walls, to ensure that all birds are moved towards the waterers.

Table 4.4 Daily water intake and water/vaccine quantities for pullets from 3-16 weeks of age.

	Units per 10,000 bird flock					
	At 20°C			At 30°C		
Wks of age	**Normal water intake (litres)**	**Water + vaccine (litres)**	**Skim milk powder (kg)**	**Normal water intake (litres)**	**Water + vaccine (litres)**	**Skim Milk (kg)**
3	300	100	0.25	400	120	0.3
4	400	120	0.30	600	180	0.5
5	550	165	0.40	800	240	0.6
6	700	210	0.50	1000	300	0.8
7	800	240	0.60	1200	360	0.9
8	900	270	0.67	1400	420	1.0
9	1000	300	0.75	1600	480	1.2
10	1100	330	0.82	1800	540	1.4
11	1250	375	0.93	2000	600	1.5
12	1400	420	1.00	2200	660	1.7
13	1500	450	1.10	2400	720	1.8
14	1600	480	1.20	2600	780	2.0
15	1700	510	1.30	2800	840	2.1
16	1800	540	1.40	3000	1000	2.4

Common problems encountered with water vaccination relate to mixing the vaccine with too small a volume of water, resulting in some birds not receiving the vaccine. Because the virus is live and multiplies in the vaccinated birds, these unvaccinated birds receive a "natural" vaccination once the vaccinated birds start to shed the virus. This situation is usually referred to as vaccination cycling or a "rolling" vaccination. Obviously the secondary "vaccination" is uncontrolled both in terms of age of bird and the quantity and virulence of the virus encountered. Another reason for poor water vaccination response is that the virus is inactivated by dirt or organic matter in the drinkers and/or water line. As previously suggested, drinkers must be cleaned, while water lines themselves are best disinfected by treating with a stock solution of 2kg citric acid/10 litres water 24h prior to vaccination.

*2) **Spray:*** Establishing good mucosal immunity in the upper respiratory tract is a logical step in helping prevent respiratory diseases such as IB and Newcastle. Most chicks are sprayed with IB vaccine at the hatchery. The major factor influencing effectiveness of such vaccines is droplet particle size. If the particle size is too small, the vaccine can get into the alveoli of the lung, and cause a severe reaction. For young birds, droplet size should be around 100µ (coarse) depending upon vaccine type, and as birds get older, the size can be reduced down to 50µ at 6-8 weeks, and down to 20µ at 12 weeks of age. As with water vaccinating, it is important that all birds are vaccinated with the spray, because non-uniform coverage can result in a "rolling" vaccination effect as birds get older. The quantity of water diluent depends upon the type of vaccine, age of bird, and applicator systems but is usually around 2 litres per 10,000 birds after 7-10d of age. Because of the small quantity of water used, it is economical to use deionized water for this type of vaccination. To ensure that the vaccine spray is not lost through the fans, the ventilation system should be turned off prior to vaccinating and then birds penned down one side of the building. With older birds, it is preferable to spray vaccinate on feed days.

d) Wing web: It is common to administer Fowl Pox and Avian Encephalomalacia vaccines, if required, by wing-web. This system involves a hand-held two needle applicator, that is immersed in vaccine and then applied to the skin web of the wing. The technique is very reliable when carried out by an experienced and conscientious vaccinating crew. Problems can arise from simply not immersing the needles into the vaccine or by having feathers deflect the injection. In order for the vaccine to be adequately picked up and released by the needles, the applicator must be held vertically and not at an angle, to both the vaccine bottle and wing.

e) In-ovo: One of the latest techniques for administering vaccines, is physical injection through the shell and into the developing 18d embryo. Currently this is most commonly carried out for application of Marek's vaccine, although vaccines for IBD are now available, and several others are under test. The main advantages of such a system are automation and the fact that the newly hatched chick more quickly develops protection against Marek's disease.

4.4 TIMING OF VACCINATION

The time that vaccines are given is critical to the development of the immune response. For breeders, the aim of the vaccination program is to *a)* protect the juvenile and adult breeder from infection and *b)* ensure optimum maternal antibodies in the offspring broiler chicks. The antibody titer levels detected in the blood follow the same type of pattern as seen in an egg production curve *ie.* there is an initial peak, followed by slow decline with age. The major peak in antibodies should coincide with the onset of maturity. This situation is achieved by careful timing of the sequence of vaccines given to the immature pullet and rooster. Initially, the breeder chick will have maternal antibodies passed on from the grandparent breeder. When these maternal antibody levels are high, there will not be a good "take" by any vaccines given to the young chick. Timing of the initial vaccine must therefore correspond with the expected decline in maternal antibodies which usually occurs in the first 7-10 days of the chick's life. The worst situation is always seen when maternal antibody levels are variable. In this situation, chicks with low maternal antibodies respond well to early vaccination, while chicks at the other extreme may be unaffected. Unfortunately for these latter chicks, their initially strong maternal antibodies quickly decline, and then these unprotected chicks will exhibit the classical "rolling" vaccination that they pick up from their vaccinated sisters. Ideally a uniform level of maternal antibodies is needed.

As previously discussed, a program for protection against any disease today usually involves a combination of live and inactivated vaccines. The timing usually means that the immune system is primed with an initial attenuated, but live, and replicating virus such that a much stronger response is seen when killed viruses are subsequently given to the older pullet. Ideally the last vaccination in the pullet house will result in a peak of antibodies corresponding to time of peak egg output. As the breeder gets older, the antibody titers will decline, and so ELISA testing is essential in order to determine the need for any re-vaccination of these older birds.

4.5 SPECIFIC VACCINE CATEGORIES

While vaccines are usually used to protect breeders against viral infections, there is currently interest in developing immunity to bacteria and protozoa challenge. The industry therefore has different types of "vaccine" available, and the following are detailed examples for each of the categories. For these descriptions, we have chosen Marek's, E. coli and Coccidiosis as examples of these vaccine categories.

A) Viral-Marek's: Marek's vaccine was first produced in the early 1970's and its development since this time is indicative of the problems facing vaccine manufacturers and poultry veterinarians. Marek's was a devastating disease to the poultry industry in the 1960's where up to 20-25% mortality was common and accommodated simply by placing proportionally more day-old chicks. The first

Marek's vaccines were an immediate success, and for a number of years, the disease was very much secondary to respiratory diseases and IBD. Over the last 10 years, so-called virulent strains of Marek's have evolved, and so vaccine programs have necessarily been modified. As with any organism, mutations evolve, and this new situation with Marek's reflects the situation that is likely to occur with our other breeder vaccines over time.

Breeder vaccines for Marek's are based on one of three serotypes:

1. Chicken based, oncogenic
2. Chicken based, non-oncogenic
3. Turkey herpes virus, non-pathogenic

The most widely used breeder vaccines to date, have been based on serotype 3 turkey herpes virus. Such vaccines induce the immune response in the breeder but cannot provide any disease threat. Serotype 1 vaccines have also been used, but because these are the lethal oncogenic (tumor forming) strains, they have to be highly attenuated. These newly developed vaccines of the early 1970's were perhaps attenuated too much, and so this speeded up their loss of activity. In Europe, Rispin's vaccine was developed which was also a serotype 1 vaccine, but the virus was of low oncogenicity. A feature of the Rispin's vaccine, was horizontal spread of the virus across the flock, a situation that did not occur with the N. American serotype 1 vaccines used at that time. Initially serotype 2 vaccines seemed to be of little use, because they were naturally non-tumor forming. In recent years with the emergence of virulent (and now very-virulent) strains of Marek's, it is found that bivalent mixtures of serotype 2 and 3, or 2 and 1, offer the best protection at this time. Bivalent and even trivalent (serotypes 1-3) vaccines have therefore been recommended for breeders in areas of very virulent Marek's. Unfortunately for the breeder industry, serotype 2 based vaccines have the disadvantage of having cross-reactivity with lymphoid leukosis (see section 4.14). Marek's vaccines that contain serotype 2 products seem to produce more lymphoid leukosis in breeder flocks that are not free of the avian leukosis virus.

Most Marek's vaccines for breeders are cell-associated, and this means that they need to be stored in liquid nitrogen. Some non-cell associated vaccines are available in regions where handling and obtaining liquid nitrogen is difficult or inconvenient. Once the vaccine ampules are thawed, the diluent must be added quickly because the freezing medium contains DMSO (dimethysulfoxide) which is toxic and so must be diluted out very quickly. Failure to handle, thaw or dilute the vaccine adequately are the major reasons for poor antibody response to the vaccine. Marek's vaccine should be diluted to give about 2-4,000 Plaque Forming

Units (PFU) per dose, and then day old chicks are given around 0.1 ml vaccine intramuscularly. With in-ovo vaccination, usually at 18d incubation, the same concepts apply although Rispin's vaccine is rarely used for this application. The advantage of in-ovo vaccinations of breeders, is that chicks will receive immunity some 3d earlier, compared to conventional vaccinations given at day of age.

Unfortunately there are no new Marek's vaccines on the horizon, and so the most "potent" prevention at this time, is the use of trivalent vaccines. Virulent Marek's appeared about 10 years after introduction of the monovalent vaccines, while very virulent Marek's appeared 10 years after bivalent vaccines were introduced. At this time, the future is unclear as to whether or not the Marek's virus will repeat its evolution and pose even greater problems in the foreseeable future.

b) Bacteria - E. coli: Bacteria also elicit the antigen-antibody reaction in the bird and so it is possible to develop vaccines for their control. Bacterial vaccines are usually killed and called bacterins. In general, bacteria are more complex organisms than are viruses, therefore vaccine production is more complex, and as a generalization, efficacy of bacterins is less than for viral vaccines - especially with long-term usage. E. coli is a ubiquitous bacteria on poultry farms, and they colonize the gut of the chick at an early age, sometimes causing colibacillosis, synovitis, omphalitis or air sac infection.

In the past, E. coli infections were treated with antibiotics such as ampicillin or chlorotetracyclin, although there is evidence of resistance developing to these products. Bacterins may therefore provide an important tool in preventing future E. coli infections. Unfortunately, as with many bacteria, there are numerous serotypes of E. coli and this makes bacterin production very challenging. There are three basic serotype groups termed O, K and H antigens. The O antigens relate to their lipopolysaccharide content, while the H and K relate to flagellar (hair-like arms) and bacterial surface coating respectively. Unfortunately there are about 140 O antigens, 90 K antigens, and 50 H antigens known. Potentially, there are well over 0.5 million potential serotypes of E. coli. Fortunately there are probably less than 100 serotype combinations that are problematic in poultry, but even this number poses problems in developing general-acting E. coli bacterins. The K antigens are associated with virulence of disease, while the flagellar H antigens are not thought to be important in this situation. However there has been recent interest in developing bacterins based on H antigens. These so-called E. coli pilus vaccines, are aimed at preventing the E. coli from adhering to or colonising the intestinal epithelium, since the bird is primed to recognize the flagella as an antigen. These bacterins consist of concentrated and purified preparations of E. coli flagella. An advantage of such bacterins is that they are not infectious to the bird. After vaccination, the bird's antibodies prevent the E. coli from adhering to the lining of the gut. These types of bacterins have been used successfully to prevent E. coli scours in young pigs and calves. To date, such pilus bacterins seem efficacious, but are no more so than bacterins prepared from whole cell cultures.

c) Protozoa - coccidiosis: The increase in drug resistance by coccidia to various anticoccidials spurred the development of live oocyst based vaccines. Four commercial vaccines are now available, namely Immucox, Paracox, Coccivac and Livacox, and all are produced from a range of live oocysts. Many breeding companies now rely entirely on such vaccines to give life-time protection against coccidiosis from a single vaccination at day-of-age.

The exact mechanisms involved in development of immunity to coccidia are not yet clear, although it seems as though both cell-mediated and humoral systems are involved. Vaccines essentially provide a very low level of infection, and it is thought that this stimulates cell-mediated thymus cells to initiate a series of events that eventually result in immunity. On the other hand, with a natural infection, which is usually of much greater intensity in terms of ingested oocyst numbers, the humoral bursal cell system developing the classical IgA, IgG etc. antibody response, is more important. The cell-associated system is perhaps most important from a vaccination view point, simply because the coccidia life cycle involves many days spent inside the host cells of the gut epithelium. The time that the coccidia developmental stages spend outside of the cell (and therefore prone to attack by the humoral defense system) is much shorter, often being a matter of minutes, and just a few hours total in the overall life cycle. To protect against infection therefore, the cell-mediated system is most important because 80-95% of the life cycle is spent in the cell, and so there is much more chance of contact with this defense system of the bird. With natural infection, it is thought that the humoral system has little chance of keeping up with infection, because the antibodies have much less chance of "catching" the sporozoites outside of the gut epithelial cells. Vaccines do prime the cell-associated system, without causing disease. As with any antibody-antigen reaction, there is specificity involved, and so the vaccine must contain oocyst types and strains specific to potential local challenge. Ongoing reformulation of vaccines for specific geographical locations, as occurs with Paracox and Immucox, is therefore a positive move in helping to prevent development of coccidia resistance.

To be economically viable, the oocyst vaccination procedures must provide uniform exposure without the need to handle individual chicks. Spray cabinets at the hatchery, adding the vaccine to drinking water, and spraying onto the feed have all been used as a method of application. More recently Immucox introduced a novel gel application system, in which a "puck" of gel containing the vaccine is simply placed in the chick box, and birds voluntarily consume this, and become vaccinated prior to arriving at the farm. Whatever system of application is used, uniform exposure to all chicks is essential because any non-vaccinated birds will be naturally infected in 5-7d as the vaccinated chicks start to shed moderate numbers of oocysts. This natural cycling is important for the vaccinated chicks, because for most Eimeria species it takes two cycles of the parasite before the bird develops complete immunity, and with E. tenella three cycles are needed. Where new litter is used, and the environment is very low in humidity, then the litter may contain insufficient moisture for efficient cycling of the oocyst. While such conditions are very rare in industry, thought should be given to careful "wetting" of such dry litter 4-7d after the initial vaccination.

Obviously the diet cannot contain any anticoccidials if vaccines are used, and especially in the first 21d after vaccination, as immunity is developing. Inadvertent inclusion of anticoccidials in starter diets will totally destroy the vaccination program. In the future, various combinations of anticoccidial and vaccination programs may be used. With continued use of coccidia vaccines, even with periodic reformulation, some resistant strains are likely to develop. Conceivably such strains could be cleaned-up by using anticoccidials every 1-2 years or as required, at any given site. Conceivably it may even be possible to develop oocyst vaccine strains that are specifically susceptible to selected anticoccidials, allowing for a very efficient system of anticoccidial/vaccine rotation.

There has also been recent interest in the potential for protecting day-old broiler chicks against coccidiosis, by ensuring transfer of maternal antibodies into the hatching egg (Smith *et al.,* 1994). Dosing breeders with 20,000 E. maxima oocysts resulted in production of antibodies which were detectable in the egg yolk and the newly hatched chicks. Antibody levels in the breeders peaked at 3-4 weeks after challenge and when their offspring were themselves challenged with oocysts, there was a 90% reduction in oocyte shedding. However chicks from eggs collected 7-8 weeks after the breeders were challenged, showed only a 50% reduction in oocyte shedding. The levels of IgG antibodies, in chicks, rather than IgA or IgM, seemed to be highly correlated with levels of maternal immunity, providing a potential basis for developing a coccidial immunization program in breeders.

4.6 BIOSECURITY

Biosecurity is a common sense approach to reducing the chance of infectious agents from coming into contact with the breeders. Obviously, therefore, the degree of biosecurity needed is influenced by the potential for disease challenge in each production region. A biosecurity program is intended to limit the potential routes of infection to the breeder flock, and in order of importance, these are: other poultry, other animals, people, farm equipment and vehicles. However it must be realized that even with the most extensive biosecurity system, there is never any absolute guarantee that breeders will not become infected. Different degrees of biosecurity will on average give varying degrees of protection for the breeder flocks. The major points to consider in developing biosecurity programs are:

1. Isolation: If breeder farms are truly isolated from other poultry, then the risk of infection is dramatically reduced. It has been suggested that a 5 km barrier between farms reduces potential for cross-infection by at least 50%. Achieving such isolation today is becoming more difficult, and there is a need to balance the isolation of a breeder site against the cost of transporting feed and eggs, and the supply of labor.

2. All-in, All-out: This system implies only one age of breeder on site, and that the site is populated at one single time. Multi-age breeder farms that are never completely depopulated will always carry a major disease threat. Less obvious sometimes is the potential problem of introducing roosters from other farms for spiking, even though hens are considered to be all-in, all-out.

3. People: Differences in how staff and visitors are challenged upon entering the breeder farm is often the most noticeable difference in biosecurity programs. The most stringent systems involve shower-in, and shower-out, where staff and visitors have no other entry to the farm other than through the shower system - this implies security fences. Such biosecurity usually implies that staff cannot own poultry of their own and visitors must not have traveled to other farms 24 hrs prior to entry. Coupled with this system are footbaths at point of entry into each breeder house, and hand washing facilities immediately inside each house. The next level of biosecurity involves merely requesting staff and visitors to use coveralls and boots supplied by the farm.

4. Other animals: It is difficult to maintain good health status in breeders, if wild birds and rodents have easy access inside the buildings. Wild birds are especially problematic, because potentially they can carry the same infectious organisms as do the breeders. Apart from the obvious advantages of a stringent rodent control program, it is now also known that rats and especially mice can be major vectors of salmonella.

5. Feed and water: Both feed and water can be vectors for bacteria and protozoa. Feed is best sanitized by pelleting and/or by inclusion of such products as organic acids and formalin where regulations allow. Studies have shown that re-contamination of feed, after it leaves the mill, is often the cause of high bacterial counts (see vehicles). On farm, this means adequate feed tank sanitation, and care in avoiding build up of mold or moisture in feed lines. Feed tanks should ideally be swept out each month, disinfected each 6 months and fumigated at the end of each crop of birds. Water should be checked at least twice each year for presence of bacteria and parasites.

6. Vehicles: Because feed and egg trucks are traveling to many farms each day, they provide a great risk for spread of infectious agents. Although it is rarely implemented, the ideal system is to have holding feed tanks at the perimeter of the farm, such that the feed truck does not have to enter the premises. The feed is then distributed to the individual breeder house by a dedicated on-farm truck or farm wagon. More often, trucks are simply sanitized as they enter the farm, by driving through disinfection tanks and being sprayed externally. In cold environments, this process is often problematic because of freezing of the water lines. Feed trucks delivering breeder feed should never be used to haul raw ingredients such as meat, fish or poultry by-product meals. If truck drivers leave their vehicles, they should be asked to wear disposable plastic boots.

7. Equipment: Moving small and large pieces of equipment from farm to farm is a weakness of most biosecurity systems. Another major concern is egg flats and egg dollies being transported to and from the hatchery. Vigilance in sanitizing such equipment at the hatchery, before it is returned to the breeder farm, is the only viable solution to minimize the risk.

8. Dead and sick birds: It is likely uneconomical to establish "sick" or "hospital" pens on breeder farms. Even with non-infectious disease, or with physical injury, such birds rarely recover sufficiently so that they can meaningfully re-establish themselves if reintroduced into the flock. The immune competence of such affected birds is likely reduced, and so they represent an easier point of establishment for pathogens. Such birds should be culled from the flock. There seems little alternative to incineration of dead birds. Freezing and re-cycling and composting may be alternatives at the broiler farm, but for breeders, the immediate destruction of dead birds is essential for optimum disease prevention.

Table 4.5 summarizes action that could be implemented at breeder farms to ensure varying degrees of biosecurity. As previously discussed, the various levels of biosecurity provide different levels of potential protection to the breeder flock, and this is obviously achieved at variable cost. In attempting to rationalize cost effectiveness of biosecurity, Gifford et al. (1986) developed a unique economic model of the cost and value of biosecurity for broiler breeders.

These workers describe three types of potential disease challenge ranging from mild through severe pathogenicity as described in Table 4.6. Obviously if a flock of breeders is exposed to ILT, then the production consequences are going to be much more severe than if MG is the problem. Conversely, biosecurity will be more valuable if ILT is the disease challenge. Gifford et al. (1986) then go on to describe three potential levels of breeder farm biosecurity, ranging from none to shower-in (Table 4.7).

TABLE 4.5. Comparison of levels of breeder farm biosecurity

	Level of biosecurity		
Consideration	**Low**	**Medium**	**High**
1. Isolation	1 km	5 km	10 km with perimeter fence
2. Other birds	Multi-age flocks	All-in, all-out, spiking males from other farms	All-in, all-out. No new males introduced
3. People	Plastic boots	Provide clean coveralls and boots	Shower-in, out. Footbaths, hand-washing facilities
4. Other animals	Rodent control	Rodent control with monitoring	Rodent and wild bird control with monitoring
5. Feed, water	Water checked periodically	Disinfect feed truck at farm. Assay water 2x/yr	Disinfect feed truck or restrict entry to perimeter. Systematic feed tank sanitation program
6. Vehicles	Insist on clean vehicles	Disinfect at point of entry	No entry
7. Equipment	Minimal transfer between farms	Disinfect all equipment between farms	No transfer
8. Dead and sick birds	Sick pens	Sick pens, incineration	Active culling and incineration

TABLE 4.6 Effect of disease on breeder performance					
			% Production consequences		
Disease category	**Example**	**Pathogenicity**	**Mortality**	**Egg Prod.**	**Hatch**
A	ILT	Severe	+10	-30	-10
B	IB	Intermediate	+5	-15	-5
C	MG	Mild	+1	-5	-1
					Adapted from Gifford *et al.* (1986)

TABLE 4.7 Procedures for various levels of biosecurity	
Biosecurity level	**Procedures necessary**
1.	None - Costs $0
2.	Restricted access to vehicles and personnel. Change-room for staff, coveralls and boots for visitors. Bird proof buildings, active rodent control and dead bird disposal. Initial capital cost 1.034/doz eggs. Annual operating cost 0.64/doz eggs.
3.	As in 2, plus shower-in for all staff and visitors. Perimeter fence. Disinfection of all trucks, egg flats and egg dollies. All equipment confined to farm. Initial capital cost 34/doz eggs. Annual operating costs 1.04/doz eggs.
	Adapted from Gifford *et al.* (1986)

Level 3 biosecurity, involving shower-in, is becoming the most common system with breeders and will obviously be the most expensive but is expected to give the greatest protection.

If a disease outbreak occurs in a region, then it is assumed that with no biosecurity (level 1, Table 4.7) there is a 100% chance of infection for the flock. In contrast with level 3 biosecurity, it is assumed that 95% of flocks will be unaffected. Using such predictions, following are the costs of biosecurity + costs associated with average production losses for these various situations involving 20,000 breeders (Table 4.8).

TABLE 4.8 Flock costs of biosecurity and disease outbreak			
Disease type	**Biosecurity level**		
	1	**2**	**3**
A *eg.* ILT	$35,000	$17,000	$3,000
B *eg.* IB	$17,000	$10,000	$3,000
C *eg.* MG	$13,900	$3,600	$2,700
			Adapted from Gifford *et al.* (1986)

With no biosecurity, and disease inevitable, Gifford et al. (1986) predict average losses for a 20,000 breeder flock at $35,000 for ILT down to $13,900 for MG. With Level 3 biosecurity, losses are a moderate $2,700 to $3,000 regardless of disease type. Obviously extreme biosecurity is no absolute guarantee of disease prevention but for birds as valuable as broiler breeders, the insurance factor of biosecurity seems irresistible. The unforseen problem with disease outbreaks in breeders of course is not merely the immediate economic loss as shown above, but more importantly the difficulty associated with procuring replacement hatching eggs or chicks, in order to service broiler customers.

4.7 DISINFECTION AND SANITIZATION

Cleaning, disinfection and general sanitizing of the breeder house, the immediate area around the house and all equipment, is an essential part of a biosecurity program. All pathogens are protected to some extent by organic material such as old litter, dust and spilled feed. Also, disinfectants and fumigants are much less effective in the presence of such organic material, and so obviously the breeder house and equipment must be thoroughly cleaned before sanitization occurs. There are five basic types of disinfectants and each has application potential for specific use.

1) Chlorine: Chlorine is relatively inexpensive and is well tolerated by birds even at 5-10x normal application rates. On breeder farms, chlorine is used primarily for the disinfection of water lines. Chlorine kills a large range of bacteria and viruses, but is quite sensitive to pH range, working best at around pH 7.2-7.4. The normal recommendation is to achieve 3 ppm chlorine at the far end of the water line and this may necessitate 5-6ppm closer to the chlorinator. At clean out, the lines should be super-chlorinated to 20-30ppm. The disadvantage of chlorine is that it is very corrosive, is of little use in presence of organic matter, and must obviously be removed from the water system when live vaccines are being administered. Regular household bleach is used most frequently as a water sanitizer.

2) Phenolic compounds: Phenols are used extensively during clean-out of breeder houses. While having limited activity against viruses, phenols are very bactericidal and unlike chlorine, work fairly well in the presence of organic material. Phenols are irritants and can be quite toxic to both poultry and humans, so care must be taken in handling and transportation. Commercial products are often mixed with a detergent.

3) Iodine: Iodine is more stable than chlorine but is still inactivated by organic matter. Used correctly, iodine compounds are one of the safest non-toxic disinfectants used on-farm, and so are useful for hand washing. Iodine is not usually considered for footbaths, because of its rapid inactivation by the organic material that usually builds up quickly in situations of heavy use.

4) Quarternary ammonium compounds (QUATS): QUATS are now used extensively for disinfection of farms and breeder equipment as well as for egg sanitation and hatchery clean-up. QUATS have the advantage of being very broad-spectrum, and are generally tasteless, odorless and less irritating to birds and humans. They also have perhaps the best residual activity of all disinfectants, although are not effective in the presence of large quantities of organic material, or against pseudomonas bacteria.

5) Formalin/Formaldehyde: Formalin liquid and formaldehyde gas are undoubtedly the most effective broad-spectrum sanitizers available. Both compounds are very irritating and toxic, and so great care must be taken in handling and application. Because of mutagenic properties, formaldehyde is now not registered for general farm or hatchery use in certain countries. Formaldehyde works even in the presence of some organic material, and can be used effectively to sterilize buildings and equipment. Both liquid formalin and formaldehyde gas are temperature and humidity dependent, and so within practical limits, their use is most beneficial with high temperature and high humidity. In brooding areas for example, after clean-out, the heat source should be turned on and the interior building surfaces and equipment saturated with a minimum of water. Formaldehyde gas is best prepared by adding formalin to potassium permanganate. For buildings, each 100 m^3 of volume can be sterilized by adding 1 litre of formalin to 250g of potassium permanganate. For large volumes, use replicate batches of formalin and potassium permanganate, rather than using one large mix. The reaction is immediate, violent and exothermic, and the procedure must only be carried out by trained personnel equipped with all necessary protective apparatus.

Clean-out, disinfection and fumigation where necessary are carried out in sequence following depopulation of the pullets or breeder flock. After removing all litter and equipment, the inside of the house needs to be thoroughly prewashed with water and a detergent. This procedure should remove the residual organic matter and then this can be followed by high-pressure application of disinfectants/ detergents. Where possible, equipment should be pre-soaked in holding tanks in mixtures of water, detergent and disinfectants such as cresylic acid which are somewhat effective in the presence of organic material. Soaking greatly reduces the time (up to 50%) needed to subsequently clean and sanitize breeder equipment. Following a disease outbreak it is advisable to fumigate the already disinfected house, and also to use disinfectants such as QUATS around the outside of the breeder house, ideally up to 5m out from the perimeter walls.

4.8 BLOOD AND TISSUE SAMPLING

Either because of concern about potential infection, or simply as a means of routine monitoring, it is sometimes necessary to obtain blood and/or tissue samples from breeders. Routine blood sampling is usually carried out from the wing veins, although experienced technicians can sample directly from the heart without any undue effects on the bird. Sampling from the wing veins can be carried out using either a needle and syringe, or simply by puncturing the vein with a needle or scalpel blade, and collecting the blood in a open tube. If blood is to be held for any length of time prior to assay, then the serum should be separated from the blood cells. This is best achieved by laying the tubes on their side for 8-12 hr at room temperature rather than in a refrigerator, and over this time, the yellow-coloured clear serum will separate from the blood cells. A 2-3 ml blood sample yields about 0.5 ml serum which is sufficient quantity for most tests. Serum, but not whole blood, can be frozen. In order to determine change in antibody status over time, serum samples collected at around 22 weeks, can be frozen and used as a benchmark for subsequent comparisons over time. For routine blood assays, about 20-30 birds per flock should be sampled.

If live birds cannot be submitted for necropsy, or if it is necessary to transport samples internationally for specialized tests, then tissues samples must be preserved. This is best achieved by fixing in 10% formalin or by freezing. It is not necessary to submit a whole organ, but rather to send slices of organs such as liver, lung or kidney etc.. The thinner the slice (2-3mm) the quicker the preservation by formalin. For organs such as the kidney, bursa and intestine, it is advantageous to open up the organ, again in order to ensure rapid fixing by the preservative. Bone samples need to be stripped of muscle and connective tissue.

4.9 ANTIMICROBIALS AND ANTICOCCIDIALS

Antibiotics: There are still a number of antibiotics available to the poultry industry that are efficacious against a range of bacteria, mycoplasma, molds and fungi. The main concern with antibiotics in general is the development of microbial resistance, which influences bird performance and potentially human health. This problem is much less acute with broiler breeders because antibiotics are not used routinely, as in the case for growth promotion with broilers, and so there is much less chance for development of resistance with this discontinuous use. Table 4.9 shows some of the most common types of antibiotics that can be added to the feed or water. Undoubtedly not all the microbial groups shown are sensitive to the antibiotics indicated in all geographical regions. The latest introduction has been the quinolones, which were initially introduced as a means of eradicating mycoplasma in breeding programs by egg dipping prior to incubation.

With prolonged use, there is likely to be some degree of resistance developing. In a recent survey in Holland, Goren (1994) indicated sensitivity of E. coli to a range of antibiotics, ranging from <5% to greater than 70% resistance. Interestingly over the last 10 years or so, with few exceptions, the development of resistance has changed little for individual antibiotics. This same study found that two-thirds of E. coli strains were resistant to more than two antibiotics. Of potential concern to human health, is the transfer of resistance from, for example, E. coli in the breeder pullet, to salmonella species that may infect humans. Such infected people could then not be treated successfully with the antibiotic in question. Such transfer has been well documented in the laboratory, although there are no clearly established epidemiological studies linking any segments of the poultry industry to major outbreaks of bacterial resistant infection in humans. The cause of such problems is more likely the continual use and abuse of antibiotics in human medicine. Long-term, however, it seems logical for the poultry industry to place less emphasis on those antimicrobials that are used in human medicine.

Probiotics: The term probiotic is used to define substances that promote microbial growth in the intestine. The basic concept of their mode of action, is that in colonizing the gut, these live beneficial microbes will displace or not allow colonization of harmful bacteria. This latter concept led to the idea of competitive exclusion. Most bacteria in breeders that have a healthy intestinal tract produce lactic acid, such as the lactobacilli and streptococci species. If this flora is adversely affected, as sometimes occurs with unrelated bacterial or

TABLE 4.9 Potential use of antibiotics

	E. coli	Mycoplasma	Staphylococcus	Cholera	Coryza	Enteritis	Necrotic Enteritis	Salmonella
Amoxycillin	✓		✓	✓			✓	✓
Sulfurs	✓		✓	✓	✓			✓
Penicillin			✓				✓	
Tylosin		✓	✓				✓	
Nitrofurans	✓							✓
Quinolones	✓	✓	✓	✓	✓			✓
Lincomycin		✓	✓				✓	
Tetracyclines	✓	✓	✓	✓				✓
Spectinomycin					✓			
Neomycin	✓					✓		✓
Bacitracin			✓				✓	

mycoplasma infection or due to stresses such as heat, transportation, handling and vaccination etc., then the balance of gut microbes changes (pH effect), and E. coli and staphylococci can quickly colonize. Probiotic use therefore goes hand in hand with products that stabilize gut pH.

Most probiotics contain lactobacilli which are non-pathogenic and are capable of producing lactic acid from the break-down of carbohydrate in the intestine. Lactic acid has been shown to inhibit the growth of E. Coli.

Lactobacilli are known to colonize the crop of the bird, and to colonize the intestine from this source as feed is stored, awaiting transfer to the proventriculus and gizzard. In the broiler chicken the crop has become quite rudimentary because with ad-libitum feeding most feed particles pass directly into the proventriculus. In the breeder however, because of our various feed restriction programs, the crop is used daily and so lactobacilli and probiotics may have greater application. It has been suggested that lactobacilli attached to the crop epithelium play an important role in inoculating incoming feed so ensuring dominance and the suppression of E. Coli. Lactobacilli have also been reported to produce an antibiotic called "acidolin" which perhaps has growth inhibiting effects against enteric pathogens.

Probiotics seem to have some use for breeders at two specific times. Firstly the use of products containing lactobacilli would seem beneficial when used in day-old chicks, so as to establish colonization of the intestine, prior to major exposure to E. coli and other pathogens. The second appropriate application would be after antibiotic use such that the lactobacilli-type probiotics would be influential in re-establishing a favorable gut microflora.

Anticoccidials: Coccidiosis is an on-going problem with breeders, and so some type of preventive program is required. Unfortunately, very few anticoccidials are cleared for use with adult breeders, and their long-term use would be cost prohibitive. It is therefore essential for the pullet to develop immunity prior to maturity and this is the reason for the popularity of vaccines as described previously. The need to establish immunity rules out many common anticoccidials because they are very efficacious and allow little chance for immunity. Amprolium has often been the anticoccidial used for growing pullets because it does allow for a build-up of immunity over time. Amprolium is also one of the few anticoccidials available as a water soluble compound, and can be used to quickly treat infection via the drinking water. There has been some research conducted on the use of high dietary levels of the anticoccidial monensin, on the reduction in feed intake of growing breeder pullets. Used at 99 ppm as an anticoccidial, monensin has little effect on feed intake. However at 200-300 ppm it does act as an anorexic, and so has been studied in this regard as a means of self-imposed growth control in pullets. At around 300 ppm monensin, the reduction in feed intake is comparable to that imposed by most feed restriction programs. Unfortunately, as with many anorexic agents, while the flock "mean effect" appears reasonable, there is increased bird variance in body weight. Apart from this loss of uniformity, the adult breeders are little affected other than showing an increase in heart size. High inclusion levels of monensin are not usually recommended for appetite suppression. There are few interactions between anticoccidials and other feed additives that are problematic to the breeder, although there is an indication of higher mortality when Tiamulin, used to treat mycoplasmosis, is used concurrently with monovalent ionophores such as monensin, salinomycin or narasin. The anticoccidial nicarbazin adversely affects reproduction in adult broiler breeders, and in fact the product contains a warning against use in breeder diets. Nicarbazin also has the unusual effect of changing shell color from brown to white. This change in shell color is almost immediate (24-48h) and the normal brown shell color returns almost as quickly once nicarbazin has been removed from the diet. Table 4.10 shows the effect of feeding graded levels of nicarbazin on egg characteristics of Leghorn breeders.

TABLE 4.10. Effect of graded levels of Nicarbazin on performance of Leghorn breeders

Nicarbazin (ppm)	Egg production after 28d (%)	Egg wt (g)	Hatchability (% fertile)
0	88.6	58.3	99.6
5	89.2	58.9	95.3
10	90.0	59.0	88.2
20	93.0	56.6	77.4
40	85.3	57.9	78.1
80	83.6	57.1	58.0*
125	65.1*	54.8*	45.2*
250	42.0*	54.6*	8.6*

***significant effect** **Adapted from Leeson *et al.* (1989)**

All birds returned to the normal level of egg production, egg size and hatchability just 28-56d after removing nicarbazin from the diet. Nicarbazin seems to adversely affect yolk development and maturation, and must be excluded from breeder diets.

4.10 MOLD AND MYCOTOXIN CONTROL

In many areas of the world, molds and associated mycotoxins are an inevitable contaminant of feed ingredients to varying degrees. The effect of most mycotoxins is additive or synergistic, and so the presence of numerous mycotoxins, even at apparently harmless levels, can be problematic to the bird. There are two types of molds, namely aerobes that most commonly occur in the field while the plant is growing, and anaerobes that most frequently flourish during storage. The growth of molds is greatly reduced if the moisture content of ingredients is less than 15%, and so simply maintaining a low level of moisture in stored grains is the first obvious step in a mold/mycotoxin control program. The molds themselves are usually not problematic to the bird (apart from some Aspergillus species that cause Aspergillosis). However many molds produce various chemicals as by-products of their metabolism which have loosely been referred to as mycotoxins. While it is relatively easy to kill the living molds, it is virtually impossible to destroy mycotoxins once they have formed. Because of the relative ease and simplicity of mycotoxin testing today, using ELISA type systems, there is no excuse for nutritionists and feed personnel to be ignorant about the mycotoxin status of ingredients and feeds.

Mold prevention starts with ensuring moisture control in stored ingredients and finished feed. During storage, this usually means adequate aeration systems, and obviously ensuring that silos are water proof. On the farm the same water proofing is essential for feed tanks, together with the implementation of routine inside sweeping, and periodic disinfection and fumigation. Molds are most easily killed, or prevented from establishing themselves in ingredients or feed, by simply creating an acidic environment through use of organic acids. Most mold inhibitors are based on propionic acid which seems to have a broad range of activity against most molds, fungi and yeasts. The quantity of organic acids needed will depend upon moisture level of the feed, ingredient composition of feed, and also its particle size. In general the smaller the particle size of the feed, the less propionic acid is needed for protection because these smaller particles ensure greater distribution of the acid within the feed, and so greater potential contact with the mold. For example having a 2-5mm vs 1mm particle size, would probably mean adding an extra 1 kg propionic acid per tonne for the coarser feed. The feed surface area also affects level of inhibitors needed. With feed pans that expose more feed to the air, there is a greater risk of infection, and there is a need for higher concentrations of products such as propionic acid. Perhaps most important of all in determining level of inhibitor needed is the ingredient composition of the diet. More acid must be added to feeds that contain ingredients that act as buffers (neutralizers) to the acid. Most of the protein ingredients, such as soybean meal, meat meal and fish meal are fairly good buffers, suggesting that high protein starter diets need more acid (+0.5kg) than do lower protein grower diets. The most active buffer is limestone, and so this means that we must add much more acid to a high calcium breeder diet than to a low calcium grower diet. In areas of high humidity where mold growth is likely, then it may be necessary to add an "extra" 2 kg/tonne of propionic acid to a 3.5% calcium breeder diet compared to a 1% grower diet.

The actual level of propionic acid used will depend on the quality of the raw ingredients and the potential for contamination on-farm. In general 1-5 kg/tonne is needed, dependent upon the conditions described previously. In many regions that import most of their grains, organic acids are now added at time of loading in the exporting country - often ingredients become heavily infested during transportation and under these conditions ingredients such as corn contain high levels of mycotoxins. The exact levels of organic acids needed to be added to finished feed should be established as a quality control procedure at the feed mill. This type of testing is necessary because there is a balance between adding just enough acid to ensure antimicrobial activity, and having two much acid which is corrosive to metal feed tanks, augers and feeders. This is most easily carried out by culturing moistened (~_ 18% moisture) feed in petri dishes maintained at 28-32°, to which are added graded levels of the acid. The lowest level of acid needed to prevent mold growth is that recommended for feed manufacturing. This type of simple test establishes precise needs for the various diets and should be undertaken ideally for all diets manufactured, or at least separately for starter-grower and breeder diets. In some countries gentian violet is still used as an effective antifungal agent, and its use is governed by factors previously described for the organic acids. Gentian violet is non-corrosive, can be added at very low levels of inclusion, and has the advantage of also being bacteriostatic.

While it is fairly easy to control mold growth in feed, it is very difficult to overcome the effects of mycotoxin contamination. Organic acids and gentian violet will not deactivate mycotoxins, and so even though plate tests show no mold growth, the breeder diets can be contaminated with mycotoxins already produced by prior mold activity. The various mycotoxins are detailed in Table 4.11, indicating that levels as low as parts per billion (milligrams per tonne) can affect breeder performance.

Mycotoxins have less severe effects on younger birds when the diets contain more protein, and so in regions of potentially high contamination it would be inadvisable to use lower crude protein levels (regardless of amino acids) in chick starter diets. Fibre can also bind some mycotoxins, and alfalfa is especially effective. However levels of 20-25% alfalfa are needed to counteract moderate levels of mycotoxins, and this is impractical in most operations. Detoxification of aflatoxin contaminated grains has received considerable attention. Treating with ammonia in an enclosed chamber does destroy aflatoxin in corn, but this

TABLE 4.11 Effect of mycotoxins on breeder health and performance		
Mycotoxin	**Problem diet concentrations[1]**	**Potential lesions and signs**
Tricothecenes (T2, DAS, DON)	1-5 ppm	Oral lesions, reduced growth, poor feathering
Ochratoxin	0.5 ppm	Reduced egg production, kidney damage, impaired immunity
Aflatoxin	<1 ppm	Liver damage, reduced egg production and hatchability
Fumonisins	100 ppm	Impaired growth
Citrinin	250 ppm	Kidney damage
Ergot	0.5% by weight	Skin necrosis, nervousness
Zearalenone	500 ppm	Impaired shell quality
[1]Young birds are more sensitive, and overall effects much worse with combinations of mycotoxins.		

is obviously a costly and specialized procedure. More recently there has been interest in using sodium calcium aluminosilicates to bind mycotoxins, making them unavailable to the bird. Depending upon source, 5-10kg aluminosilicates per tonne of feed will effectively counteract the effects of up to 5ppm aflatoxin. The aluminosilicate binds with aflatoxin, by incorporation into its complex tetrahedral configuration. Ideally, aflatoxin contaminated corn is not recommended for use in breeder diets, yet where its use is necessary or sometimes inevitable, then aluminosilicates seem a reasonable protective strategy. There has been considerable research and claims for the potential of aluminosilicates to bind mycotoxins other than aflatoxin. Results are often variable, possibly because the structure and composition of aluminosilicates is variable. It seems likely that aluminosilicates, or similar synthetic structures will eventually be developed that have potential to bind a range of important mycotoxins.

4.11 INSECT CONTROL

Flies, Northern Fowl Mite (NFM) fleas and darkling beetle are the main insect problems occurring on breeder farms. Flies are rarely a problem to the breeders themselves, but are a nuisance factor for neighbors, can cause fly-specks (defecation on eggs) and can transmit some diseases. Flies are more problematic in caged breeders, especially where there is a deep-pit manure system. However the major insect problem for breeder managers is caused by infestation with NFM.

Northern fowl mite: Mites are blood-sucking parasites that tend to migrate to the vent area of the bird. With heavy infestation the vent area has a dirty black/grey appearance caused by the mites themselves and their feces, together with egg clusters and upon close examination the mites can be clearly seen moving around on the feathers and skin. Loss of 7 eggs per breeder with increase in feed cost of 3¢/doz eggs has been reported as a consequence of heavy infestation. Mites will often bite workers in the breeder house or those handling eggs from infected birds. After hatching, all life cycle stages of the parasite must feed by sucking blood, and so NFM cannot usually survive for any long period of time off of the bird. The mite can develop from an egg to an egg-laying adult in 7 days, and a whole flock of breeders can potentially become infected within 30 days from a single infected bird. Prevention relies on biosecurity applied to movement of equipment and personnel between flocks. Early detection is critical, and this can only be accomplished by routine (monthly) inspection of up to 20 birds in a flock - this is most easily accomplished by inspecting birds during routine weighing. If infestation occurs, then birds must be treated immediately. Two treatments are usually necessary, because a bird that is inadvertently missed, or treated inadequately, provides a reservoir for subsequent infection. With floor managed birds, there is no alternative but to handle and treat birds individually. With caged breeders, the first approach is to spray insecticide up through the bottom of the cage such that the vent area is saturated. If in-cage spraying is unsuccessful, then breeders must be removed and treated individually. Many insecticide products are available as spray or dust. Following are some of the more common insecticides used to treat NFM infected breeders (Table 4.12).

TABLE 4.12 Northern Fowl Mite treatments

Pesticide	Application
Cabaryl - Liquid	Mix 10g/litre water and spray at rate of 45ml/bird
(Sevin®) - Dust	5 kg dust per 1000 breeders applied to vent area
Malathion - Liquid	Mix 1 litre/100 litres water, apply at 45 ml/bird
- Dust	5 kg dust per 1000 breeders applied to vent area
Permethrin - Liquid (Disvap®)	Dilute to produce a 0.05% solution and spray at 45 ml/bird
Permethrin - Liquid (Ectiban®)	Mix 200 ml/100 litres water and apply at 45 ml/bird
Note: Not all products are available or registered in all countries. Follow label instructions to ensure exact final concentrations as recommended by manufacturers.	

The sprays and dust products should be applied directly to the vent area. Most pesticides are harmful to humans, and so operators must wear appropriate protective apparatus and clothing. Unfortunately, mites are becoming resistant to many pesticides and so shuttling of products each year is recommended. A key step in control of NFM is to prevent reinfestation, since some birds may not have been treated adequately, and mites can live off the bird for up to 25d in extreme situations. About 10d after pesticide application, birds from different regions of the breeder house should be inspected, and if mites are found, it may be necessary to re-treat the birds. Under conditions of extreme mite persistence, as sometimes happens with caged birds, it may be necessary to dip all birds in a bath of the appropriate insecticide.

Periodically NFM leave the breeders in large numbers, and at these times, the mites are most noticeable in the nests and on the eggs. When mites leave the birds, there is the greatest chance for infecting other flocks, especially via carry-over on eggs, egg-trays and egg dollies. Devaney and co-workers at College Station Texas have probably been the most active group in developing mite control programs, and for this particular situation, these researchers suggest fumigation of breeder equipment with methyl bromine which is commonly used as a grain fumigant. Using methyl bromine under carefully controlled conditions at 32g/cubic meter for 24h seems 100% effective in killing NFM on breeder equipment. (Note methyl bromine should only be handled by licensed operators).

Flies: Manure management is the key to fly control in breeder houses. Flies are most problematic in cage breeder houses, but can also be of concern with partially slatted floor operations. The flies do not spend any time of their life cycle on the live bird, rather they lay eggs and pupate in the manure, and in this respect manure moisture is very important. There are basically four methods of fly control available, namely topical insecticide spray, treated granular fly baits, feed systemic larvicides or biological control through seeding parasitic wasps or other insects. Insecticide sprays including permethrin and carbaryl have limited use for long term fly control. They can be used effectively as part of an integrated pest management system but are generally ineffective in controlling the breeding sites. Most insecticides have only limited effectiveness when applied to manure, and with breeders on slats, it is often difficult to achieve good coverage of the fly breeding sites in the manure. Insecticide sprays play a role in controlling fly numbers in feed rooms, egg rooms etc. However, care must be taken in applying insecticides close to eggs, or "wetting" egg trays or egg carts. A more controlled method of using such insecticides, is application of granular baits, that are usually yellow or orange in colour for ease of visibility by the operators. Again such baits are useful in egg and feed rooms etc., but not actually in the immediate vicinity of the birds.

Some 10 years ago a number of insect growth regulators were developed, that could be applied via the feed of the breeder - in essence, the products were continually excreted in the manure, and so this was a simple means of ensuring contact between the fly and the larvicide. Although not registered in all countries, Larvadex® kills the larval stage of the house fly. There have been some reports of resistance build-up, and as with many chemical-based treatments, systemic insecticides should be part of an integrated and balanced fly management program. Toxicity of products such as Larvadex® to the breeder are not a serious problem, because levels of even 200x the normal recommended level of 1.5 ppm of the breeder diet, seem to have no long term effect on reproduction.

However, because of the problems of insect resistence to persistent use of chemical insecticides, and the fact that it is becoming more difficult to justify even minute concentrations of these compounds in eggs, biological control programs have gained in popularity. A number of pupal parasites are often present in manure pits of breeder facilities, and these help to maintain some balance of larval growth. Seeding manure with large numbers of the more aggressive larval parasites has proven to be an effective system of biological control. These larval parasites, which are usually specially selected species of wasps, are now available commercially. The effectiveness of any fly control program is best monitored by either observing the number of flys caught on sticky fly strips, or more easily by observing fly specs (which are fecal and regurgitated material from the fly) on white file cards, replaced weekly at 5-6 positions throughout the breeder house.

Fleas: Periodically fleas will become a problem in adult breeder houses, where workers complain of bites during egg collection, because fleas are not host-specific and so are continually seeking new nest sites. Flea control involves regular nest management, including changing of litter, and where necessary, spraying the empty nest monthly with 0.125% permethrin or similar insecticides. Insecticides applied to the nest as dusting powders also seem effective and perhaps have more long-term control over flea numbers.

Darkling Beetle: Darkling beetle, also known as the lesser meal worm, or litter beetle is a serious problem in many breeder houses, especially in warmer climates. The 2mm beetle is easily seen moving through the litter, where it survives on spilled feed. The beetles and larvae can be vectors for Salmonella, E coli, Aspergillus, Streptococcus and the Marek's/Leukosis virus. With heavy infestation, the beetles migrate into the structure of the building and are especially destructive to insulation material. Because they migrate to cracks and crevices in the building, clean-up and eradication are very difficult. The life cycle from egg to adult beetle is about 60 days depending upon environmental temperature, and adults can live for up to 1 year. Reproductive rate is most active between 20-38°C. Outside of these temperatures there is little egg-laying activity, and most developmental stages in the life cycle are killed at temperatures below 5°C. The greatest number of adult and larvae are found at litter moistures of 20-30%, and so initial populations are often found around drinkers. The adult beetle and the larvae can be killed by a number of common insecticides, although ensuring complete contact is always difficult. With heavy infestations, the litter should be sprayed immediately (hrs) after depopulation before any litter is removed, in order to prevent migration into the building structure. Litter should be spread immediately, away from the breeder house, or piled to ensure composting with heating. The building should then be sprayed, and where possible, fumigated. The main challenge in eradication is treating beetles and larvae that are in the insulation, or are behind wall and ceiling cladding etc.

Treatment of the litter while the breeders are still in the house is a more logical approach to prevention and/or treatment. In the past, new litter was treated with insecticides prior to placing birds in the house. However boron containing insecticides are now more commonly used, being based on products such as sodium octaborate or orthoboric acid. Top dressing such boron products at about 0.2 - 1 kg/10m^2 litter area, seems to provide a reasonably effective preventive treatment. There has been some concern about the toxicity of boron to breeders, because they could easily pick this product up from the litter. Breeder hens continuously fed 250ppm boron showed normal egg production and hatchability. However, there was an indication of such treated males showing more damaged sperm cells, although fertility was not affected. Most vendors of these products do warn against top dressing of boron products when birds are present, because out of curiosity they could consume a toxic level of this mineral.

4.12 INTERNAL PARASITES

The main internal parasites are worms that can reside in the digestive tract or respiratory system. The more common intestinal worms are debilitating to the bird, and with heavy infestation, can lead to nutrient deficiencies. Worms are classified as nematodes (roundworms) or cestodes (tapeworms) and they are particularly prevalent in breeders because of litter management systems and the relatively long 64-69 week breeder cycle. Some worms require an intermediary host, such as earthworms, snails, insects etc., and consequently preventing contact with these invertebrates is an obvious step in control and prevention. The use of concrete floors in breeder houses is probably the single most important contribution to eradication of internal parasites, since it is now uncommon for birds to come in contact with these intermediary hosts. However a number of the round worms can reproduce without passing through such other animals, and it is these parasites that are now of concern in the breeder industry. The cestodes, or tapeworms, are therefore not usual parasites of breeders because they must use snails, slugs or insects as an intermediary host. The most common tapeworm of breeders is Davainea proglottina, which is a flat ribbon shaped worm made up of short "independent" body segments that are continually breaking off and pass out with the feces. Eggs from the segments are picked up by snails or slugs, and after 7-14d are in a stage that can infect the bird should it eat the snail. Mature tapeworms can be up to 25cm in length, and the continual shedding and regrowing of body segments, leads to a continual drain on the nutrient reserves of the bird. Control over infection simply relies upon breaking the reproductive cycle of the tapeworm, by eradicating the intermediary hosts. Slug and snail bait, usually containing metaldehyde, must therefore be applied around the perimeter of the house. Chemical treatment of infected birds is possible, but a number of these require 24h prior starvation of the bird, and so this naturally disrupts egg production in mature birds. Products such as praziquantel are effective against tapeworms, while most of the common chemical treatments used for roundworms are ineffective.

The nematodes or roundworms are the most common internal parasites of breeders. These include Ascaridia galli (intestine) Heterakis gallinarum (ceca) and various Capillaria species (crop→intestine) found through the digestive tract, and Syngamus trachea or gape worm found in the lungs and trachea. As a group, the nematodes are characterized by being long spindle shaped worms varying in color from off-white to creamy yellow. When viewed under the microscope, they have transverse grooves running across the body, but unlike the tapeworms they do not physically segment and so only the complete worms are found in the intestine or feces. Female worms produce eggs which are deposited in the feces. Earthworms can be a carrier, but are not a necessary transition, because eggs can "mature" in the feces and reach an infective stage in 10-12 days. Ascaridia galli is perhaps the most common of the round worms, being found most frequently in the small intestine. Birds will eventually develop some resistance/immunity to infection, and so young birds are most susceptible. However if birds are infected at a young age, then a resident infective population can remain inside the bird through the complete adult breeder period. With very heavy infestation, the worms can break through the intestine and are found in the body cavity - infrequently they arrive at the oviduct, and then find their way into the shelled egg. Alternatively they pass out of the cloaca, and then immediately travel up the adjacent oviduct.

It is the larval stage of the life cycle that actually does damage to the intestinal mucosa of the bird, and that can cause signs of poor growth, lethargy etc. In the early stages of infection therefore, birds may show clinical signs of depression and loss of pigmentation etc., without there being adult worms apparent in the feces. The traditional worming compounds, used in the feed or water, have been piperazine and hygromycin. Hygromycin is usually used at around 750g/tonne feed, while piperazine use is at 2-3kg/tonne feed. Birds can also be treated individually if desired, with about 100mg piperazine. The traditional wormers are narcotics, that paralyze, but do not kill the worm. The worms lose their attachment, and are passed out with the feces. At this stage, the eggs can still be infective, and so effective treatment must involve 2 or 3 dosages of the wormer, each some 7-10d apart. Depending upon the degree of infestation, a single deworming operation at the time of move to the breeder house may be sufficient. Newer compounds such as flubendazole are effective against all worms, including tapeworms.

The gapeworm is an unusual parasite, in that it burrows through the intestinal wall and then makes its way to the respiratory tract. As the degree of infestation increases, worms travel up the trachea, causing partial blockage, and birds then show the characteristic gaping (or gasping) with an outstretched neck. Gape worms are classically controlled by treating birds with thiabendazole at 2-4kg/tonne feed.

4.13 RODENT CONTROL

Control over populations of rats and mice has always been an important part of any health management program, and now assumes even more importance with the realization that mice especially can be major vectors of salmonella. Rodents are capable of both mechanical and biological transmission of bacteria responsible for leptospirosis, erysipilas, salmonellosis and fowl cholera, as well as the virus for fowl pox. Most recently, mice have been shown to be common carriers of Salmonella enteriditis. Apart from these direct health problems, rodents consume and contaminate the feed and water, destroy insulation material and pose a real fire hazard by gnawing on electrical cables.

Rodents living in the breeder houses are most active at dusk and dawn. Mice feed sporadically, taking up to 20-30 meals each day, most of which are usually consumed within 10m of their nest. Rats on the other hand eat only one or two meals per day and are prepared to travel up to 50m or so from the nest each time. While mice can survive a number of days without water, rats must drink daily, and so are more likely to be found close to a source of water. Without seeing the rodents, the main differentiation is in size of the droppings, since mice have rice-sized fecal pellets, while rats produce raisin sized pellets. Each of these rodents can produce up to 20,000 fecal pellets in a year, which is about their average life span.

Because of their prodigious reproductive rate, rodent populations can quickly increase. Mice are mature at about 8 weeks of age, and from that time can produce up to 8 litters per year, each with 5-6 offspring. It has been calculated that a single pair of mice could potentially yield a population of 20 million animals in three years. Reproduction in the rat is similar to that of the mouse.

It becomes more difficult to control rodent populations once they are established in the breeder house because of the abundance of feed, water and nesting material. Sanitation around the perimeter of the breeder house is one of the best deterrents to initial infestation. Removing debris, old equipment etc., and keeping grass and weeds at 3-4 cm height reduces chances of infestation. Once rodents are inside the breeder house then trapping and/or use of rodenticide baits are the only options. Glue boards placed in strategic locations can catch a number of mice, although in most breeder houses, dust makes them ineffective in a few days. Multiple traps are also effective for mice, although they do need constant supervision.

Rodenticide baits are the most common means of controlling both mice and rats. Baits are usually anticoagulants, the most widespread products being based on warfarin. Anticoagulants destroy the animals ability for blood clotting and so they bleed to death internally. Most of these baits are very slow acting, often taking 4-6 days before rats and mice consume enough of a lethal dose. Rats are more wary than are mice of new objects such as bait stations, and often take 3-7 days to accept these and start eating the poison. Because anticoagulants act over time, the baits must be continually replaced. A single rat will eat about 30g per day while mice consume about 3g feed per day. Rats also consume up to 60ml water each day, and some pest control companies place water stations close to bait stations when rat populations are particularly problematic. Some of the new anticoagulant baits, such as bromadiolon and brodifacoum are much faster acting than warfarin, and can kill with just one feeding. Non anti-coagulant baits are products such as bromethalin, cholecalciferol and zinc phosphide. Cholecalciferol, or vitamin D is highly toxic to rodents at large doses. Most of the non-anticoagulant poisons can be lethal after just one feeding, but also act cumulatively if rodents take small quantities over time. These baits are also usually effective in killing rodents that have become resistant to warfarin. Most baits are poisonous to humans, other animals and the birds themselves, and so must be located in specialized bait stations. Brodifacoun is especially toxic to dogs. Well designed bait containers provide both safety to farm staff etc. and also protect the bait. One of the best containers for mice is constructed of a "⊥" shaped 5 cm PVC black plastic pipe, about 60 cm high and 30 cm along the base. The base is positioned along wall-floor joints, and bait simply poured into the top of the vertical tube.

4.14 MAJOR HEALTH MANAGEMENT CONCERNS WITH BREEDERS

Coccidiosis

Coccidiosis continues to be one of the major diseases affecting breeders worldwide. The various Eimeria species protozoan parasites invade and eventually destroy the epithelial lining of the intestine. With severe infection birds will die, and with mild infection, there can be permanent reduction in their ability to absorb nutrients. Occurrence of coccidiosis is of particular concern with replacement breeder candidates, because the condition is accentuated by management systems that impose restricted feeding programs. When infected, pullets and roosters will not gain weight, and then quickly become smaller than their uninfected siblings. Being smaller, they have greater difficulty in competing at the feeder, and subsequently consume proportionally less feed and anticoccidial. The coccidial infection gets worse and is often associated with secondary infections such as Clostridium perfringens causing necrotic enteritis. Most of the common Eimeria species infect breeders, including acervulina, maxima and necatrix which invade the small intestine, and tenella which infects the ceca. Even with so called subclinical infection, there will likely be loss of uniformity of the pullets and roosters.

Unfortunately the oocysts can survive outside of the bird for up to 1 year under ideal conditions, and are easily spread from farm to farm by personnel, equipment and trucks. There are likely few breeder farms that are free of oocysts, and so any preventative programs rely on controlled exposure so as to allow a build up of immunity. Unfortunately immunity is species specific, and so infection with E. tenella, confers no protection against subsequent infection with E. necatrix and vice versa.

Unlike the situation with the broiler chicken, for breeder candidates it is not ideal to simply prevent coccidiosis by using very efficient anticoccidials such as nicarbazin or ionophores. Instead, the management program must allow immunity to develop, because most anticoccidials today are not cleared for use in adult breeders. Controlled low level infection is therefore desirable, and signs of lesions in 4-6 week old birds is likely an indication of developing immunity. Such controlled infection can be managed through use of selected anticoccidials or vaccination programs.

Anticoccidials: Skip-a-day feeding adds a major complication to coccidiosis control programs that rely on dietary anticoccidials. After 6-8 weeks of age, the bird may have feed/anticoccidial in the gut for only a few hours each 48 hrs and so there is non-uniform exposure to the oocysts. This is particularly important with the ionophores, because their anticoccidial activity relies on contact with the oocyst, and there is no residual effect if the gut is empty. There are basically two choices of chemotherapeutics because the intent of the program is not to kill all oocysts, but rather to allow a low level of recycling through the litter. Most modern anticoccidials, at normal therapeutic levels, do not allow this recycling to occur, because in general they have been developed for the commercial broiler industry, where total eradication is ideal. One choice therefore is to use one of the older coccidiostats, such as amprolium. Amprolium rarely gives complete protection against Eimeria, because over the last 20-30 years, immunity has developed against this product. However because it is rarely used in commercial broilers today, many strains are again "susceptible" to amprolium. Even with susceptible strains of Eimeria, there will never be complete destruction of all oocysts, and some will survive to recycle through the litter. This recycling is essential for build-up of immunity, because some Eimeria strains require one or two such cycles in order to activate immunity.

An alternate approach to using these older chemical anticoccidials, is to use modern ionophores, but at the lowest levels recommended such that "leakage" occurs. For example; 99-120ppm of monensin will not likely allow much immunity to develop, whereas 60ppm if allowed by feed regulations, will likely allow sufficient leakage for immunity to develop.

Vaccines: Vaccination is now becoming very popular with breeders, because it provides a controlled exposure to a known species mixture of Eimeria. There are a number of vaccines now available based on live-oocyst cultures. These vaccines are given in the drinking water, sprayed onto the feed, and most recently administered through a novel gel that is placed in the chick box at the hatchery. Many breeding companies now rely 100% on such coccidial vaccines to give life time protection from a single day-old vaccination. As with the chemical anticoccidials, resistance can develop to the vaccines, and so the more astute vaccine manufacturers are continually adjusting their oocyte strains, and sometimes develop novel vaccines for specific geographical locations.

The key to successful vaccine use, is conscientious administration at day of age, coupled with knowledge of in-house conditions that are conducive to oocyst recycling. Because full immunity only occurs after two cycles with most Eimeria, and three cycles with E. tenella, then litter conditions must be ideal for oocyst sporulation. In extremely dry conditions, it may be necessary to slightly moisten the litter 10-12d after vaccinating. As with any live vaccine, the oocyst mixture must be handled and stored under ideal conditions so as to protect its cellular integrity. Dead oocysts confer little or no immunity to the bird. With poor vaccination technique, clinical coccidiosis may occur in previously unvaccinated birds that receive large doses of oocysts from their siblings that start to shed oocysts. Obviously anticoccidials cannot be used in the feed for at least 21d post vaccinating, and in fact there should be no need for their use at any time after vaccinating. However there have been some reports of success in using shuttles of vaccine and anticoccidials in successive flocks, so as to prevent resistance build-up to either product. In reality, it may be necessary to use anticoccidials, such that shuttles of the products can provide very long term control programs. Of all the vaccine programs available today, Danforth (1997) suggests the gel delivery system as introduced by Immucox7 to be one of the most effective.

Avian leucosis

Avian leucosis or "big liver disease" has continually re-curred as a problem in the poultry industry over the last 40 years. In the late 1960's, leucosis was a major problem for most table egg birds, where subgroups A and B caused up to 20% mortality in growing pullets and in mature birds in the early part of lay. Fortunately blood tests were developed that allowed identification of infected or carrier breeders, and so these could be removed from the hierarchy of the breeding programs. Heavy meat breeders were never as severely affected by subgroup A and B leucosis, and infected birds often showed none of the classic tumors commonly found in the Leghorn birds. While these leucosis sub-groups have now almost become history in Leghorn stock, a new subgroup, known as J-virus, emerged in the 1990's and has been of particular concern in heavy breeders.

J-virus was first isolated by Dr. Payne in the UK in the mid 1980's and now many of the major strains of breeding stock are infected. Unlike the older classical lymphoid leucosis, which affected mainly lymphoid tissue such as the bursa, the new J-strain is a myeloid leucosis which affects primarily the bone marrow. Signs of J-virus proliferation are tumors on the ribs and keel although sometimes the virus spreads to the kidney and spleen. The tumors are often soft and friable, and there may be multiple tumors grouped together on the bone surface. Care must be taken in differentiating between tumors caused by Marek's and J-virus.

Although the bird either inherits the virus from its parents, or becomes infected at an early age, problems are often not seen with the breeders until after egg production starts. The occurrence of tumors and associated loss in egg production and increase in mortality are greatly influenced by secondary stressors. For this reason, infected sister flocks may show 2 vs 20% mortality from 25-35 weeks caused by differential degrees of secondary stressors.

A major complication with the J-virus is that it can infect birds both vertically (parent→chick) as well as horizontally (chick→chick). There is also the added complexity of the virus existing as a "normal" part of the bird's genetic makeup (endogenous) or as a regular field infection (exogenous). The exogenous virus can also be transmitted vertically. These different types of J-virus and their potential modes of infection mean that within a flock, a number of different serotypes may be present. Variable serotypes mean it is much more difficult to isolate carriers for the endogenous and exogenous leucosis virus.

The avian leucosis virus contains a protein core whose composition is controlled by a specific gene group. This gene (group specific antigen) is used in sophisticated laboratory diagnosis. This protein core is itself encapsulated with another protein coating, the development of which is again controlled by another gene group within the bird. Unfortunately the viron core can replicate and integrate itself within the bird's own DNA sequencing. The endogenous virus can therefore replicate itself, and the bird can shed the virus. However because the viral protein is part of the bird's own DNA, it is not recognized as "foreign" and so there is no antibody produced.

The normal exogenous virus can be transmitted vertically or horizontally. Horizontal transmission, caused by bird-to-bird contact occurs quite quickly, especially in young chicks. The chicks have a transient period when the virus can be detected in their blood but then antibodies quickly develop and there are rarely clinical signs of leucosis. However these chicks, if potential breeders, can subsequently pass on the virus to their offspring. This leads to the potential for vertical transmission from breeder to offspring. Such transmission can occur at any level of the breeding program and so grandparent chicks can be infected by pure line parents, and parent breeder chicks themselves infected from grandparent carriers etc. At each level, breeders can shed exogenous leucosis virus from the oviduct into the albumen of the developing egg. This transmitted virus usually, but not always, infects the chick. Males can also pass the virus through the semen. This infected semen rarely causes infection in the chick, but obviously causes horizontal transmission to any breeder hens that he mates with. Chicks infected by this vertical transmission, develop immune tolerance (don=t recognize the virus as being foreign) and do not produce antibodies to the virus. These chicks, when subsequently mature, are those most at risk from exhibiting leucosis tumors during early egg production. Such vertical transmission therefore provides the on-going source of the J-virus infection in the breeding industry. The breeding companies now have to clean-up the various lines for both endogenous virus, and also the congenital exogenous virus that may have affected the breeders. Unfortunately this is a very costly and time consuming procedure, but obviously one that must eventually be undertaken.

The J-virus can be found in the feces and albumen of fresh eggs and also in the feather pulp as well as body tissues. An ELISA test is now available for the virus, usually determined using cloacal or vaginal swabs. Unfortunately it is difficult to differentiate between positive results due to genetic material from the endogenous gene in the bird's DNA and the presence of exogenous infection. Ideally the breeders would like to be able to identify, and remove the carriers of the endogenous gene only, because long-term (2-3 generations) this should eliminate the problem, because most exogenous viruses start from this source. In the short-term therefore, breeders are faced with selecting out "false" positives.

While the long-term solution resides with the breeding companies, commercial breeders are still faced with the short term problem of managing infected flocks. There is little doubt that tumor development is greatly influenced by general immune status of the birds, biosecurity and day to day management procedures. Such variation accounts for the drastic range of clinical leucosis seen in breeders that carry the virus. Simply minimizing the stress on the bird, especially during transport to the breeder house is of importance. Signs of J-virus are much more common in birds where Marek's programs have failed, especially in areas where very virulent forms of Marek's are found. Appropriate vaccine selection and scheduling is therefore critical in these situations. The breeder will show more tumors and higher mortality if other immunosuppressant viruses are present, such as IBD, reovirus and chick anemia agent. Many mycotoxins impair immune response and so can trigger increased mortality if birds carry the J-virus. Because the disease can be strain specific, or at least occur with higher incidence in some genetic lines, then it is reasonable to consider separate sex grow out of pullets and roosters where strain crosses are used commercially. Birds seem to be more prone to horizontal transmission of the virus up to about 4 weeks of age, consequently keeping sexes separate at least until 6-8 weeks is recommended to stop the spread of disease from a potentially infected to non-infected sex. During vaccination, needles should be changed more frequently, and different needles used for the pullets and roosters. Tumor incidence is also known to be worse in the presence of reticuloendothelial virus, which in the past has been shown to be a contaminant of some live vaccines (fowl pox for example) that were manufactured by culturing in contaminated embryos. Biosecurity in general must be optimized for these susceptible breeders.

The effect of J-virus on commercial broilers has not been extensively documented. Certainly the endogenous ev21 gene, associated with the fast-feathering gene and that encodes for lymphoid leucosis, has been implicated in poorer breeder performance. However the effects of the endogenous J-virus *per se* on breeder performance independent of tumor production and mortality, has not been clearly established. There is some anecdotal evidence for slightly poorer uniformity and higher early mortality in commercial broilers hatched from infected flocks.

Lameness

In a recent survey conducted in N. America, lameness due to a number of different causes, was the major (20%) reason for culling and/or mortality in broiler breeders. Viral arthritis and staphylococcal infection are among the two most common causes. Viral arthritis is caused by a reovirus infection, and this happens most frequently in very young birds in the first few weeks of life. At the time of initial infection, there are often few signs displayed by the chicks, and resistance quickly develops over time. However the early infection results in viral migration to the tendons in the leg, and most problems are seen when the pullets are moved to the breeder house. The physical move, the increase in weight gain, and the extra stress imposed on the tendons by the bird jumping onto and off of the slats or nests, places an extra strain on the weakened tendon that will eventually rupture. Once the tendon has torn or ruptured, the bird assumes the classical hock-sitting position. The physical changes are not reversible, and so the bird quickly loses condition within the competitive environment of the breeder house.

The long term solution may reside with a vaccination of the GP's or parent chicks at day of age, depending upon the local reovirus challenge. Maternal antibodies, produced by vaccinating the grandparents is often sufficient to protect chicks in low challenge areas. In high challenge areas where reovirus-induced lameness is a recurring problem in young breeders, then it is advisable to vaccinate the day old commercial breeder chicks. The breeder pullets themselves can also be vaccinated in order to confer maternal antibodies to the commercial broilers. Spread of reovirus infection is mainly horizontal, but vertical transmission through the egg can occur, which provides a potential reservoir of infection.

Staphylococcal infection, caused by S. aureus, is another major cause of lameness in breeders. Unlike viral arthritis, this bacteria can infect any age of breeder, although there are similarities in that occurrence is most obvious in younger adult breeders - again because of associated stress on the tendons at this time. Infection is most likely to occur when the immune status of the breeder pullet is compromised, such as at the time of beak trimming, moving, etc. Day old toe clipping of birds can also provide a route of entry for the bacteria. Staphylococci have a tendency to become associated with bruises or injury, meaning that general management conditions and equipment maintenance carried out to reduce physical injury are important. Signs are somewhat similar to those caused by reovirus infection, although with staphylococci infection there is usually more initial swelling of the joint which is warm to the touch. Staphylococci infection can be treated with antibiotics such as streptomycin, chlortetracycline and novobiocin. Because of bacterial resistance, drug sensitivity should be determined prior to treatment. Feeding relatively high levels of antibiotics (100g/tonne novobiocin or 185g/ tonne erythromycin) for the first 14-21d has been used successfully in some areas as a preventative treatment, while bacitracin at 50g/tonne through rearing is another possible preventative measure. Giving antibiotics in the drinking water for 1-2 days prior to, and 1-2 days following vaccinations and beak trimming is also recommended where staphlococci infection is a major cause of leg problems. Staphylococci also seem to become more easily established following an outbreak of coccidiosis or other enteric disorders such as necrotic enteritis. If breeders exhibit a high incidence of staphylococcus infection, then at flock termination, the house must be thoroughly cleaned and disinfected with cresylic acid based disinfectants, and then ideally fumigated with formaldehyde.

Regardless of the infective agent, leg problems in breeders are usually more severe when slatted floors are part of the management system. Birds jumping onto slats and moving over feeder lines etc., seem to place more stress on their joints and tendons. Slats should be no more than 60 cm high, and even at this height it may be advantageous to install ramps for birds to gain easier access to the slats. In order to discourage nesting underneath such access ramps, they should be constructed so as to be totally enclosed.

Mycoplasma iowae infection, which is more common in turkeys than in chickens, has been shown to cause rupture of the tendon in broiler breeders. Leg problems can also be caused by a variety of nutritional deficiencies, since most minerals and vitamins are involved in skeletal or cartilage development. Deficiencies of manganese, zinc, calcium and phosphorus as well as vitamins D_3, biotin, riboflavin and pyridoxine have all been implicated in leg problems. In a number of situations, such deficiencies are induced by interaction with other nutrients or antinutrients, and so diagnosis can be quite difficult based on simple diet analyses. Muscular dystrophy has been reported in breeders, and the condition seems to relate to selenium metabolism. Breeders are usually fed diets containing 0.2-0.3 ppm selenium, and this fortification usually prevents occurrence of muscular dystrophy. Where problems have occurred involving diets containing apparently adequate levels of selenium (and where the condition is responsive to extra selenium) then the deficiency is often traced to the use of copper sulfate as an antifungal. High levels of copper can increase the need for a number of other minerals including selenium.

Foot pad lesions can be a problem with both hens and roosters. In addition to causing problems of movement for the bird, severe cracking of the pad provides a route of entry for bacteria such as staphylococcus. Birds fed biotin-deficient diets show a characteristic foot pad dermatitis and the condition is obviously responsive to biotin. However even in diets well fortified with all vitamins, foot pad dermatitis still occurs sporadically, and seems to be largely a factor of litter condition. With wet and caked litter, regardless of the diet, some birds will develop foot pad lesions. There is some concern over the use of ingredients such as soybean meal, where manure composition or its consistency seems to accentuate the foot pad problems. Soybean meal contains high levels of potassium, and so this effect may simply relate to litter moisture, or alternatively, undigested oligosaccharides may be causative agents. Caged birds show a much higher incidence than do floor managed birds, therefore physical abrasion to the foot pad seems to be a factor. The major predisposing factor is litter condition, and so even within a single breeder house, the occurrence of dermatitis can vary from one end of the building to the other depending on the ventilation system etc. Initially, the foot pad becomes cracked and encrusted with manure. Swelling of the foot pad and reluctance to move are likely a result of secondary bacterial infection. When comparing incidence of foot pad lesions in different flocks, the only associated factor is often simply litter moisture content.

E. coli Infections

E. coli infections are one of the most common causes of mortality and morbidity in breeders, although ironically the bacteria is rarely a primary disease producing organism. In adult breeders, infection usually manifests itself as peritonitis of the ovary and inflammation of the oviduct, a condition usually termed salpingitis. In newly hatched chicks, the problem is omphalitis or yolk sac infections, and in growing birds the condition known as colibacillosis sometimes complicates other respiratory infections.

E. coli is fairly heat sensitive, being killed by exposure to about 60°C for just 20 minutes, and possesses no unique characteristics that make it resistant to any chemical disinfectants. Adequate chlorination of drinking water at 2-3ppm is usually effective against E. coli. However large numbers of E. coli are often present in the small intestine of even normal healthy birds. At the body temperature of the chicken, one E. coli organism is capable of generating a colony of 250 x 10^{18} within 24h. As the flock grows, the environment becomes progressively more contaminated, and dust in the air can contain as many as 10^{6} bacteria per gram. Horizontal transmission is the main means of infection, although vertical transmission can occur. It is not known if such egg-borne transmission occurs via true *in ovo* contamination (as occurs with salmonella) or by the bacteria gaining entry to the hatching egg through the shell. Potential infection in the hatchery is of great concern, because E. coli can quickly become the predominant bacteria in the gut, and so septicemia is more likely. In healthy chicks, gram negative bacteria such as E. coli have more difficulty in establishing themselves in the presence of other gram positive bacteria. Therefore even though colonization with E. coli is inevitable on-farm the bacterial numbers are kept in balance by the general gut flora, and this more manageable E. coli population is tolerated with no ill effects. Maternal antibodies from immunized GP's, also give some protection to the young breeder chick for 14-21d. However, the major problems with E. coli usually occur in the immunosuppressed bird.

With omphalitis, or yolk sac infection, the chicks have a characteristic distended abdomen and inflamed purple/blue colored navel. Affected chicks should be culled because they present a reservoir of infection to other chicks, and they themselves will likely lead to reduced uniformity should they eventually recover.

In adult breeders, a common cause of mortality (up to 1% per week) is salpingitis caused by E. coli invasion of the reproductive tract. The condition is sometimes loosely referred to as egg peritonitis. Such affected flocks may show extended feed clean up time together with flushing or diarrhea. In immature birds, infection of the ovary and oviduct is often a consequence of air sac infections, and IB virus is sometimes involved. In mature birds, the route of infection is reverse flow of bacteria from the cloaca up through the oviduct and possibly to the ovary. Eggs and yolks in various stages of decomposition are usually found in the oviduct and/or body cavity.

Many field isolates of E. coli are now resistant to a number of commonly used antibiotics, although unfortunately there are few treatment options available other than judicious shuttling of antibiotics and antimicrobials. At the present time, the newly introduced fluoroquinolones are the most effective antibiotics, although over time the effectiveness of these compounds, if used continually at one site, will likely diminish. Vaccines, or E. coli bacterins (see section 4.5) have not generally been accepted because of the large number of serotypes occurring naturally available. However E. coli bacterins can play a useful role in areas of specific localized infection with antibiotic resistant strains. Such bacterins need to be tailored to the specific infection.

Barnes (1994) describes E. coli infection as a "threshold disease" meaning that below a certain level of bacteria the bird is generally unaffected by the microbial load. The threshold level of E. coli however changes with age of bird, and most certainly with the general health status of the bird. Long term an E. coli prevention program has to involve minimizing the degree of exposure, and so this concept again relates to carefully prescribed programs of sanitation, disinfection/ fumigation and biosecurity. In the future we may see more use of E. coli bacterins coupled with competitive exclusion.

Fowl cholera

Cholera is caused by the bacteria Pasteurella multocida and unfortunately is a fairly common pathogen of breeder flocks. Cholera is less frequently seen in broilers or even growing breeder pullets, and so long-term chronic exposure to the bacteria may be involved in infections. Rats and mice are major vectors of cholera, and preventative measures must involve a comprehensive rodent eradication program. Because Pasteurella is a bacteria, there is the option of using antibiotics as well as bacterins for treatments or prevention respectively.

Cholera manifests itself as an acute form causing high mortality or as a more chronic form where birds are little affected. The reason for change in virulence of the bacteria is not fully understood, although may relate to whether or not the cell is encapsulated (virulent). With acute infection, signs are often present for only a few hours before death. These signs include feed refusal, ruffled feathers and mucous discharge from the mouth. With chronic infection, the signs are more localized, such as swollen wattles etc., and there is no generalized septicemia. Vaccination programs are common in areas of high potential exposure, and combinations of dead and inactivated bacterins are used. It is not ideal to use live vaccines close to time of moving pullets to the breeder house because the vaccine causes some clinical signs and these can be accentuated with the stresses imposed during the move. It is ideal to use a killed bacterin followed by a live attenuated dose, although this second vaccination should be completed at least 14-21d prior to transport of the birds. Studies have shown that vaccination programs producing ELISA antibody titres ($\log_{10}$) greater than 6.0 at 20 weeks, usually provide sufficient protection for breeders through to 64 weeks of age.

Salmonella

Salmonella is a ubiquitous bacteria, present as many different serotypes. Because of its widespread distribution in the environment, complete eradication will be very difficult, and so control measures are designed to limit any incidence of contamination. For the poultry industry, salmonella pose two threats, namely, as an infectious disease of the bird, and also as a potential cause of food poisoning in humans. It is this latter concern that is now the impetus for salmonella control systems. Unfortunately salmonella can be ovarian (vertically) transmitted, and so broiler breeder flocks are a meaningful route of infection for the commercial broilers.

Salmonellosis in poultry can be caused by S. typhimurium S. pullorum, S. enteriditis or S. gallinarum (typhoid). Pullorum disease was common in the poultry industry prior to the introduction of stringent blood testing procedures initiated by the breeding companies in the 1950's. Virtual eradication of S. pullorum and S. gallinarum in commercial breeders today shows that individual serotypes of salmonella can successfully be eliminated. However there are over 2,000 serotypes of salmonella, and the breeders are merely one route of potential infection for commercial broilers.

Starting with a brand new broiler breeder farm, what are the potential routes of infection for these birds? As previously indicated, the chicks themselves must be negative for salmonella, and this means that they are hatched from a salmonella-free GP flock, and/or eggs are cleaned up prior to incubation. The transovarian rate of transfer in birds is exceptionally low, being in the order of 1 in 1,000 to 1 in 10,000 eggs. For a flock of 5,000 breeders therefore, the mean chance of transovarian infection is merely 1 chick! However this one chick can then potentially infect many others by horizontal transmission. Having salmonella free chicks is therefore an essential element in a "control" program.

Feed is another potential major route of infection. It is very difficult to detect salmonella in mixed feed because the rate of contamination is again often quite low, being in the order of just 1-2 organisms/kg feed. Since only a small quantity of feed is sampled for salmonella assays, then it is very easy to be complacent about false negative results. In reality, multiple sampling and testing of feed often shows the same serotypes as found in the birds. Animal proteins, such as meat and fish meals, are always likely to be the most frequently and heavily contaminated ingredients, but many samples of vegetable proteins and cereals also test positive. Production of salmonella-free feed is possible, at extra cost, and must be considered as part of a control program.

On farm, the general biosecurity procedures are going to be instrumental in reducing stress on the bird and allowing either entry of salmonella onto the farm or proliferation of salmonella already present in low numbers. Rodents, and especially mice, are almost always infected with the same serotypes as those found in infected birds.

As previously discussed, salmonellosis as a disease in poultry today is quite rare, mainly because of eradication of critical serotypes, but also because poultry are often little affected by low-level contamination of many serotypes. Periodically there are reports of S. pullorum or S. typhimurium infection, and these are usually traced back to breeders at some level. For example in commercial broilers an outbreak of S. pullorum was diagnosed in over 100 flocks and the source traced back to 22 breeder flocks. Further investigation indicated a single flock of GP males was the original source for vertical transmission through to the commercial rooster chicks. Similarly an outbreak of S. typhimurium in broilers in Mexico was traced back to infected breeders.

Detecting salmonella in breeder flocks is not always easy, although recently introduced ELISA tests make the procedure more manageable on a large scale. ELISA tests have been developed for B, C, and D serotypes and this includes S. typhimurium (B) and S. enteriditis (D). Identification of these two serotypes is important because these now represent the majority of human food poisoning cases caused by salmonella. The ELISA test accurately diagnoses the seronegative samples, although seropositive results should be confirmed by more detailed bacteriological culture procedures. Cloacal swabs are often used for bacteriological testing, although recent studies suggest that sampling of cecal droppings gives a better chance of identifying carrier birds.

There seem to be meaningful correlations between the salmonella status of breeder flocks, and a number of very common management situations. In one recent survey, about 20% of breeder flocks blood tested in the southern USA were positive for salmonella. Most of these positive flocks were found to have a common series of management problems, one of which was increased incidence following vaccination for fowl cholera (perhaps due to cross reaction with blood test). There was also a definite relationship with heat stress since breeders subjected to environmental temperatures of around 35°C had 22.5% incidence, while at 25° and 29°C, the incidence was 4.5 and 9% respectively. It seems likely that salmonella, often present in the bird at very low levels, proliferates when the bird is subjected to major stress as occurs at high temperature. In a more recent epidemiological study of over 100 breeder flocks in Europe, it was found that flocks with good biosecurity programs that involved footbaths etc., and where feed was from a large feed mill, were 50 times less likely to have salmonella contamination compared to flocks with no biosecurity or footbaths and where feed was from small local suppliers. In this European study all feed was pelleted, and so this indicates that pelleting *per se* is not always a guarantee of "clean" feed. In many surveys, the lowest levels of salmonella contamination are found in caged rather than floor managed breeders.

Salmonella control programs rely on conscientious biosecurity and managing breeders under minimal stress situations. Because feed is a major potential route of infection, then ingredient selection, feed manufacture, and feed delivery must be carefully scrutinized. There are two basic approaches to producing salmonella-free feed. Firstly, there is the option of using only salmonella-free ingredients, while the second approach is to worry less about raw ingredients, but rather to ensure destruction of salmonella during feed manufacture. Sourcing salmonella-free ingredients is very difficult, but in the future microbial loading of ingredients may become a factor in pricing. Because animal proteins have a much higher chance of microbial contamination than do other ingredients, then their use in breeder diets must be seriously questioned. Using vegetable protein ingredients alone however does not ensure salmonella-free status of the feed. Salmonella are fairly heat sensitive, and the most economical way to sanitize feed is heat treatment and/or pelleting. Treating feed with steam to establish 80°C for 3 minutes is usually sufficient to kill all salmonella. Feed exiting the pellet mill is likely to be clean, but can quickly become recontaminated in cooling bins, augers and delivery trucks. Cleanliness during post-pelleting feed storage and distribution is critical in a salmonella control program. Adding 2-2.5kg propionic acid per tonne feed post-pelleting is a useful way of preventing recontamination.

Competitive exclusion (CE) holds great potential for reducing salmonella colonization of the young breeder chicks. Systems have been developed for spraying CE cultures onto boxed chicks at the hatchery, similar to the system used for infectious bronchitis. At 7-10d of age, CE treated chicks, challenged with salmonella, had around 10 organisms/g cecal content, compared to 10^6 salmonella/g cecal contents for control chicks. If CE is used, it must occur very early after hatch, so as to exclude salmonella colonization. Because many breeder chicks are transported long distances prior to placement, then CE treatment at the breeder farm is usually too late. When competitive exclusion is used, extra care has to be taken in subsequent selection and use of antibiotics. Indiscriminate use of antibiotics or antimicrobials will influence the gut microflora, perhaps killing the CE organisms and so allowing salmonella to proliferate. This situation sometimes occurs with breeders at 25-30 weeks during early lay, where following stress of transportation and relocation, birds are given antibiotics. In order to prevent this problem, a two stage CE program has been suggested. This involves CE treatment at the hatchery, followed by antibiotic treatment two days prior to moving to the breeder house and then a second CE treatment at day 1 in the breeder house. Undoubtedly such programs will be modified over time as more sophisticated and balanced cultures of microbes are used in CE preparations.

Floor eggs pose a serious threat to a salmonella control program, and they should not usually be sent to the hatchery or even handled with the same equipment used for nest eggs. Washing and sanitizing of eggs is subject to some controversy. Such cleaning should remove any surface salmonella on the egg, although the severity of the washing and sanitizing can lead to removal of the cuticle and subsequent entry of bacteria through the pores of the shell. If eggs are contaminated with salmonella post-laying, then it usually occurs in the first few minutes as the egg is cooling and before the cuticle hardens. Nest hygiene is therefore the only solution to salmonella control at this critical point. If salmonella invade the egg, they can sometimes by-pass the protective systems of the albumen and penetrate the embryo. Just as problematic, is the reproduction of salmonella on the shell or in the pores during incubation, and contamination of the chick during hatching. This situation has led to research on effective sanitation and fumigation processes that have minimal deleterious effects on hatchability. Treating eggs with 1% formalin solution is very effective against salmonella. Best results are obtained by placing eggs in warm water (clean) at 40°C for about 5 minutes and then immersing in 1% formalin at 4°C for 2 minutes. As the egg cools, the formalin is drawn into the pores, so increasing the level of sanitization both inside and outside the shell. Similar treatments have been developed using hydrogen peroxide, QUATS and alkylated phenol disinfectant dips following hot water pre-treatment. Hypochlorites and QUATS seem to do little damage to the cuticle.

Sometimes at the grandparent level, and less frequently with commercial breeders, antibiotic dipping of eggs is used as a means of salmonella eradication. Dipping in products such as gentamycin or quinolones is very effective in killing salmonella, although hatchability is sometimes affected and long-term there will likely be antibiotic resistant strains developed. In order to overcome the problem of reduced hatchability, antibiotics can be injected into the egg at 18d incubation.

The other potential for salmonella control is vaccination. Vaccines would obviously need to be serotype specific although bivalent or trivalent mixtures of serotypes have not been too useful to date. A limitation of vaccination programs for breeders is the introduction of a false positive test for S. pullorum.

Initiating a salmonella eradication program, or handling flocks that become positive requires special consideration. McIlroy *et al.* (1989) recently outlined a management program used to eradicate S. enteriditis from infected breeder flocks in an integrated broiler operation in Europe. A number of breeder flocks were found to be carriers, but were clinically normal. All flocks were treated with 200 ppm furazolidone in the drinking water for 7 days and then 400 ppm furazolidone added to the feed. All floor, dirty and cracked eggs were discarded and hatching eggs treated with formaldehyde both at the farm and again at the hatchery. Eggs from suspect breeders were kept separate from eggs from all other breeder flocks. Egg trucks were cleaned, disinfected and fumigated after visiting the flocks. All eggs were set in separate machines, and these chicks pulled only after all other chicks had been removed. Broiler chicks were sent to dedicated company farms and chicks given feed medicated with furazolidone. At the end of the breeder cycle, litter was removed and piled for 6 months prior to spreading as a fertilizer. Houses were cleaned and disinfected with 10% solution of iodophores and then fumigated with formaldehyde, twice over a 24 hr period. The water system was drained and disinfected with iodophores. Any wooden nests or slats were destroyed and the top 15 cm of soil from the immediate vicinity of the houses was removed and replaced with stone. The feed mill management procedures were re-evaluated and systems changed so as to ensure heating to 70°C for 1 min. prior to pelleting.

Salmonella control will become of increasing importance in the poultry industry, as governments use microbial status as a means of regulating or controlling imports of meat, hatching eggs and breeding stock. Because of the potential for both true ovarian and egg-borne contamination, it will be essential for the breeder industry to implement stringent control programs. As discussed, such programs involve biosecurity, ELISA testing, feed quality control and maintenance of general health status of the bird.

4.15 OTHER POTENTIAL DISEASES

1) Infectious Bronchitis

Infectious bronchitis is an acute highly contagious respiratory disease where the causative agent is a filterable virus. The disease spreads rapidly in a flock and air-borne transmission can readily take place.

In young chicks the characteristic symptoms are nasal discharges, gasping, rales and coughing. The chicks crowd close to a source of heat in order to keep warm and wet eyes and swollen sinuses may be seen. While some of the above symptoms may be seen with adult breeders, a noticeable drop in production and rough and soft shelled eggs will also be noted. While the flock may recover in several weeks, poor quality eggs may continue for some time, and albumen quality (thinner albumen) may persist sporadically for the life of the flock.

The best prevention is vaccination in conjunction with strict isolation and rearing chicks away from adults.

2) Newcastle Disease

Newcastle is a highly infectious viral disease that can affect birds of all ages and cause heavy mortality. The disease can appear suddenly and spreads rapidly through a susceptible flock. In chicks the most common sign is gasping, coughing and hoarse chirping. Increased thirst and huddling are often seen. Nervous disorders include partial or complete paralysis of the extremities, muscle tremors and spasms. Lateral deviations of the head are associated with abnormal movements such as somersaulting, walking in circles and falling. Delayed growth and permanent stunting is a variable consequence of the disease.

For adult breeders, the disease occurs suddenly and respiratory distress of varying severity with coughing and gasping by sometimes just a few but often many birds, is noted. These symptoms are identical with bronchitis and closely resemble those seen with laryngotracheitis. Egg production may drop to near zero. Nervous symptoms may appear as with chicks but is much less common. Production of poor shelled eggs is noted during an outbreak and can persist beyond apparent recovery of the flock. Poor albumen quality is also noted and this can be a permanent feature with a flock. The normal spread of the disease is mainly through exudates, and excreta of infected birds with the digestive and respiratory routes being the main channels of entry.

While complete isolation is a logical method for preventing the spread of the disease, it is common practice today to initiate a good vaccination program. Treatment of the flock as a means of eradicating the disease is usually not economical or effective. Newcastle is a reportable disease in many countries.

3) Infectious Laryngotracheitis

The causative agent is a filterable virus which has a distinct specificity for chickens, although pheasants may also become infected. The natural route of infection is by way of the respiratory tract. The disease spreads rapidly in a flock and most of the birds eventually become infected. The common symptoms are gasping, rales and coughing, while birds appear listless and may spend considerable time sitting on the floor. In severely infected individuals coughing is frequent and often results in bloody mucous being expelled. An accumulation of inflammatory exudate and blood in the larynx and trachea are often seen. In breeder flocks a variable drop in production is noted.

Sound management practices are needed to prevent the disease from coming onto a farm. A thorough clean up of the farm and buildings may ensure the next flock will not be infected. However, where problems have often reoccurred or if one is in an area where the disease has appeared, an appropriate vaccination program must be used. Vaccinated birds shed the virus, and so the program must be an "all or none" situation.

4) Avian Encephalomyelitis (Epidemic Tremor)

Avian encephalomyelitis is a viral infection affecting primarily young chickens and symptoms seen are mainly ataxia and tremor of the head and neck. Flocks hatched from susceptible parents may become infected from just several chicks infected via the egg. Natural outbreaks usually occur when chicks are 1 to 3 weeks of age. Birds will appear listless which is followed by ataxia or incoordination of the leg muscles. Eventually the chicks show a tendency to sit on their hocks.

While infection has been reported in adults, with a notable drop in egg production, typical signs as seen with chicks do not occur. It appears that once a flock has had an outbreak of the disease no further evidence of the condition is noted. Vaccination programs are now available to protect breeder flocks which in turn will prevent the spread of the disease to their progeny through egg transmission.

5) Marek's Disease

This disease is caused by a lymphotropic herpes virus which can vary widely in it's ability to produce disease. The condition was often referred to as range paralysis or polyneuritis. The disease attacks mainly young pullets and roosters around 2 to 5 months of age but can be seen much earlier. Losses can range from 5 to 25% of a flock. Clinical signs of the disease are partial paralysis of the leg, wing or neck, while blindness or gray, pearly fish eyes may also be noted. Anatomic features of the disease are localized diffuse soft swelling of the femoral portion of the sciatic nerve trunk.

Visceral lymphomatosis, or big liver disease can also be seen in breeders. However, this usually occurs after or later than the nerve or eye type lesions and more often during the laying period. With this variant, the comb becomes pale and shriveled and then darkened as in cyanosis. Eventually loss of appetite, weight loss and diarrhea may develop.

No therapeutic measures are available to combat the disease. Birds showing clinical symptoms should be culled. While complete isolation and the use of genetically resistant stock can give some protection, it is now almost universal to vaccinate chicks at day of age or at 18d incubation. However, occasional outbreaks appear from time to time mainly due to poor vaccination practices, poor house disinfection, or new virulent strains of the virus.

6) Chick Anemia Virus (CAV)

The condition is caused by a small, heat resistant virus that can be transmitted horizontally by direct contact with other birds or contaminated material, and also vertically through embryonated eggs. CAV will be transmitted vertically as long as the hen is viremic (1 to 3 wk). Maternal antibodies generally protect chicks from the disease, but do not prevent infection. Immunosuppressive agents such as other viral diseases can reduce the effectiveness of the maternal protection, and problems are more severe where IBD is also involved.

The disease is seen mainly in young chicks that appear listless and pale. Feed consumption is markedly depressed and birds become anemic with packed cell volume less than 27. There is no specific treatment however, secondary bacterial infections respond to antibiotic treatment. Vaccines are available which allow for maternal protection for chicks.

7) Infectious Bursal Disease (IBD, Gumboro Disease)

The disease is caused by a highly contagious viral infection of young chicks. Infections before 3 weeks of age are usually subclinical but result in marked immunosuppression. Consequences of infection depend on age of bird, breed and virulence of the virus, and may be divided into subclinical and clinical infections. Early subclinical infection is the more serious form of the disease as it causes long-lasting immunosuppresssion, due to destruction of lymphocytes in the bursa of Fabricius, thymus and spleen. These birds do not respond well to vaccination against other viral diseases, thus severe economical losses can occur with clinical infections. Onset of the clinical disease is sudden with chicks showing severe prostration, loss of balance, watery diarrhea and inflammation of the cloaca. There is no known treatment for the disease and depopulation and rigorous disinfection has only met with limited success. Vaccination of breeders provides some protection to chicks via maternal antibodies deposited in the egg.

8) Egg Drop Syndrome (EDS)

The condition is caused by an adenovirus and is widely distributed in both wild and domestic ducks and geese although it does not seem to spread directly from waterfowl to chickens. Although all breeds and ages of birds are susceptible to the disease it appears to be more severe in broiler breeders and brown egg layers. Breeding stock can transmit the virus vertically through eggs.

The virus can often remain latent until the bird reaches sexual maturity when it is excreted in the egg or in manure. In flocks without detectable antibodies the first signs noted are loss of color in brown eggs, followed by soft-shelled and then shell-less eggs. Due mainly to shell-less eggs, which are not collected, egg production can drop 10 to 40%. EDS can be distinguished from other viral diseases by the absence of any apparent illness. There is no treatment, however, the classical form of the disease has been eliminated from most primary breeders. The endemic form can be controlled by strict sanitation, including washing and disinfecting plastic egg trays. Vaccines are now available, and should be used in regions where EDS is common in breeders or egg layers.

9) Avian Influenza (Fowl Plague)

Avian influenza is a viral disease of domestic and wild birds with symptoms ranging from almost no clinical signs to very high mortality. There are a number of virus strains involved and these can grow rapidly in embryonated eggs. In severely affected birds, greenish diarrhea, cyanosis and edema of the head, comb and wattles may be noted.

While vaccines are available their effectiveness is complicated by the antigenic variability of subtypes that may be responsible for the disease. Treatment of infected flocks with antibiotics to help control secondary bacterial infections may help reduce mortality.

10) Avian Rhinotracheitis (Swollen Head Syndrome)

Rhinotracheitis is caused by a pneumovirus affecting birds from around 10 days of age to end of lay. Initial signs are sneezing followed by swelling of the glands in the head and wattle area especially when E. coli is present. While adult breeders are often affected, the signs are less severe than with younger birds. A small percentage of an adult flock may show mild respiratory problems followed by a small portion of the flock showing swollen heads. These swollen heads can lead to difficulty during feeding with narrow grill systems ($\simeq$ 43 mm). In breeders, reduced egg production and hatchability have been reported.

There is no really effective treatment available but good general management practices are helpful in controlling the disease. There are now several vaccines available which show promise in controlling the disease.

11) Fowl Pox

This is a slow spreading viral infection characterized by lesions on the skin or by yellow plaques in the upper GI and respiratory tracts. Mosquitoes and other biting insects can serve as mechanical vectors. Transmission in a flock can be rapid. Extensive infection in a breeder flock results in a decrease in egg production and mortality can be high in the generalized diphtheritic form.

There are good vaccines available that should be used in order to protect birds against the disease. Because the disease is usually slow in spreading, vaccination is often helpful in limiting spread of the problem in an already infected flock.

12) Fowl Cholera (Pasteurellosis)

The causative agent is a small, gram negative bacteria. The condition can develop into a mild infection or a severe septicemia resulting in sudden, high and long lasting mortality. With acute cholera, dead birds may be the initial indication of the disease. Fever, listlessness, anorexia, mucous discharge from the mouth, ruffled feathers, diarrhea and respiratory signs may be seen as the disease progresses through a flock. The signs and lesions are generally related to localized infections.

Good management practices are essential in preventing the disease. Bacterins can also be used and are usually effective. Live vaccines are available and these can induce immunity against different serotypes of the Pasteurella bacteria. For treatment of an infected flock sulfonamides and antibiotics are commonly used.

13) Salmonellosis

The disease is caused be several species of salmonella bacteria. For poultry Salmonella pullorum, gallinarum, arizona and typhimurium can cause a variety of problems.

Pullorum: An outbreak can result in high mortality in young chicks and occasionally in adult birds. Although it was once a very common disease it has now been eradicated from most commercial flocks through extensive blood testing of breeding stock.

Transmission is usually through the egg but can also be by direct or indirect contact. Infection resulting from egg transmission results in mortality during the first few days of life. Birds will huddle, do not eat, are sleepy and show a whitish fecal vent pasting. Lesions usually include unabsorbed egg yolks and necrosis of the spleen and liver. Adult carriers often have no gross lesions but pericarditis, peritonitis or distorted ovarian follicles may be noted. Acute infections in mature birds can be similar to that seen with fowl typhoid. Several antibacterials are available which are effective in reducing mortality but do not eliminate the infection from a flock.

Fowl Typhoid (S. gallinarum): Since the causative agent is similar to that of S. pullorum these are often considered as one. Infection is now rare in many countries. Although the condition is egg transmitted and produces lesions in young birds similar to that of S. pullorum it has a tendency to spread more in growing and adult flocks and mortality can be high for all ages. Older birds may be dehydrated and have enlarged, friable and often bile stained livers, enlarged spleens and perhaps anemia and enteritis. Treatment is similar to that for pullorum although bacterins are available which have been successful in controlling mortality.

Paratyphoid Infections: These can be caused by a number of non-specific salmonella species, however, S. typhimurium is the most common. All ages of birds are susceptible to the infection but the incidence is higher in younger flocks with mortality usually seen mainly in the first few weeks of age. Lesions may include enlarged livers with necrotic areas sometimes noted, as well as unabsorbed egg yolks. Infections can localize in the eye or synovial tissues.

There are several antibacterial agents that are capable of preventing mortality but do not prevent flock infection. Strict sanitation in hatcheries helps to prevent transmission between successive flocks. Fumigation of hatching eggs is recommended to prevent shell surface penetration of the organism although infection from true egg transmission is rare. The heat generated during pelleting feed is reasonably effective in destroying salmonella in feed. Good, strict management procedures and exclusion of wild birds and pets from the breeder house will help to control transmission of the disease. Several methods are available for determining the salmonella status of a breeder flock. Periodic culturing of samples of litter, dust, water, hatchery debris, etc. is recommended for early detection of infection.

14) Staphylococcus Infections

Staphylococcus aureus is the predominate species which can appear as an opportunistic infection in all ages of poultry. It can remain viable on inanimate objects for months. While this coagulase-positive species can gain entry into the body through any type of injury that breaks the epithelial surface, the respiratory tract can also be a major route of infection. These organisms can pass from the respiratory tract into the blood or lymphatic systems. Colonization of the liver, spleen and synovial fluids can then result.

Clinical signs include reluctance to walk, drowsiness, emaciation and a greenish type diarrhea. Infection can occur in any age of bird and is often seen in breeders as they mature. Vaccination is not directly successful in reducing the infection. Good breeder house management, nutrition and handling conditions that prevent stress or injury are important factors in reducing the occurrence of staphylococcus infection.

15) Colibacillosis

This is a common systemic disease which can infect all birds, resulting in acute fatal septicemia, or subacute pericarditis and airsacculitis. While there are a large number of coliforms present in most poultry houses and on birds themselves, Escherichia coli is the species responsible for most of the serious coliform infections. While initial exposure to this organism can readily occur, systemic infection requires some other predisposing factor such as other viruses or bacteria or poor air quality or other adverse environmental and handling conditions.

Clinical findings and lesions vary with age, the organs involved and concurrent diseases. Young birds dying from acute septicemia may have few lesions except for enlarged and hyperemic liver and spleen along with increased fluid in the body cavity. Yolk sac infection can be caused by E. coli infection although other bacteria like bacillus and staph can also be involved. These bacteria can result in toxemia resulting in death on the hatching trays or in the first few days of life. Losses cease after approximately one week of age.

Egg peritonitis is a disorder arising from infection of the ovary or oviduct. E. coli, along with other bacteria can cause septicemia resulting in mortality especially during early lay.

16) Viral Arthritis (Reovirus infection, Tenosynovitis)

The condition is caused by a reovirus which is egg transmitted and is of short duration except when lateral transmission takes place in a flock. Respiratory and digestive infections can occur but are of short duration, however, the virus survives in tendon sheaths for quite some time. The arthritic form of the disease (tenosynovitis) usually occurs in 4 to 8 week old birds with swelling of the tendons of the shank and above the hock. Birds walk with a stilted gait and in severely infected flocks rupture of the gastrocnemius tendon is often seen. Mortality can be 2 to 10% while morbidity is 5 to 50%.

There is no known treatment for the disease, however, parental antibodies prevent early infection in chicks and reduce and perhaps prevent egg transmission. Since egg transmission is the principal means of contamination, it is essential to have breeder flocks protected by adequate vaccination programs.

17) Mycoplasmosis

There are several Mycoplasma species that affect breeders. These are fastidious bacteria like organisms, which lack a cell wall and do not survive long outside the host and are susceptible to common disinfectants.

Mycoplasma gallisepticum (MG): MG infection is commonly called Chronic Respiratory Disease (CRD) in chickens and infectious sinusitis in turkeys. MG is the most pathogenic avian mycoplasma, however, strains differ markedly in their virulence. The disease is egg transmitted, although degrees of transmission are highly variable, ranging from 30 to 40% during the first two months of infection of a susceptible breeder flock, to 0-5% during the latter part of egg production. Most breeder flocks are MG-free, however, outbreaks can occur due to lateral transmission from other infected flocks.

Affected birds have varying degrees of respiratory distress with difficulty in breathing, while coughing and sneezing are often noted. Morbidity is usually high while mortality can be low. E coli infections are often noted along with MG resulting in severe air sac thickening and turbidity.

Since many field cases of MG are complicated by other pathogenic bacteria, effective treatment must also control the secondary invaders. Most strains of MG are sensitive to a number of antibiotics. Eradication of MG from breeder flocks is now common for most breeding companies. For primary breeding stock, treating eggs with tylosin or heat treatment can be used to eliminate egg-transmission with infected birds. Vaccines are now available that have been used with some success.

Mycoplasma synoviae (MS): The condition is often referred to as Infectious Synovitis and was first recognized as a chronic infection in chickens which produced tendonitis and bursitis. However, MS now occurs frequently as a subclinical upper respiratory tract infection. MS is egg transmitted but the rate is low, usually less than 5%. Lateral transmission is similar to that for MG but the rate of spread is much more rapid.

Outbreaks of MS occur most commonly in chickens 4 to 6 weeks of age. Lame birds tend to sit and are found around feeders and waterers. Morbidity is 2-15% and mortality 1-10%. When infecting the respiratory tract, airsacculitis usually occurs especially when the birds are stressed with other viral infections or poor ventilation. During the early stages of infection, the liver can be enlarged and sometimes appears green, while the spleen and kidneys may also be enlarged and pale. A yellow-gray viscous exudate is present in all synovial structures. Serological testing and isolation similar to those for MG have resulted in eradication of the infection from most primary breeders. Various antibiotics can be successful in treatment or prevention of synovitis, however, medication of a breeder flock is of little value in preventing egg transmission.

18) Aspergillosis

The condition is caused by the inhalation of spores from various fungi, with Aspergillus fumigatus being the main species involved. Chicks may be infected by inhaling spores in contaminated hatchers or from contaminated litter. Sugarcane bagasse litter is notorious for its mold count.

Poor appetite, emaciation, increased thirst and signs of nervous involvement may be seen. In birds up to 6 weeks of age the lungs are usually involved with cream coloured plaques noted. Plaques may also be seen in the air sacs , air passages , intestines and occasionally the brain. Strict sanitation procedures are necessary to prevent or minimize outbreaks. Contaminated eggs should not be used for incubation since they could explode thus spreading spores throughout the hatchery. Avoiding moldy litter is a critical step in preventing outbreaks in birds. Treatment of infected birds is usually without effect.

19) Sudden Death Syndrome

A syndrome specifically associated with broiler breeders was first described in Australia some 10 years ago. No evidence of respiratory infection or any other disease symptoms are noted. The problem commences when flocks reach around 5% production and can persist until 20 to 30% production is reached. Mortality can range from .5 to 2% per week with most of the birds dying at feeding time.

There is some evidence that the condition is due to a mineral imbalance associated with low blood potassium as the flock matures. It seems more common where diets contain high levels of meat and bone meal as occur in Australia. The addition of potassium carbonate to the diet has been reported to reduce the incidence of the problem. More recently, the magnesium status of birds has been questioned, and there seem to be certain breeder strains that are more susceptible to the condition. (This condition is not to be confused with Acute Death Syndrome or "Flip-overs" which is a common occurrence with certain broiler flocks). Adding 1-2kg potassium magnesium sulfate to the feed has been reported to reduce mortality in susceptible flocks.

BIBLIOGRAPHY

Barnes, H.J., 1994. Colibacillosis in Poultry. Pfizer Veterinary Practicum. Publ. Veterinary Learning Systems.

Danforth, H.D., 1997. Use of live oocyst-based vaccines in avian coccidial control. Proc VII Int. Coccidiosis Conf. Peble College, Oxford, UK. Sept. 1-5.

Gifford, D.H., S.M. Shane, M. Hugh-Jones and B.J. Weigler, 1986. Evaluation of biosecurity in broiler breeders. Avian Diseases 31:339-344.

Goren, E., 1994. Bacterial resistance is still a major problem. World Poultry 10(4), 53.

Leeson, S., L.J. Caston and J.D. Summers, 1989. The effect of graded levels of nicarbazin on reproductive performance of laying hens. Can. J. Anim. Sci. 69:757-764.

McIlroy, S.G., 1995. Coccidiosis control programs in broiler breeders. Zootechnia Int. May 1995, pp 40-44.

McIlroy, S.G., R.M. McCraken, S.D. Neill and J.J. O'Brien 1989. Control, prevention and eradication of S. enteriditis infection in broiler and broiler breeder flocks. Vet. Record 125:545-548.

Smith, N.C., M. Wallach, C. Miller, R. Morganstern, R. Braun and J. Eckert, 1994. Maternal transmission of immunity to E. maxima. Am. Soc. Microbiol. 62:1348-1357.

SUGGESTED READING

Compendium of Veterinary Products. N. American Compendiums Ltd. Hensall, Ontario, Canada.

Calnek, B.W. et al., 1997. Diseases of Poultry. 10th Rev. Edition. Iowa State Univ. Press.

Jordan, F.T.W. and M. Pattison, 1996. Poultry Diseases. 4th Rev. Edition. Saunders.

CHAPTER 5. NUTRITION AND FEEDING

The challenge of feeding broiler breeders relates to tempering their growth potential in order to realize adequate reproductive performance. As discussed in Chapter 1, there is a negative correlation between growth rate and reproduction, and so this means that we cannot allow either the hen or the rooster to exhibit genetic growth potential, because reproduction in these very large birds is uneconomical. Feeding programs therefore involve conscientious formulation of appropriate diets, and perhaps more importantly, a schedule for feed restriction aimed at control over growth rate. With commercial breeders, the weight of the birds at maturity is very similar to that potentially achieved at 5-6 weeks with free choice feeding. At this time, there is no viable alternative to physical feed restriction. Although such restriction does impose major management problems, use of anorexic agents or fillers are of no practical use. In the past, attempts have been made to control growth with amino acid imbalanced diets or use of unusual fatty acids in the diet, and while these programs do seem to reduce feed intake, there is tremendous loss in uniformity of growth. For example, average weight of a flock of pullets can be controlled by simply limiting the salt level of the diet. As salt level is reduced, there is a linear decline in growth. Unfortunately some pullets seem to grow quite well on low salt diets, whereas others become severely runted. It is this variance in nutrient needs that make these so-called "qualitative" restriction programs of little commercial use. Likewise, the use of diet fillers, such as fiber, merely add to manure build up, wet litter and increased trucking costs of the bulky feed. Currently, we have no real alternative for simple physical feed restriction throughout the entire life of the breeder flock. Criteria used in assessing the effectiveness of the feeding program, are initially, body weight and uniformity during rearing, and coupled with these factors, are those related to reproduction such as egg production and egg size for the adult breeders.

Energy, calcium and protein or amino acids are the most critical nutrients for the breeder. Energy is the most critical of all nutrients, and undoubtedly balancing supply with needs often means the difference between good and average breeder performance. Because of high maintenance needs associated with a relatively large body size, the energy needs of the breeder hen are proportionally much greater than for the Leghorn bird, even though peak egg production is less with the heavier breeder birds. Complicating the adult feeding program is the influence of environmental temperature because this has a dramatic effect on maintenance energy needs. Perhaps the most challenging situation for the nutritionist and breeder manager is development of diets and feeding programs for breeders at peak production in very hot climates. As will be discussed later in this Chapter, heat stress actually increases the energy needs of the hen, and so we are faced with the challenge of stimulating energy intake at a time when the breeder voluntarily wishes to reduce its feed intake. Maintaining energy intake under a range of environmental conditions is the key to optimizing performance of today's breeder hens.

5.1 DIET SPECIFICATIONS

Diet specifications are obviously an important part of breeder nutrition, but they must always be viewed in relation to guidelines for feed intake. However, it is important for the nutritionist to provide well balanced diets that can be part of a comprehensive feed management program, and so it is important to critically review the feed specifications. Reviewing the management guides from the various commercial breeding companies shows a fairly consistent pattern of diet specifications (Tables 5.1-5.4). However there are some significant differences

TABLE 5.1 Nutrient specifications for Starter diets (Management Guide Data)

	Hubbard	Shaver	Cobb	Ross	Arbor Acres	Avian	Hybro
Metabolizable energy (kcal/kg)	2865	2850	2915	2860	2855	2875	2800
Crude protein (%)	17.5	17.5	19.0	20.0	17.5	18.5	18.5
Calcium (%)	0.97	1.0	0.95	1.0	0.95	0.95	1.0
Av. Phosphorus (%)	0.43	0.47	0.45	0.45	0.47	0.48	0.48
Sodium (%)	0.19	0.17	0.19	0.18	0.19	0.22	0.18
Linoleic acid (%)	1.25	1.30	1.20	1.0	1.0	1.25	1.5
Methionine (%)	0.36	0.40	0.46	0.45	0.35	0.36	0.42
Meth + cystine (%)	0.71	0.70	0.76	0.73	0.74	0.70	0.80
Lysine (%)	0.94	0.90	1.00	1.10	0.95	0.89	1.00
Tryptophan (%)	0.19	0.18	0.24	0.28	0.18	0.18	0.18
Vitamin A (TIU/kg)	7.26	12.0	4.0	4.6	11.0	9.9	12.5
Vitamin D3 (TIU/kg)	3.3	2.0	1.25	1.6	3.3	3.0	3.8
Vitamin E (IU/kg)	33	30	20	25	22	25	30
Vitamin K3 (mg/kg)	2.4	2.0	1.5	1.0	2.2	2.0	3
Thiamine (mg/kg)	4.4	3.0	1.2	1.0	2.2	2.2	2.5
Riboflavin (mg/kg)	5.5	6.0	5.0	2.8	5.5	8.8	8
Pantothenate (mg/kg)	11.0	14.0	6.0	7.0	11.0	16.5	15
Niacin (mg/kg)	53	40	30	16	33	44	35
Pyridoxine (mg/kg)	3.3	6.0	1.8	1.0	1.1	4.4	3
Choline (mg/kg)	660	500	186	550	440	660	400
Folic acid (mg/kg)	1.0	1.5	1.0	0.45	0.88	1.0	1.0
Biotin (mg/kg)	0.11	0.20	.06	0.12	0.11	0.20	0.25
Vitamin B12 (Fg/kg)	11	30	20	10	13	16.5	15
Manganese (mg/kg)	80	80	90	30	120	100	100
Zinc (mg/kg)	80	50	75	25	100	80	50
Iron (mg/kg)	66	60	20	30	40	30	40
Copper (mg/kg)	9	8	3.6	4	8	3.0	6
Iodine (mg/kg)	1.1	0.6	1.5	0.23	1.1	0.74	0.5
Selenium (mg/kg)	0.30	0.30	0.13	0.10	0.30	0.30	0.15

TABLE 5.2 Nutrient specifications for Grower diets (Management Guide Data)

	Hubbard	Shaver	Cobb	Ross	Arbor Acres	Avian	Hybro
Metabolizable energy (kcal/kg)	2865	2700	2860	2860	2750	2840	2700
Crude protein (%)	15.5	15.2	15.0	15.0	15.3	15.5	15.0
Calcium (%)	0.92	0.95	0.93	1.0	0.87	0.90	1.0
Av. Phosphorus (%)	0.40	0.44	0.45	0.40	0.41	0.45	0.42
Sodium (%)	0.19	0.16	0.19	0.16	0.19	0.22	0.16
Linoleic acid (%)	1.1	1.0	1.2	1.0	1.0	1.25	0.8
Methionine (%)	0.31	0.35	0.26	0.35	0.33	0.30	0.28
Meth + cystine (%)	0.59	0.60	0.52	0.60	0.58	0.57	0.52
Lysine (%)	0.68	0.72	0.65	0.75	0.65	0.67	0.70
Tryptophan (%)	0.16	0.16	0.14	0.19	0.18	0.17	0.15
Vitamin A (TIU/kg)	7.3	10.0	4.0	4.5	11.0	9.0	10.0
Vitamin D_3 (TIU/kg)	3.3	1.5	1.25	1.6	3.3	3.0	3.0
Vitamin E (IU/kg)	33	20	20	20	22	22.0	20
Vitamin K_3 (mg/kg)	2.4	1.5	1.5	1.0	2.2	2.0	2.5
Thiamine (mg/kg)	4.4	2.0	1.2	1.0	2.2	2.2	2
Riboflavin (mg/kg)	5.5	4.0	5.0	2.75	5.5	8.8	6
Pantothenate (mg/kg)	11.0	10.0	6.0	7.0	11.0	16.5	10
Niacin (mg/kg)	53	35	30	16	33	40	30
Pyridoxine (mg/kg)	3.3	4.0	1.8	1.0	1.1	4.0	2
Choline (mg/kg)	660	200	186	450	440	600	350
Folic acid (mg/kg)	1.0	1.3	1.0	0.45	0.88	1.0	0.8
Biotin (mg/kg)	0.11	0.15	0.06	0.09	0.11	0.18	0.1
Vitamin B_{12} (μg/kg)	11	20	20	10	13	16.5	10
Manganese (mg/kg)	80	80	90	30	120	100	70
Zinc (mg/kg)	80	50	75	25	110	80	50
Iron (mg/kg)	66	60	20	20	40	30	40
Copper (mg/kg)	9	8	3.6	3	8	3	6
Iodine (mg/kg)	1.1	0.6	1.5	0.23	1.1	0.74	0.5
Selenium (mg/kg)	0.30	0.30	0.13	0.10	0.3	0.30	0.10

TABLE 5.3 Nutrient specifications for Pre-breeder diets (Management Guide Data)

	Hubbard	Shaver[1]	Cobb	Ross[1]	Arbor Acres	Avian[1]	Hybro
Metabolizable energy (kcal/kg)	2865		2860		2855		2750
Crude protein (%)	17.5		16.0		16.0		18.5
Calcium (%)	1.3		1.35		1.62		1.4
Av. Phosphorus (%)	0.40		0.45		0.41		0.40
Sodium (%)	0.19		0.17		0.18		0.16
Linoleic acid (%)	1.1		1.5		1.38		1.6
Methionine (%)	0.38		0.32		0.31		0.33
Meth+cystine (%)	0.71		0.58		0.62		0.60
Lysine (%)	0.87		0.74		0.83		0.75
Tryptophan (%)	0.17		0.16		0.17		0.16
Vitamin A (TIU/kg)	8.8		11.0		15.4		15.5
Vitamin D3 (TIU/kg)	3.3		1.75		3.3		3.8
Vitamin E (IU/kg)	33		40		33		30
Vitamin K3 (mg/kg)	3.3		5.0		2.2		3.0
Thiamine (mg/kg)	4.4		2.5		2.2		2.5
Riboflavin (mg/kg)	8.8		10.0		9.9		8
Pantothenate (mg/kg)	15.5		20.0		13.2		15
Niacin (mg/kg)	53		45		44		40
Pyridoxine (mg/kg)	3.3		5.0		5.5		5
Choline (mg/kg)	660		186		330		500
Folic acid (mg/kg)	1.0		1.25		1.65		1.5
Biotin (mg/kg)	0.22		0.20		0.22		0.25
Vitamin B12 (Fg/kg)	11		20		13		20
Manganese (mg/kg)	80		90		120		100
Zinc (mg/kg)	80		75		110		50
Iron (mg/kg)	66		20		40		40
Copper (mg/kg)	9		3.6		8		8
Iodine (mg/kg)	1.1		1.5		1.1		1
Selenium (mg/kg)	0.30		0.13		0.30		0.15

[1]No specifications given

TABLE 5.4 Nutrient specifications for Breeder diets[1] (Managemenet Guide Data)

	Hubbard	Shaver	Cobb	Ross	Arbor Acres	Avian	Hybro
Metabolizable energy (kcal/kg)	2865	2750	2860	2860	2855	2870	2750
Crude protein (%)	15.5	15.8	16.0	16.0	16.0	16.3	17.0
Calcium (%)	3.2	3.3	2.9	3.0	3.2	3.2	3.0
Av. Phosphorus (%)	0.40	0.44	0.45	0.40	0.41	0.47	0.40
Sodium (%)	0.17	0.16	0.17	0.16	0.18	0.20	0.16
Linoleic acid (%)	1.25	1.30	1.5	1.25	1.5	1.5	1.8
Methionine (%)	0.35	0.36	0.35	0.35	0.31	0.33	0.34
Meth + cystine (%)	0.58	0.65	0.64	0.61	0.62	0.64	0.62
Lysine (%)	0.71	0.75	0.78	0.83	0.82	0.74	0.75
Tryptophan (%)	0.17	0.17	0.17	0.21	0.17	0.17	0.16
Vitamin A (TIU/kg)	8.8	13.0	11.0	5.45	15.4	9.9	15.5
Vitamin D3 (TIU/kg)	3.3	3.0	1.75	1.6	3.3	3.0	3.8
Vitamin E (IU/kg)	44	40	40	45	33	33	30
Vitamin K3 (mg/kg)	3.3	3.0	5.0	2.0	2.2	2.0	3
Thiamine (mg/kg)	4.4	3.0	2.5	3.0	2.2	2.2	2.5
Riboflavin (mg/kg)	8.8	10.0	10.0	5.5	9.9	8.8	8
Pantothenate (mg/kg)	15.5	16.0	20.0	7.0	13.2	16.5	15
Niacin (mg/kg)	53	45	45	18	44	38	40
Pyridoxine (mg/kg)	3.3	6.0	5.0	2.0	5.5	4.4	5
Choline (mg/kg)	660	350	186	450	330	600	500
Folic acid (mg/kg)	1.0	1.5	1.25	0.90	1.65	1.0	1.5
Biotin (mg/kg)	0.22	0.25	0.20	0.20	0.22	0.20	0.20
Vitamin B12 (Fg/kg)	11	30	20	20	13	16.5	20
Manganese (mg/kg)	80	100	90	30	120	100	100
Zinc (mg/kg)	80	70	75	40	110	80	50
Iron (mg/kg)	66	80	20	30	40	30	40
Copper (mg/kg)	9	8	3.6	4	8	3.0	8
Iodine (mg/kg)	1.1	0.8	1.5	0.46	1.1	0.74	1.0
Selenium (mg/kg)	0.30	0.30	0.13	0.10	0.30	0.30	0.15

[1]Phase I, if more than one diet recommended

for certain critical nutrients and managers must decide on the relevance of these subtle changes relative to any differences in requirement known to exist for certain strains. The breeding companies obviously have the best estimate of diet specifications for their strains, and these should be followed if possible. For smaller operations that utilize a number of different strains, there is often the question of the need for strain specific diets, because this obviously imposes more work at the feed mill, and with trucking of many different diets. In these situations, it is advised to compare the nutrient specifications for the two or three strains used, and to develop a compromise specification that will meet the maximum need for any strain specific critical nutrient. This type of calculation can be applied to nutrients such as calcium, available phosphorus and the trace minerals and vitamins. For amino acids the situation is a little more complex, because in reality the quantity of amino acid per unit of protein and/or per unit of energy should be considered, rather than simple percentage levels as shown in most management guides. Table 5.5 shows calculations of important amino acid needs expressed per unit of crude protein and per unit of energy.

The quantity of amino acid per unit of crude protein is perhaps the least important of these numbers, because unless crude protein levels are very low (<14% CP) then protein *per se* is not likely to be an issue in the nutrition of the bird (as will be discussed later, high CP diets are in fact detrimental). Assuming normal levels of CP, the quantity of amino acid per unit of energy is the most important criteria. Table 5.5 suggests that in adult breeder diets the Shaver strain has the highest methionine and methionine + cystine requirement in this regard, while the Arbor Acre strain has the lowest need. In feeding those two strains a common diet therefore, it would be advisable to feed at the highest level, as dictated by the Shaver specifications.

In comparing nutrient specifications for the different breeds, it is also important to consider feed intake, because daily nutrient intake is merely a factor of feed intake x diet concentration. This situation is perhaps most critical in the early breeder phase where different primary breeding companies dictate quite different levels of feed intake for their specific strains. Data in Table 5.6 shows daily nutrient intakes for the various breeder strains at 28 weeks of age.

Taking into account feed intake together with diet specifications shows a fairly consistent pattern of recommendations for the various strains, and so this type of information provides confidence for those managers who wish to feed a single diet to more than one strain of bird. In reality, a single compromise diet for multiple strains is manageable, and specific strain anomalies can probably best be met by adjusting the daily feed intake.

TABLE 5.5 Starter and Breeder diet specifications for amino acids expressed per unit of protein or per unit of energy

	Hubbard	Shaver	Cobb	Ross	Arbor Acres	Avian	Hybro
STARTER							
Methionine							
(g/kg CP)	20.6	22.2	23.9	22.9	20.0	20.0	22.7
(g/Mcal)	1.26	1.40	1.48	1.40	1.22	1.35	1.50
Meth + Cys							
(g/kg CP)	40.6	38.8	41.1	41.1	42.2	36.5	43.2
(g/Mcal)	2.48	2.46	2.53	2.51	2.59	2.47	2.85
Lysine							
(g/kg CP)	53.7	50.0	51.6	51.4	54.2	50.5	54.1
(g/Mcal)	3.28	3.15	3.19	3.15	3.33	3.41	3.57
Tryptophan							
(g/kg CP)	10.9	10.0	11.1	12.6	10.3	10.5	9.7
(g/Mcal)	0.66	0.63	0.69	0.80	0.63	0.71	0.64
BREEDER							
Methionine							
(g/kg CP)	22.5	22.5	22.2	21.3	19.4	20.6	20.0
(g/Mcal)	1.26	1.39	1.20	1.19	1.09	1.17	1.24
Meth + Cys							
(g/kg CP)	37.4	40.6	40.0	36.3	38.8	38.8	36.5
(g/Mcal)	2.02	2.36	2.20	2.03	2.17	2.19	2.25
Lysine							
(g/kg CP)	45.8	46.9	48.8	50.0	51.3	46.3	44.1
(g/Mcal)	2.47	2.73	2.68	2.80	2.87	2.61	2.72
Tryptophan							
(g/kg CP)	10.9	10.6	10.6	11.3	10.6	11.3	9.4
(g/Mcal)	0.59	0.62	0.58	0.63	0.60	0.63	0.58

Breeder managers are often concerned about the ingredient make up of the diet, and in particular any changes that will occur as a result of ongoing least cost formulation. There is no good scientific evidence available to suggest that regular changes to ingredient composition of a diet have any detrimental effect on breeder performance. However most conscientious managers are able to detect such diet changes, often in terms of subtle changes in such factors as water intake, manure consistency, feed clean up time etc. Regardless of the scientific evidence, it is not normal practice to least cost reformulate on a regular basis (as occurs with broiler

TABLE 5.6 Daily intake of selected nutrients for breeder strains at 28 weeks of age

	Hubbard	Shaver	Cobb	Ross	Arbor Acres	Avian	Hybro
Energy (kcal)	458	468	469	478	463	458	453
Crude protein (g)	24.8	25.6	25.8	26.7	25.9	25.9	28.0
Calcium (g)	5.1	5.1	4.7	5.0	5.2	5.2	5.0
Av. Phosphorus (mg)	640	720	724	668	664	761	660
Methionine (mg)	560	576	563	567	502	534	561
Meth + Cys (mg)	928	1040	1030	967	1004	1004	1023
Lysine (mg)	1136	1200	1256	1336	1328	1199	1238
Feed intake (g)	160	170[1]	161	167[1]	162	162	165
B.Wt (kg)	3.10	2.99	3.13	3.15	3.09	3.31	3.18

[1]Estimated from management guide data

diets for example) but rather to accept either a fixed formula, or only gradual changes to ingredient use over time. Such formulation is undoubtedly more expensive than true least costing, but this situation is accepted by most breeder managers. Certainly for pure line and GP breeders, fixed formulas are considered "cheap" insurance against adverse bird reaction to diet ingredient change. Even within a fixed formula, there are usually guidelines for maximum inclusion of certain ingredients. These limitations are based on expectations of problems such as manure consistency, feed refusal, changes to diet texture, etc. that can influence breeder performance. Table 5.7 summarizes ingredient constraints for inclusion in breeder diets.

5.2 FEEDING PROGRAMS FOR GROWING PULLETS AND ROOSTERS

Feed represents about 55% of the cost of placing birds into the breeder house and so feed efficiency must be optimized over this period. However, it is essential to provide optimum nutrition because any inadequacies that occur during rearing will inevitably have to be corrected early in the breeder house. Most managers agree that it is very difficult to correct body weight or uniformity problems in the breeder house prior to maturity.

TABLE 5.7 Maximum ingredient inclusion levels for formulation of breeder diets

Ingredient	Maximum inclusion (% diet)
Yellow corn	70
Wheat (+enzyme)	25(50)
Oats	25
Barley (+enzyme)	15(30)
Rice (rough)	20
Wheat bran	20
Wheat shorts	20
Wheat screenings	20
Rice bran	20
Rice polishings	20
Milo	50
Triticale	10
Bakery by-product	10
Molasses	3
Dehydrated alfalfa	10
Canola meal	7
Full-fat canola	10
Soybean meal (48%)	30
Full fat soybean	15
Corn gluten meal (60%)	10
Corn gluten feed (20%)	10
Cotton seed meal	10
Peanut meal (groundnut)	10
Peas	10
Safflower meal	10
Sesame meal	10
Sunflower meal	10
Lupins	10
Flax	10
Meat meal	6
Fish meal (60%)	8
Blood meal	2
Feather meal	2
Dried whey	8
Animal fats	5
Vegetable oils	5

Diet specifications as shown in Tables 5.1 and 5.2 will be allocated essentially on the basis of body weight and uniformity of weight. Monitoring body weight and its uniformity within the flock should be used to dictate needs for regular changes in feed allocation. It is generally recognized that each commercial strain of bird has an optimum weight at the time of approaching sexual maturity - for most strains, this is around 2.2 kg at 22 weeks of age. With the potential to influence nutrient intake with both diet formulation and level of feed restriction, it is obvious that target weights can be achieved by various means, and these will influence rearing (feed) costs. Over the years, both qualitative and quantitative nutrient restriction programs have been proposed to realize these goals.

Qualitative feed restriction - By modifying the "quality" of the diet, growth rate can theoretically be controlled. For example, diets that are deficient in protein or an essential nutrient should limit growth, and hopefully formulation can be adjusted to manipulate growth up to mature body size. In most instances, these programs have failed since all birds in a flock do not have identical nutrient requirements. For example, reducing the methionine content of the diet by 25% may well lead to a 15-20% reduction in mean flock weight. Unfortunately, those birds with a high inherent methionine requirement will be very light weight, while those birds with an inherently low methionine requirement will be little affected by the diet and grow at a normal rate. Therefore, while mean flock weight can often be manipulated with qualitative feed restriction, uniformity of flock weight is usually very poor, often being at only 30-40% compared to 80% under ideal conditions (% of birds ± 15% of flock mean weight). For example, our studies with salt deficient diets indicated that mean flock weight could be quite accurately controlled by regulating the level of salt added to a corn-soybean meal based diet. Unfortunately, flock uniformity at 20 weeks was very low, and consequently many birds were over or underweight in the breeder house, and egg production and fertility were both impaired. Similar attempts at qualitative feed restriction have been made with manipulation of fatty acid and amino acid levels in the diet. Adding 30 kg propionic acid/tonne feed also controls feed intake, yet this is very expensive and the acidic diet is very corrosive. In some countries, very low energy high fiber diets are used for growing breeder pullets. It is difficult to fully control growth rate with low energy diets alone because the breeder pullet is able to increase its feed intake quite dramatically in an attempt at normalizing its energy intake. However low energy diets can be used to help reduce the stress of quantitative feed restriction programs. As a generalization, each 10% dilution of the diet, results in about a 30% longer feed clean up time in pullets up to 12-15 weeks of age. However low energy high fiber diets are expensive to transport and store because of low bulk density, and cause wetter litter and greater manure production. Total production costs per unit of energy consumed must be calculated with such programs.

Physical feed restriction - Some form of physical feed restriction is now universal with broiler breeders of all ages. With mechanical weigh scales attached to automatic feeders, it is relatively easy to realize accurate feed allocation under commercial conditions. A typical feed restriction program is shown in Table 5.8.

TABLE 5.8 Skip-a-day and daily feed restriction programs for juvenile breeders (diet at 2900 kcal/kg)

Age (weeks)	Pullets (g)		Cockerels (g)	
	Skip-a-day	Daily	Skip-a-day	Daily
1	Ad-lib		Ad-lib	
2	Controlled 25/day		Controlled 27/day	
3	Controlled 30/day		Controlled 32/day	
4	65	32	80	36
5	75	35	90	40
6	85	39	100	45
7	95	44	110	50
8	100	46	115	53
9	105	48	120	55
10	110	51	125	58
11	115	53	130	60
12	120	55	135	63
13	125	57	140	65
14	130	60	145	66
15	137	62	150	68
16	145	65	160	71
17	155	70	170	75
18	168	75	180	80
19	175	80	190	85
20	185	85	200	90

Actual feed intake will obviously depend upon nutrient density and environmental conditions, yet these values can be used as guidelines. The concept of feeding to body weight, and the regulation of body weight will be discussed more fully in a subsequent section. Table 5.8 indicates a restricted feeding program for both pullets and cockerels to be started at 4 weeks of age. Prior to this, "controlled" feeding should be practiced so as to acclimatize birds to a limited feed intake. Controlled feeding should be adjusted to ensure that birds are cleaning up their feed on a daily basis within 4-6 hours.

Because different strains of birds have different growth characteristics, then initiation of controlled and restricted feeding must be flexible in order to control body weight. For strains with inherently fast initial growth rate, true restricted feeding on a daily basis may be necessary as early as 7-10 d of age. For other strains, ad-lib feeding to 3-4 weeks is possible since they have a slow initial growth rate.

For growing birds, feed is eaten in a very short period of time, being from 30 minutes - 2 hrs. depending upon age and frequency of feeding. Feeding and drinking are the major activities of the immature bird. Most producers will feed growing pullets and roosters early in the morning, especially in warm or hot climates. Digested feed is not utilized with 100% efficiency, and a consequence of such inefficiency is heat production in the bird's body. In most situations, this extra heat (sometimes called heat of metabolism, specific dynamic action, or heat increment), peaks about 4-6 hours after feed is eaten. Because of the restricted feeding program, feeding time is short and predictable, and so the heat of metabolism will consistently peak 4-6 hrs. after feeding time. In hot climates, peak environmental heat load occurs in the early afternoon, and so there is a distinct disadvantage to having extra heat generated in the bird's body at this time. For this reason, we have the common practice of feeding birds at 6-7 a.m.

With such early morning feeding, the heat load of nutrient metabolism occurs before the early afternoon daily high temperature. Alternatively, growing birds could be fed in late afternoon or early evening. However this latter situation does not work well with short daylengths for growing birds.

When using mechanical feeders there is a tendency to feed birds even earlier, sometimes at daylight or when artificial lights are switched on. There are two disadvantages to very early morning feeding. Firstly, feeding often occurs before staff are present to observe feeding activity and bird distribution. Under these conditions, it is impossible to know if feed is being evenly distributed and if all birds have access to the feed. The second problem, which becomes more acute as birds get older, is the condition of choking, which occurs with a small percentage of older birds, especially on skip-a-day feeding. This problem can often be resolved by switching on drinkers for at least one hour before feed is available. This is obviously impossible to accomplish if birds are mechanically fed at first daylight or when artificial lights are switched on - pullets seldom drink in the dark period. The ideal feeding time for growing pullets and roosters therefore is early morning, when staff can observe feeding behavior, and after birds have had access to water for up to 1 hour.

With the skip-a-day program shown in Table 5.8, birds are given these quantities of feed only every other day. The concept behind this program, is that with every other day feeding, birds are offered a considerable quantity of feed and this is easier to distribute around the pen so that even the smallest, most timid bird, can get a chance to eat. The usual alternative to skip-a-day feeding, is feeding restricted quantities every day. For example at 12 weeks of age, pullets could be fed 60 g each day. The problem with every day feeding, is that feed is eaten very quickly, and so all birds within a flock may not get adequate feed. With such small quantities of feed, and using slow speed feed chains or auger delivery, it is not unheard of for birds to "keep up" with feed delivery close to the feed hoppers, and reduce effective feeder space. With every day feeding, birds may well consume their daily allocation within 45 minutes, and so adequate feeder space is essential with this type of program. However, there are some real advantages to every day feeding. The previous statement that every day feeding at 12 weeks means that birds should get 60 g/day, since skip-a-day birds get 120 g every-other-day (Table 5.8) is in fact incorrect. In practice, birds will become overweight if regular skip-a-day allowances are halved in order to calculate every-day allowances. Unfortunately this error is made by most breeding companies, since they invariably make this statement in their management guides. The reason for this error, is that birds will utilize their feed 10-15% more efficiently when fed every day, rather than skip-a-day. When fed skip-a-day, the bird must store nutrients (body fat and some body protein) which must be utilized by the bird for growth and maintenance the following day when it has no access to feed. Unfortunately this deposition and re-utilization of nutrients is not 100% efficient. Results from two experiments where birds are fed identical quantities of feed are shown in Table 5.9, indicating every day feeding to be about 6% more efficient than skip-a-day feeding.

As shown in Fig 5.1, there are major differences in heat production (energy expenditure) of birds fed every day vs skip-a-day, with the latter showing major differences on feed vs off feed days. The mean difference in heat production for these birds was around 10% in favour of every-day feeding. These data suggest that if every day feeding can be made to work under commercial conditions, then there should be a saving of up to 10% in feed required to produce a pullet of 2.3 kg body weight. Such adjustments to skip-a-day standards are shown for the every day schedule in Table 5.8.

Time of introduction of restricted feeding needs to be flexible, according to the growth potential of the strain of birds used. However, as shown by Wilson *et al.* (1989), trying to control mature 24 wk body weight by later, more severe feed restriction, results in a very large increase in feed:gain, delayed maturity, and loss of chicks per breeder (Table 5.10).

TABLE 5.9 Effect of providing equal quantities of feed by skip-a-day or every-day feeding on growth of pullets and roosters					
Pullet weight[1] (g)			19 wk Rooster weight[2] (g)		
Age (wks)	Skip-a-day	Every day	Diet Treatment	Skip-a-day	Every day
8	530[b]	790[a]	2850 ME, 15% CP	2410	2530
11	950[b]	1010[a]	2850 ME, 20% CP	2320	2510
14	1190[b]	1290[a]	2000 ME, 15% CP	1960	2150
17	1540[b]	1630[a]	2000 ME, 20% CP	1920	2040
20	1890[b]	1980[a]			
					[1]Adapted from Bennett and Leeson (1989)
					[2]Adapted from Vaughters *et al.* (1987)

Figure 5.1 Heat production of breeder pullets.

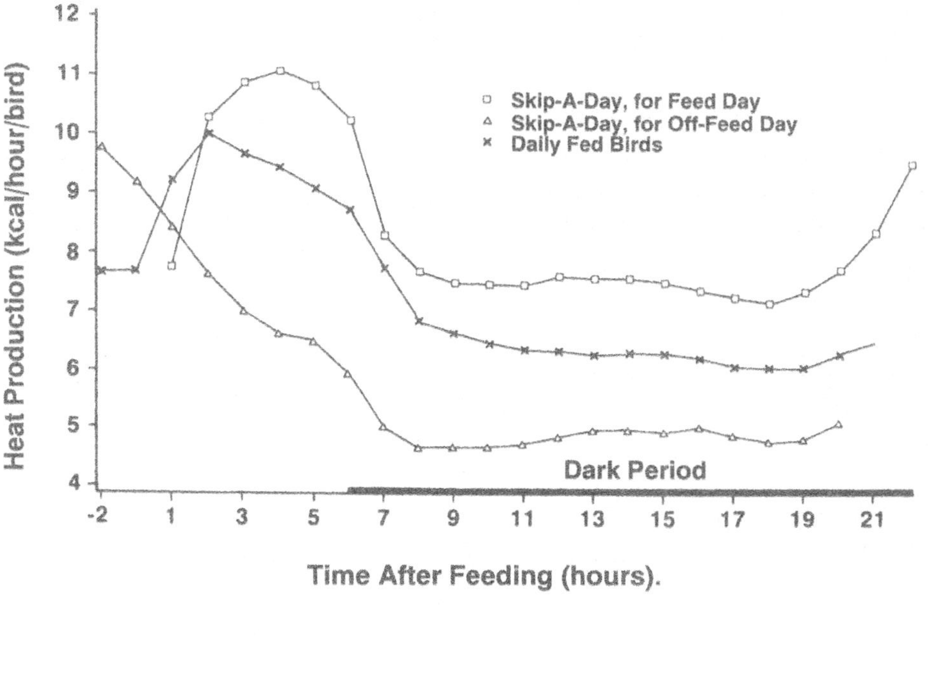

TABLE 5.10 Effect of time of starting skip-a-day feeding on breeder performance

Age at starting skip-a-day restriction	Body wt (kg)		Feed:gain	Age at maturity	Chicks per hen
(wks)	8 wk	24 wk	8-24 wk	(days)	24-64 wk
2	0.8	2.4	6.0	204	129
4	0.9	2.5	6.1	204	128
6	1.1	2.5	7.0	211	125
8	1.6	2.5	10.1	215	116

Adapted from Wilson *et al.* (1989)

In general, "concave" growth curves are more desirable then "convex" growth curves, if only on the basis of reduced feed for maintenance energy requirements. Each day of delayed maturity increases growing costs by about 1%. A question often asked is why the need to delay maturity until 23-24 weeks, when "mature" weight is easily achieved much earlier simply by increasing feed allocation. For example we have grown birds on conventional restricted quantities of feed, or +5, +10 or +20% extra feed (Table 5.11). Pullets mature much earlier with the greater feed allocation, yet there is little persistency of peak production, and so hatching egg numbers are greatly reduced. It seems as though the pullets have to obtain a given weight and age, prior to maturity, and problems are often seen if one of these parameters is not achieved. As birds will necessarily be restricted in their nutrient intake at some time during rearing, one may question industry practice of utilizing starter diets with high protein/amino acid levels. For example, starter diets with 18-20% CP with appropriate levels of methionine and lysine will lead to rapid early growth in most strains of birds. After this initial starter period, one is then faced with the difficult task of tempering growth so as to meet weight guidelines by 6-8 weeks of age. There seems no logical reason to enforce rapid early growth when this must necessarily be followed by severe feed restriction, which imposes considerable management problems.

A more logical approach is to initiate a much slower initial growth, such that subsequent restriction is less severe, and so less stressful.

TABLE 5.11 Effect of feed allocation on early breeder performance					
		Feeding schedule (4-25 weeks)			
		Control	**+5% extra feed**	**+10% extra feed**	**+20% extra feed**
Body wt 8 wks (g)		1005	1050	1100	1170
Body wt 20 wks (g)		2340	2400	2440	2620
Age at maturity (d)		161	150	147	140
Age peak egg prod (d)		205	196	189	179
Persistency of peak (d)		35	14	10	7
Egg wt:	21 wk (g)	-	-	-	46.9
	22 wk (g)	-	42.0	42.0	51.4
	24 wk (g)	46.9	51.9	50.0	52.6
	30 wk (g)	60.0	59.2	59.7	57.6
Adapted from Leeson and Summers (1983)					

Our studies have indicated that offering breeder pullets diets of very low protein (13-15%) in the starter period will aid in controlling early growth (Table 5.12). Protein levels as low as 13-14% are not usually recommended for commercial use, because amino acid balance becomes more critical, feathering is often adversely affected, and periodically these diets are more expensive to formulate than are diets with less severe protein restriction. However few problems are seen with starter diets of 15-16% CP under ideal conditions and in fact these can very successfully be used in single stage starter-grower programs for breeder pullets to 18-20 weeks of age. The reason for the success of this simple program is the flexibility afforded by feed allocation. However, if low protein starter diets are used, then fatter pullets can be expected at 3-5 weeks of age. Similarly, reduced growth rate caused by lower protein diets is associated with reduced shank length (Table 5.13).

TABLE 5.12 Effect of starter diet protein level on body weight of broiler breeder pullets with a common 16% CP grower diet from 21 days (g)

Crude protein in diet 0-21d (%)	Days of age						
	7	**14**	**21**	**49**	**77**	**105**	**161**
20	110	259	477	881	1285	1714	2688
19	110	256	461				
18	109	252	476	875	1280	1703	2648
17	108	250	455				
16	101	236	442				
15	98	196	387	843	1243	1692	2657
14	92	199	382				
13	86	173	337	810	1216	1661	2643

TABLE 5.13 Shank length of breeder pullets (cm)

Crude protein in diet 0-21d	Days of age				
%	**7**	**21**	**49**	**105**	**161**
20	3.7	6.6	8.7	11.2	11.3
19	3.7	6.6			
18	3.7	6.6	8.8	11.3	11.5
17	3.7	6.6			
16	3.6	6.5			
15	3.6	6.1	8.5	11.4	11.4
14	3.5	6.1			
13	3.5	5.8	8.4	11.2	11.4

However, both shank length and carcass composition appear to be normalized by 18-20 weeks of age. As shown many times with Leghorn birds, it is around 12-14 weeks of age that such mature characteristics seem to be established. Thus if shank length was adversely affected at around 12 weeks, then this would likely be carried through for the remainder of the breeder cycle. A question often raised concerning lower protein starter diets is the immune competence of the bird.

Breeder pullets are subjected to an extensive vaccination program, and so immune competence is of vital commercial importance. While critical organ weights are reduced at 21d of age when chicks are fed lower protein starter diets, these organ weights subsequently normalize during the growing period, and it seems that immune competence is not affected if diet protein is maintained above 10%. While low protein diets can therefore be used to temper early growth rate, and so delay the onset and severity of quantitative restriction, continued use of low protein diets fed ad-lib during rearing has met with only limited success.

For example, pullets fed 10% CP diets ad-lib will likely be 0.6-0.7 kg heavier at 20 weeks than birds fed a 14% CP diet on a restricted basis. Low protein starter diets are therefore only designed to temper very early growth rate, and some form of restricted feeding will become essential at 2-6 weeks depending upon the strain of bird. Lower crude protein starter diets regardless of amino acid levels, are not recommended for cockerels.

Restricted feeding provides absolute control over the bird's nutrient intake. Unfortunately, many producers use the primary breeder's feed intake guidelines without considering the energy level of their feeds - this can obviously lead to differences in energy intake, and therefore differences in fat deposition of the pullet. In recent studies, pullets were fed quantities of feed according to the breeder's recommendations, although energy level for the feed varied considerably (Table 5.14). In this study, all pullets matured at about the same time, but had vastly different body weight and composition. Overly fat birds will likely have more reproductive problems, while too lean a bird may not carry sufficient energy reserves to take it through peak egg production. In agreement with other researchers, the data shown in Table 5.14, indicates a relatively constant fat free mass at time of first egg, and this seems more highly correlated with maturity than either body weight or fat content at this age.

Whatever system of feed restriction is used, and regardless of diet specifications, birds must be fed according to body weight and condition. As previously discussed, it is not essential to promote rapid early growth in the young pullet, because this usually means that subsequent feed restriction is imposed early and/ or more severely. Early slow growth rate is therefore recommended and in fact, there are economic advantages to early slower growth rate. Feeding lower nutrient dense starter diets followed by regular or increased severity of restriction means that smaller birds have reduced maintenance costs. However, feed allocation must be adjusted according to body weight, such that the pullet is at the breeder's target weight by 15-16 weeks of age. This is to ensure that the bird will be of correct weight at maturity. Therefore, if pullets are fed low protein starter diets "catch up" growth must occur at least 5-6 weeks prior to sexual maturity. This is essential as it seems as though pullets cannot exhibit catch up growth at the same time that they are expected to start producing eggs, and start to show increased egg size necessary for production of settable eggs. Underweight birds at sexual maturity most often show a characteristic loss in production immediately after peak egg production.

TABLE 5.14 Effect of diet energy level on breeder pullet development and carcass characteristics at first egg

	Low energy diet	Standard energy diet	High energy diet
Age at first egg (days)	185	180	181
Body weight at week 20 (g)	1907a	2059b	2208c
Body weight at first egg (g)	2679a	2872b	3130c
Carcass fat (g)	395a	501b	624c
Carcass protein (g)	543a	565a	607b
Carcass fat free mass (g)	2284a	2371a	2506b

After 14-15 weeks of age, feed allowance becomes quite large, and problems with "choking" (excess feed intake by some birds) starts to occur. If there is adequate feeder space, then birds can be started on alternate restriction programs that entail different sequencing of feed. The idea behind these alternate feeding schedules is to give birds less feed each day, but more feed in total, relative to every day feeding. Changing to one of these programs also helps in transition from skip-a-day to every day feeding. A rule of thumb for change from skip-a-day, is when the feed allowance reaches that expected at peak production. For example, in Table 5.8, if birds are to be peaked on 145 g feed daily, then this is reached with skip-a-day feeding at 16 weeks in this schedule, and so this is the time to change the feed program. Following is an example of various feeding programs where the standard is skip-a-day fed birds consuming 100 g at each feeding or 50 g/day equivalent (Table 5.15).

Whatever system is used, there needs to be flexibility related to status of the flock as affected by various management decisions. For example, some live vaccines, and the physical transportation of birds, cause a 1-2 day delay in growth rate. These periods of known stress should be counteracted by extra feeding. For example, if skip-a-day fed birds are scheduled to be moved on day 6 (Table 5.15 non feed day), then birds should be given feed this day regardless of the preplanned schedule.

TABLE 5.15 Comparison of feed restriction systems for breeder pullets

	Grams per bird per feeding each day									
System	**1**	**2**	**3**	**4**	**5**	**6**	**7**	**8**	**9**	**10**
Every day	50	50	50	50	50	50	50	50	50	50
Skip-a-day	100	-	100	-	100	-	100	-	100	-
3-1-2-1	70	70	70	-	70	70	-	70	70	70
6-1	58	58	58	58	58	58	-	58	58	58

Up to 20 weeks of age, the pullets and cockerels should consume around 7.6 and 9.0 kg feed respectively, assuming diet specifications similar to those shown in Tables 5.1 and 5.2. On this basis, it is possible to calculate corresponding guidelines for intake of energy and amino acids (Table 5.16).

TABLE 5.16 Total feed and nutrient intake to 20 weeks of age

	Pullet	**Cockerel**
Feed (kg)	7.6	9.0
Energy (Mcal)	22	25
Protein (g)	1150	1400
Methionine (g)	28	33
Methionine+Cystine (g)	47	56
Lysine (g)	57	67

Model predicted nutrient requirements: While starter and grower diet specifications are shown in Tables 5.1 and 5.2 respectively, the exact nutrient requirements of the growing pullet have not been clearly established. In large part, this situation is due to a lack of experimentation aimed at clearly establishing nutrient needs. Such experiments, unconfounded with other diet or environmental treatments are time consuming and very expensive to perform. An alternative approach, that is gaining in popularity, is the development of so-called "models" that mathematically describe nutrient needs in terms of growth and maintenance. For breeder pullets, Waldroup *et al.* (1976) used a number of equations for estimation of energy and protein/amino acid needs of pullets (Tables, 5.17 and 5.18 respectively). In recent years, there have been other prediction equations developed, and these agree quite well with these earlier predictions made by Waldroup *et al.* (1976). The major advantage of such simple models is that more exact needs can quickly be established, dependent upon the changing circumstances of a particular flock. For example, energy intake will be influenced by any change in environmental temperature (Table 5.17) and likewise amino acid needs will vary dependent upon weight for age and growth rate at any one time.

TABLE 5.17 Model predicted energy needs of breeder pullets as affected by environmental temperature (kcal/bird/day)[1]

		Temperature			
Weeks of age	**B. wt (g)**	**18°C**	**24°C**	**29°C**	**35°C**
2	77	-	-	95	92
4	417	-	134	125	115
6	720	170	156	143	131
8	1003	188	172	156	140
10	1249	204	185	167	148
12	1476	216	195	175	155
14	1684	227	205	182	160
16	1870	236	212	188	165
18	2084	243	218	193	168
20	2190	250	224	198	171

Adapted from Waldroup *et al.* (1976)

[1]Based on model of Combs (1968)

$ME = (1.78-0.12T)\ (1.45W^{.0653}) + 3.13\Delta W + 3.15E$

Where T = °C; W = weight in grams; ΔW = change in weight in grams and E =daily egg mass in grams

Coccidiosis is an ever present problem for those involved with rearing breeder pullets on litter. Because anticoccidials are not usually allowed in adult breeder diets, the bird must develop a degree of immunity during rearing. Such immunity does not develop with anticoccidials commonly used for commercial broilers, and especially the ionophores. This means that if ionophores are used during rearing of breeder pullets, they will most likely prevent clinical coccidioisis, but these birds may develop symptoms as soon as they are transferred to the breeder house.

If an anticoccidial is used during rearing, then products such as amprolium are more advantageous.

TABLE 5.18 Model predicted amino acid needs of breeder pullets

		Amino acid (mg/pullet/day)				
Weeks of age	CP1 (g)	Lysine	Tryptophan	Methionine	Meth +Cyst	Threonine
2	5.0	386	43	98	192	211
4	5.3	356	45	117	208	219
6	5.6	341	50	136	228	231
8	5.6	315	52	151	241	237
10	5.7	298	55	166	255	245
12	5.8	280	58	179	266	251
14	5.9	266	60	191	279	258
16	6.0	253	62	202	289	263
18	6.0	238	64	211	297	267
20	6.1	227	65	219	305	273

Adapted from Waldroup *et al.* (1976)

[1]Based on Protein model of Hurwitz and Bornstein (1973)

$CP (g/d) = 1.858W + (0.21x\Delta W) + (0.174xE)$

W = body weight in kg; ΔW = daily change in weight in grams;
E - daily egg mass (g)

Amino acids from model of Hurwitz and Bornstein (1973) and Leville *et al.* (1960.)

Compounds such as amprolium usually prevent acute clinical symptoms, while at the same time allowing some build up of immunity. In certain countries, depending upon feed regulations, amprolium can be used throughout the life cycle for the bird. An alternate approach, and one that requires superior management, is to use non-medicated feed during rearing, and to treat birds as soon as clinical symptoms occur. Since treatment must be immediate, only water dispensable products are recommended. The most recent development in coccidial control is use of attenuated vaccines (see Chapter 4). These vaccines can be given in the drinking water, or sprayed on the feed when chicks are 2-3 days of age. The latest idea is a vaccine within a gel puck placed in the chick box at the hatchery or spraying chicks at the hatchery such that chicks arrive at the farm already vaccinated.

Controlling water intake - As part of the general management program for feed-restricted pullets and cockerels, it is common to implement some form of water restriction. With feed restriction, birds can consume their feed in 30 mins to 2 hrs depending upon the system and age of bird, and so it is thought that given the opportunity, these birds will consume excessive quantities of water simply out of boredom or to satisfy physical hunger. There are considerable strain differences in water intake. Certainly birds given free access to water seem to have wetter litter, and there is no doubt that a water restriction program is necessary in order to maintain good litter quality and to help prevent build-up of intestinal parasites and maintain foot pad condition. Various water restriction programs are used and there are no universal guidelines that should be adhered to. Pullets develop normally when given as little as ½ hr access to water each day, although longer periods than this are usually recommended. It seems advisable to give birds ½ hr to 1 hr access to water prior to feed delivery, especially with skip-a-day feeding. The reason for this is prevention of a sudden death type syndrome that occurs with a small proportion of birds that invariably have grossly distended crops full of dry feed. The exact cause of death is unknown although it is possible that the sudden intake of a large volume of dry feed acts as a "sponge" to normal body fluids and so upsets the bird's normal water/electrolyte balance. Giving birds access to water prior to feed delivery often seems to resolve this problem. Table 5.19 gives a general recommendation for water access.

These values should be considered as guidelines only, and during periods of heat stress or during disease conditions and around the time of moving etc., longer water access times should be given. With skip-a-day feeding, it is usual to more severely limit water access on off-feed days, based on the assumption that birds tend to drink more water on this day (due to boredom or need to meet physical satiety) since they are without feed. However, studies suggest that breeder pullets drink most of their water on feed days, and seem generally uninterested in water on off-feed days (Table 5.20).

TABLE 5.19 Suggested water access time for growing breeder pullets and cockerels

	Feed-Day		**Off-feed Day**	
	am	**pm**	**am**	**pm**
Skip-a-day feeding	2-3 hr, starting 1 hr prior to feeding	1 hr	1 hr	1 hr
Every-day feeding	2 hr, starting 1 hr prior to feeding	1 hr	-	-

TABLE 5.20 Water consumption of 13 week old skip-a-day or daily fed birds with free or restricted access to water (litres/1000 birds/day)					
		Skip-a-day fed birds			
		Water restricted each day	**Water restricted on feed days**	**Free access to water**	**Daily fed birds, free access to water**
Feed day		192	196	273	205
Off-feed day		122	122	37	217
Average		157	161	155	211
	Water:feed	2.38	2.44	2.35	3.20
Bennett and Leeson, (1989)					

When birds are fed daily and given unlimited access to water, there is a fairly consistent pattern of water intake. With skip-a-day feeding and free access to water, pullets surprisingly consume very little water on an off-feed day. For these birds, the largest water intake occurs on the feed day. However, it is the exceptionally high water intake on the feed day (273 g, Table 5.20) that quickly leads to wet litter, and so the need for water restriction programs. These data suggest that the major emphasis on water restriction of skip-a-day fed birds should occur on the feed day rather than the off-feed day.

These results are perhaps not too surprising in view of the well established relationship between the intakes of water and feed. Water consumption guidelines for pullets are shown in Table 5.21. Actual intake on feed days, but not off feed days, will be influenced by diet salt level.

Feeding the immature rooster: Males can be grown with the hens or grown separately, but in both situations they will almost exclusively be fed starter and grower diets designed for the female birds. This poses no major problem, because there are no large differences in nutrient requirements of the sexes up to the time of maturity, and we can manage with a "compromise" situation. Where males and females are grown together, the onset of restriction programs and general feed allocation systems are usually dictated by progress in hen weight and condition. Male growth and condition cannot be controlled as well under these situations, and this has to be an accepted consequence of this management decision.

TABLE 5.21 Daily water consumption of pullets on skip-a-day feeding (litres/1000 pullets)		
Age wks	**20°C**	**35°C**
4	70	145
6	105	175
8	115	192
10	130	220
12	145	240
14	160	270
16	175	290
18	190	320
20	205	345

Growing males separately provides the best opportunity to dictate and control their development. As with commercial broilers, the male breeders will respond more to high protein starter diets or to more prolonged feeding of these diets. The opposite situation also applies, in that male breeder chicks will be more adversely affected by low protein or low amino acid starter diets. For example, under ideal conditions, a well-balanced 15% CP diet can be used as a starter for female chicks and this results in slower early growth rate with the added advantage of delay in introducing restricted feeding. Male chicks can also be grown on such diets, although it is not usually recommended, because there will be poorer early feathering and perhaps more uneven growth rate. These problems resolve themselves over time, but as a general rule it is better to start male breeder chicks on a 17-18% CP diet. The male breeder chick is also more sensitive to the effects of low protein diets that contain anticoccidials, such as monensin. Again, poor feathering will result if starter diets contain much less than 18% CP. Poor early feathering has no long lasting effect on subsequent breeder performance, although the chicks obviously look different and they may suffer more from early cold stress.

Male chicks will usually be started on a controlled feeding program at around 3 weeks of age. The starting time for a skip-a-day program is based upon body weight. As with the female chicks, it is important not to have birds overweight early, because this is costly on feed, and subsequent attempts at bringing birds back "on to standard" are usually associated with loss of uniformity. Starting at 3 weeks of age, groups of 10 chicks can be weighed together to give an idea of body weight and controlled feeding started. Starting at 4 weeks of age, sample birds should be weighed individually, just as occurs with the hens, and mean weight and uniformity plotted to give a visual image of flock progress. Ideally, feed allocation will be increased on a weekly basis, although this should be dictated by the weekly body weight measurements. Changes in environmental temperature or unprogrammed changes in diet energy (due to ingredient variability, etc.) will affect nutrient needs, feed intake and/or growth rate. Usually the body weight and uniformity of the birds represents their true feed needs at that time and so there needs to be flexibility in feed allocation to account for these variables.

Skip-a-day feeding is usually the preferred system up to time of transfer to the breeder house. However in some situations, choking can occur with males (and females) after 14-16 weeks of age, and this is caused by rapid and excessive feed intake on feeding days. Such choking causes 0.5% mortality per day in extreme situations, but can sometimes be resolved by ensuring that water is available for at least 1 hour prior to feeding. Where this technique fails to correct the problem, it may be necessary to change to a 5:2 or even a 6:1 feeding program (see Table 5.15). These programs provide the same amount of feed on a weekly basis, but this is given as smaller quantities, more often. There seems to be less gorging when birds eat smaller quantities of feed more often. A potential problem with changing to 5:2 or 6:1 feeding programs is loss of uniformity, because daily feeding time will be very short. If males are grown separately from females, then this uniformity problem can sometimes be resolved by changing to a lower nutrient density diet, and giving proportionally more feed so as to maintain normal nutrient intake (however under these conditions, daily feed intake will still be less than with skip-a-day feeding). Whatever feeding system is used, it is essential to provide adequate feeder space such that all birds can eat at one time.

5.3 PREBREEDER NUTRITION

While most companies provide nutrient specifications for pre-breeder diets, there is considerable variation in their commercial application. Using a prebreeder or prelay diet is based on the assumption that the bird's nutrient requirements change in this critical period of the bird's life at around 19-23 weeks of age. There are certainly major changes occurring in the bird's metabolism, hopefully related to ovary and oviduct development, and so this is the basis for a specialized diet at this time. With egg laying stock, prelay diets most often involve a change in calcium level, in order to establish the bird's calcium reserves necessary for rapid and sudden onset of eggshell production. The same situation can be applied to heavy breeders today, because with flocks of uniform body weight and with good light management, the subsequent synchronization of maturity leads to rapid increase in egg numbers up to peak production. However, most often prebreeder diets are used in an attempt to "condition" or correct growth and/or body composition problems that have arisen during the 14-18 week growing period. In these situations managers are perhaps ill-informed of the expectations that result from merely changing diet specifications at this time.

Although there is no specific prebreeder "period", most breeder managers consider the 19-23 week period to be the major transition time for sexual development of the bird. During this time (4 weeks) the pullet is expected to increase in weight by about 570 g. This is somewhat more than the growth expectation of around 350 g for the previous 4 weeks (15-19 week) or growth of around 450 g for the 4 weeks from 23-27 weeks of age. It is expected that a significant proportion of this growth spurt will be as ovary and oviduct, which are developing in response to light stimulation. However there is little evidence to suggest that high nutrient dense diets and/or feed allocation has any meaningful effect on ovary or oviduct development. Studies suggest that the protein requirement of the bird at this critical time is only around 10 g/bird/day, which is much less than is provided by most prebreeder diets. There is some evidence to suggest that excess protein fed during the late growing/prebreeder period causes an increase in plasma uric acid levels, and especially 2-3 hr after feeding. Plasma uric acid levels in such birds are compatible with birds showing articular gout, and so there is concern about excess protein contributing to the potential for leg problems in these young breeders.

A practical complication of this sexual development, is that it invariably coincides with moving the pullets from grower to breeder facilities. Under adverse conditions, such as transportation over long distances, heat stress, etc., birds can lose up to 100 g of body weight at this critical time. If weight loss is characteristic of such transportation, then pullets should be given an extra feeding. For example, pullets should be moved on an "off-feed" day, but they should nevertheless be fed that day in the breeder house after all birds are housed. Weight loss cannot be allowed at this critical time, and so the question to be answered is - do prebreeder diets help in this physical move, as well as prime the bird for sexual maturity? Development of the ovary and oviduct require both protein/amino acids and energy (fat accretion). Nutrients of interest, therefore, are protein and energy, together with an increase in calcium for early deposition of medullary bone. It has never been clearly established that such nutrients need to come from a specially fortified diet versus simply increasing the feed allowance of the grower diet or breeder diet that is introduced prior to maturity. Following are factors to consider in feeding the bird in the pre-breeder transition period.

a) Calcium metabolism

Prebreeder diets can be used to pre-condition the pullet for impending eggshell production. The very first egg represents a 1.5-2.0 g loss in calcium from the body, the source of which is both feed and medullary bone reserve. Breeder hens today are capable of a sustained long clutch length which is necessary to achieve potential peak production at 85-87%. Calcium metabolism is, therefore, very important for the breeder. With Leghorn hens the consequence of inadequate early calcium balance is cage layer fatigue. Breeders do not show such signs, because they naturally have more exercise, and also have a readily available alternate source of diet calcium in the form of their flockmates' eggs. Hens have an innate ability to select out calcium, and so improperly fed breeders will eat litter and eggshells in an attempt to balance their diet. However inadequate calcium in the diet does lead to disruption of ovulation, and so these birds stop laying until their meager calcium reserves are replenished. In a breeder flock, it is the larger bodied, early maturing pullets that are disadvantaged in this manner.

Commercially, three different approaches are used in prebreeder calcium nutrition. Firstly, is the use of grower diets that contain just 0.9-1.0% calcium being fed up to 5% egg production. This is the system that was used many years ago, and unfortunately is still sometimes used today. At 5% egg production, 100% of the flock is not producing at 5% egg production - rather closer to 5% of the early maturing heavier pullets are producing at almost 100% production. Pullets can produce just 2-3 eggs with a diet containing 1% calcium. After this time they will eat litter and/or eggs as previously described, or more commonly, they simply shut down the ovary. With this approach, the flock may in fact be at 10-15% production before the breeder diet is introduced, since no farm system allows for instantaneous change in feed supply because feed tanks are hopefully never completely empty. There is no justification, therefore, for this old system of feed management, as it will be very detrimental to life-time productivity of today's genetic strains.

The second system involves the classical prebreeder diet containing around 1.5% calcium, which is really a compromise situation. It allows for greater medullary bone reserves to develop, without having to resort to the 3.0% calcium as used in a breeder diet. However 1.5% calcium is still inadequate for sustained eggshell production - with this diet the breeder can produce 4-6 eggs before the ovulation pattern is affected. If a prebreeder diet is used, therefore, and a moderate calcium level is part of this program, then the diet must be replaced by the breeder diet before egg production starts. A good rule of thumb is to change from prebreeder to breeder when the very first egg is noticed, because this occurs usually around 10 days before 1% egg production.

The third option is perhaps the most simple solution, and involves changing from grower to breeder at first egg (10 days before 1% production). Having the breeder diet in place before maturity, ensures that even the earliest maturing birds have adequate calcium for sustained early egg production. Proponents of prebreeder diets suggest that breeder diets introduced early provide too much calcium, and that this contributes to kidney disorders, because the extra ingested calcium must be excreted in the urine. There is an indication that feeding adult breeder diets for 10-12 weeks prior to maturity can adversely affect kidney function, especially if birds are also challenged with infectious bronchitis. However feeding "extra" calcium for two to three weeks prior to maturity has no such effect. It is also interesting to realize that most roosters today are fed high calcium breeder diets, which provide 4-6x their calcium needs, yet kidney dysfunction is quite rare in these birds.

b) Body weight and size

Body weight and body condition of the bird around the time of maturity, are perhaps the most important criteria that will ultimately influence breeder performance. Body weight and body condition should not be considered in isolation, although at this time we do not have a good method of readily assessing body condition. Each strain of bird has a characteristic mature body weight that must be reached or surpassed for adequate egg production and egg mass output. In general, prebreeder diets should not be used in an attempt to manipulate mature body size. The reason for this is that with most flocks it is too late at this stage of rearing to meaningfully influence body weight - all too often prebreeder diets are used as a crutch for poor rearing management.

However, if birds are underweight when placed in the breeder house, then there is perhaps a need to manipulate body weight prior to maturity. Under controlled environment conditions, this can sometimes be achieved by delaying photostimulation. If prebreeder diets are used in an attempt to correct rearing mismanagement it seems as though the bird is most responsive to energy. This fact likely fits in with the effect of estrogen on fat metabolism, and the significance of fat for liver and ovary development at this time. While higher nutrient density prebreeder diets may be useful in manipulating body weight, it must be remembered that this late growth spurt (if it occurs) will not be accompanied by any meaningful change in skeletal growth. This means that in extreme cases, where birds are very small in weight and stature at 16-18 weeks of age, the end result of using high nutrient dense prebreeder diets may well be development of pullets with correct body weight, but of small stature. These short shank length breeders seem more prone to prolapse/pick-out, and so this is another example of the limitations in use of classical prebreeder diets.

Use of high nutrient dense prebreeder diets to manipulate late growth of broiler breeder pullets does, however, seem somewhat redundant. The reason for this is that with restricted feeding programs, it is more logical to increase feed allowance than to add the complexity of introducing another diet. The only potential problem with this approach is that in extreme cases, feed intake is increased to a level that is in excess of the initial allowance of the breeder diet at start of lay. This can be a potential problem because breeders should not be subjected to a step down in feed allocation prior to peak production.

c) Body composition

While body composition at maturity may well be as important as body weight at this age, it is obviously a parameter that is difficult to measure. There is little doubt that energy is likely the limiting nutrient for egg production, and that at around peak production, feed may not be the sole source of such energy. Labile fat reserves at this time are, therefore, essential to augment feed sources. These labile fat reserves become critical during situations of heat stress or general hot weather conditions. Once the bird starts to produce eggs, then its ability to deposit fat reserves is greatly limited. Obviously if labile fat reserves are to be of significance, then they must be deposited prior to maturity.

d) Egg weight and hatchability

It seems as though egg size is ultimately controlled by the size of the yolk that enters the oviduct. In large part this is influenced by body weight of the bird, and so factors described previously for body weight can also be applied to concerns with egg size. There is a general need for as large an early egg size as possible. Increased levels of linoleic acid in prebreeder diets may be of some use, although levels in excess of the regular 1% found in most diets produce only marginal effects on early egg size. From a nutritional standpoint, egg size can best be manipulated with diet protein, and especially methionine concentration. It is logical, therefore, to consider increasing the methionine levels in prebreeder diets. For these diets, DL-methionine and analogue products such as Alimet® are comparable and both promote maximum early egg size. Early egg size can also be increased by more rapid increase in feed allocation early in the breeder house. Lilburn and Myers-Miller (1990) fed birds from 16 weeks so as to attain peak feed allowance of 159 g/day at either 24, 26 or 28 weeks of age. More rapid increase in feed resulted in much earlier maturity and about a 4 g increase in egg size up to 28 weeks. However such rapid increase in feed was associated with a dramatic increase in production of double yolked eggs (11.1% vs a mean of 4% for the other treatment groups).

For breeders we must also consider egg composition as it relates to early hatchability success. Eggs from young breeders seem inherently to have a hatchability problem and perhaps this is one of the reasons that we wait for egg size to increase before shipping eggs to the hatchery. The reason for this early hatch problem is not fully resolved, but most likely relates in some way to maturity and development of embryonic membranes and their effect on transfer of nutrients from the yolk to the embryo. There may also be a problem of inadequate transfer of vitamins into the egg although simply increasing vitamin levels in prebreeder diets does not seem to resolve this problem. For a number of critical B-vitamins, their concentration in successive eggs does not plateau until after 7-10 eggs have been laid. The effect of prebreeder nutrition on these factors warrants further study, but at this time these problems cannot be resolved by simply over-fortifying prebreeder diets with vitamins, certain fatty acids or amino acids.

Prebreeder diets can successfully be used as part of a feeding program aimed at maximizing production potential in young breeders. However any desired increase in nutrient intake prior to maturity can most easily be achieved by simply increasing the feed allowance of either grower or adult breeder diet at this time. If prebreeder diets are used, then 19-23 weeks seems the most ideal time, assuming 1% production will occur at around 24 weeks of age.

5.4 FEEDING PROGRAMS FOR ADULT HENS

As with the growing bird, adult breeders must be given restricted quantities of feed in order to control body weight. After 20 weeks, regardless of rearing program, all birds should be fed on a daily, rather than skip-a-day program. There is little doubt that optimum breeder performance will only be seen following successful rearing management. Data from flocks around the world, housed under various conditions and fed varying types of diet indicate that better performance is invariably achieved when body weight gain is optimum through the late rearing, prebreeder, early breeder transition period. The key nutrient under these conditions is most likely energy, because as with the Leghorn pullet, the broiler breeder is in a somewhat delicate balance regarding energy input and energy expenditure. There is considerable variation in suggested energy requirements for the breeder at this time of early egg production. In fact, reported values vary from 220-440 kcal/bird/day.

Energy - In attempting to rationalize this obvious range of recommendations, energy requirements were calculated for a commercial strain of broiler breeder (Table 5.22).

TABLE 5.22 Comparison of calculated energy requirement and feed allowance for the breeder pullet. Units are kcal ME equivalents

Weeks of age	Body wt (kg)	Total maintenance (kcal)	Growth (kcal)	Eggs (kcal)	Total daily energy req. (kcal)	Highest feed allowance (kcal)
20	2.07	235	85	-	320	250
21	2.17	245	85	-	330	315
22	2.27	255	105	-	360	330
23	2.39	260	105	-	365	350
24	2.67	290	110	10	410	380
25	2.80	300	90	20	410	420
26	2.91	305	75	40	420	440
27	3.00	310	50	60	420	470
28	3.06	315	30	80	425	480

In these calculations, values for maintenance net energy requirements were extrapolated from our work with breeders. A subsequent factor of 0.82 was used in conversion to ME. An arbitrary 35% activity allowance was included, while growth was assumed to require 5.8 kcal ME/g (50:50, fat:muscle). As shown in Table 5.22, there is concern over the calculated energy requirement in relation to feed allowance, even at the highest feeding level recommended by the breeder. These results suggest that the breeder is in a very precarious situation with regard to energy balance at the critical time of sexual maturity.

As shown in Table 5.23, the major factors influencing energy needs are body weight and environmental temperature.

The problem of energy availability may well be confounded by the nutritionist's overestimation of that portion of diet energy available to the broiler breeder. Most energy levels of diets and/or ingredients, when assayed, are derived using Leghorn type birds. Work at Guelph indicates that broiler breeders are less able to metabolize diet energy, than are Leghorn birds (Table 5.24). Regardless of diet specifications, it would appear that broiler breeders metabolize about 2.5% less energy from feeds than do Leghorns. This relates to some 70 kcal/kg for most breeder diets. Deficiencies of energy around the time of peak egg production will likely reduce egg production at this time, or as often happens in commercial situations, production will decline some 2-3 weeks after peak, when a characteristic "dip" in production is seen.

TABLE 5.23 Model predicted energy needs of breeder hens as affected by environmental temperature

			Temperature				
At weeks of age	**B.wt (g)**	**Egg Mass (g/d)**	**14°C**	**18°C**	**24°C**	**29°C**	**35°C**
22	2320	-	284	256	229	201	175
24	2450	3.5	300	272	254	215	187
26	2565	18.0	350	320	290	260	235
28	2665	44.3	439	409	379	348	320
30	2758	53.7	475	444	413	382	352
40	3100	53.6	490	456	423	390	357
50	3310	48.0	482	445	411	376	341
60	3425	41.0	464	428	393	357	322
70	3500	34.0	445	410	373	337	302

Adapted from Waldroup *et al.* 1976)
(See Table 5.17)

TABLE 5.24 Diet ME determined with Leghorn and broiler breeder pullets

	Diet ME (kcal/kg)		
Diet type	Leghorn	Broiler Breeder	Δ
20% CP, 2756 ME	2805	2736	-2.5%
14% CP, 2756 ME	2847	2806	-1.5%
16% CP, 2878 ME	2976	2906	-2.4%
15% CP, 2574 ME	2685	2622	-2.4%

Spratt and Leeson 1987

It is concluded that optimum breeder performance will occur when the bird is in positive energy balance, and sufficient energy is available for production. With energy intakes of 325, 385, or 450 kcal ME/bird/day, the following partitioning of diet energy intake during a 24-40 week laying period was observed (Table 5.25).

Energy intake and energy balance are therefore critical to breeders that are expected to consistently peak at 82-85% production. This concept reinforces the statement made earlier regarding optimum body weight and optimum body condition of birds at start of lay. The fact that birds seem to do better when they are on the heavy side of the breeder's weight guide is likely a factor of such increased body mass acting as a source of additional energy in order to meet the bird's requirements at this time. It is undoubtedly true that any flock that does not gain some weight each week through peak production, will give inferior egg production and hatchability.

TABLE 5.25 Energy partitioning of broiler breeders (24-40 weeks)

	Daily energy intake (kcal/bird)		
	450	**385**	**325**
Input: Feed (kcal)	60,000	51,000	32,000
Output:Body fat (kcal)	21,300	14,700	12,100
:Body protein (kcal)	0	1,900	2,400
:Eggs (kcal)	11,000	10,000	8,000
% ME into growth	36	32	33
% ME into eggs	18	20	18

Adapted from Spratt and Leeson (1987)

Data from controlled studies suggest that the maintenance energy need of the breeder at 20°C is around 100 kcal ME/day/kg body mass. For a 3.2kg bird at peak, this equates to 320 kcal for maintenance. A total of around 450 kcal/d is calculated when activity, growth and egg production are factored in. Burke and Jensen (1994) recently showed the importance of feeding breeders just this level of energy (Table 5.26).

Protein/amino acids - Protein and amino acid needs of the breeder hen have not been clearly established. In general, most breeder flocks will be over fed, rather than under fed crude protein, because it is difficult to justify much more than 23-25 g protein per day. With a feed intake of 165 g daily, this means a maximum protein need of only about 15% (Table 5.27).

TABLE 5.26 Effect of energy allotment on breeder performance (21-61 wks)			
	Peak energy allotment (29-34 wks)		
	450 kcal	424 kcal	396 kcal
Eggs per hen	165	149	141
Fertility (%)	92.6	89.8	87.2
Chicks per hen	123	116	102
Egg weight (g)	66.1	66.5	66.7
Adapted from Burke and Jensen (1994)			

TABLE 5.27 Model predicted protein and amino acid needs of breeder hens						
		Amino acid (mg/hen/day)				
Weeks of age	CP (g/d)	Lysine	Tryptophan	Methionine	Meth + Cyst	Threonine
22	7.2	282	79	258	362	320
24	7.4	282	84	275	382	335
26	9.8	400	110	341	485	428
28	13.2	608	153	450	652	580
30	15.1	742	183	530	770	690
40	15.5	722	187	552	809	695
50	14.4	625	173	528	750	650
60	13.2	542	160	495	698	600
70	12.5	497	152	480	664	570
Adapted from Waldroup *et al.* (1976). See Table 5.18						

Studies have been carried out involving very low protein diets where levels of methionine + cystine and lysine are kept constant. Diets were formulated at 0.82% lysine and 0.59% methionine + cystine in 10, 12, 14 or 16% CP diets. All diets contained the same level of energy and all other nutrients, and quantities fed daily were as suggested by the primary breeder. All roosters were separate fed a 12% CP male diet. Breeders fed 10% CP performed remarkably well, and although they did not have the highest peak, their better persistency meant no difference in overall egg production (Fig. 5.2).

Fig. 5.2 Egg production of broiler breeder hens from 25 to 60 weeks of age. (From Lopez and Leeson, 1993).

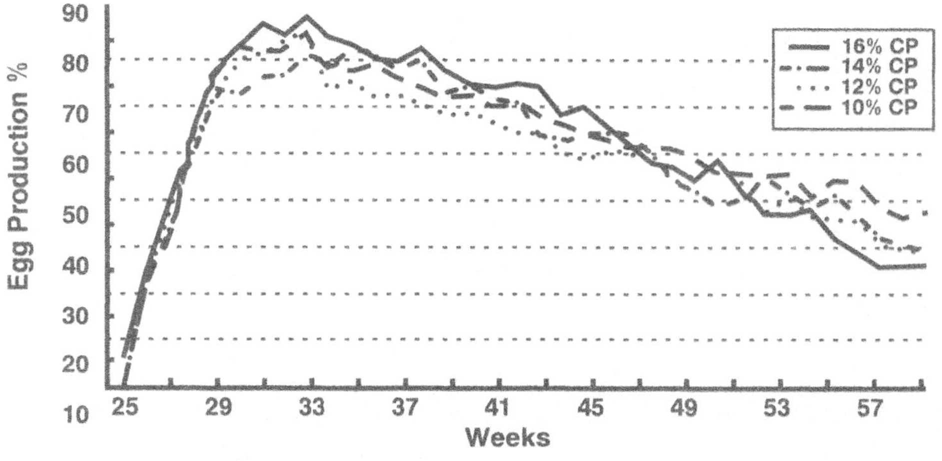

Fig. 5.3. Body weight of broiler breeder hens from 18 to 60 weeks of age. (From Lopez and Leeson, 1993).

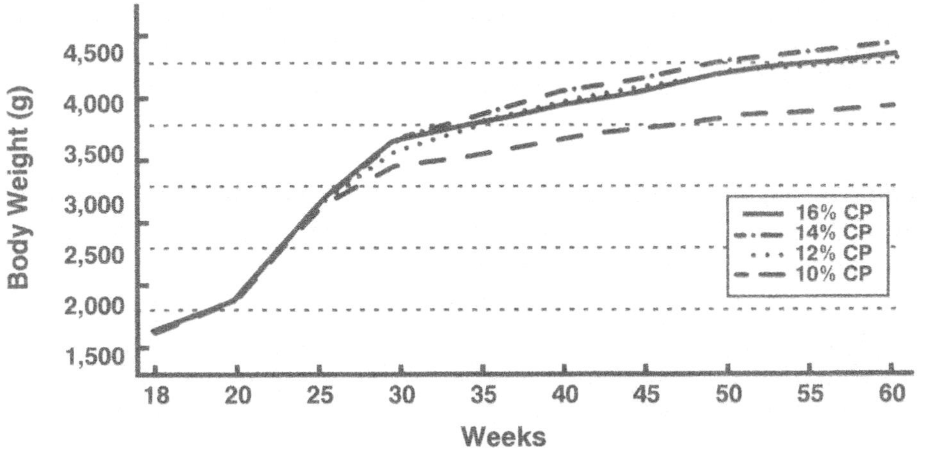

One of the most surprising results from the study, was better fertility with the lower protein diets. For example, overall fertility to 64 weeks for birds fed 10 vs 16% CP was 95.4 vs 90.6%. The reason for better fertility is thought to be due simply to the fact that these birds gained less weight (Fig 5.3), because there is a negative correlation between obesity and fertility. These data suggest that protein/amino acid intake of the breeder hen is related to weight gain, and that excessive weight gain occurring after peak egg production is not merely a factor of energy balance. The results from this study were therefore somewhat unexpected, because birds fed the lowest level of protein produced the most chicks. Although 10% CP diets for breeder hens are not advocated, this data shows that lower, rather than higher levels of protein could be used, assuming that adequate amino acid balance is maintained.

Feed intake during early egg production should be governed by: a) egg production (egg mass); b) body weight; and c) feed clean up time. All three of these factors are important in the feeding of breeders. The following discussion sections on each of these factors should not be considered in isolation, but rather all three taken into account prior to increasing or decreasing a feed allocation.

Feeding to egg production - Considering the large nutrient output in each egg, it is essential to lead-feed for egg production. It must be remembered that birds are continually producing yolk material, and so a bird at 10% production, should in fact be fed as though it is at 30-40% egg production. Failure to lead-feed for egg production, results in the bird utilizing its body fat reserves to supplement the nutrient supply in the feed. If this scenario continues for long enough, all labile energy reserves are utilized, and the bird shows a characteristic loss or stalling in weight that immediately precedes loss in production. This scenario assumes that the bird has body energy reserves to utilize at this time. An example of a lead-feeding schedule according to egg production is shown in Table 5.28. Although metric is used throughout this book, we have also included a column in imperial units for Table 5.28 because we realize that producers in many countries still use this measure in describing feed intake of breeders.

This schedule means that if breeders are uniform then they should be at peak feed allocation by the time they reach 35% egg production. Obviously the figures should be used as guidelines, and if local conditions dictate the use of higher or lower energy density etc., then allocations must be modified accordingly. Also if separate male feeding is not practised, then allowances may need to be increased by 5-10% in order to accommodate over consumption by males. For non-uniform birds, the move to peak feed must be slower (Table 5.28). High and sustained peak egg production can only be achieved with uniform breeder flocks fed to meet their nutritional requirements. With 85-88% peaks now possible, it is obvious that we have to carefully plan and execute a feeding program tailored to meet the breeder's nutrient needs. Under- feeding results in very short term peaks, of only 3-4 weeks, and these are usually associated with the classical sign of loss or stall out in body weight for 1-2 weeks. On the other hand, overfeeding, especially with energy, will result in excessive weight gain, and while peak production may be little affected, there will be precipitous loss in egg production through 34-64 weeks of age. The basis of feed allocation at this critical time is obviously to allow genetic potential for increases in both egg numbers and egg size, and also to allow for modest weekly gains in body weight. Managers should consider "challenge feeding" as part of their feed management system at this critical time.

TABLE 5.28 Lead-feeding schedule for breeder pullets up to time of 50% egg production assuming diet provides 15.56% CP and 2850 kcal ME/kg

	Daily Feed Intake			
	Body weight Uniformity 85% (±15%)		Body weight Uniformity 70% (±15%)	
Egg Production (%)	(g)	(lbs/100)	(g)	(lbs/100)
1	135	30	128	28
5	140	31	132	29
10	145	32	136	30
15	150	33	140	31
20	155	34	144	32
25	160	35	148	33
30	164	36	152	33.5
35	168	37	156	34
40	↓	↓	160	35
45			164	36
50			168	37

Challenge feeding involves giving the hens extra feed 2 or 3 days each week, based on need, without changing the base feed quantity scheduled for the flock. For example, a flock may receive 168 g/bird/day at peak, with an additional "challenge" of 7 g/bird/day given three days each week. The challenge feed is, therefore, equivalent to 3 x 7 g ÷ 7 d = 3 g/bird/day. In reality birds receive the equivalent of 168 g + 3 g = 171 g/bird/day. The immediate question is why bother with this more complicated system, rather than just giving the flock a base feed allowance of 171 g/bird/day? The advantages of challenge feeding, rather than simply increasing the base allocation are:

- On days of challenge feeding, feeding time will increase, and this helps to improve overall flock uniformity.

- It is easier to make adjustments to nutrient intake based on day-to-day change in needs as may occur with changes in environmental temperature.

- Birds become accustomed to change in feed allocation, which will be important once feed withdrawal is practised after peak.

- Ease of tailoring nutrient needs to individual flocks. For example, a base feed allocation of 165g/bird/day may be standardised across all flocks, with individual flock needs at peak being tailored with the quantity and/or frequency of challenge, depending upon actual production, environmental temperature, etc.

The actual quantity and timing of challenge feed must be flexible if it is to be used efficiently. In practice the challenge should not represent more than 5% of total feed intake, and most often the quantity will be 2- 4%. On the other hand, the quantity of the challenge should be large enough to meaningfully contribute to the factors listed previously. For this reason there needs to be a balance between the quantity of feed given, and the frequency of this feeding. For example, a daily challenge of 3 g/bird/day given daily will be much less effective than 7 g/bird/day given 3 times each week. In both instances birds are receiving 21 g/week as a challenge, but in the later example the challenge quantity is more meaningful and we are more likely to see a bird response in terms of egg output. Challenge feeding should start when birds are at 60-70% production, and should be discontinued after peak, when egg production falls below 80%. For most flocks, therefore, we can expect to practice challenge feeding from about 29 through 40 weeks of age. The idea of challenge feeding is to more closely tailor feed allocation to breeder hen needs, and so there should be no standardised system. Managers must be given flexibility to alter challenge feeding based on fluctuating needs. In most instances the challenge will be used to help lead birds into a sustained peak. Because the concept of challenge feeding is to more closely tailor feed allocation to needs, then it is usual practice to alter the quantity and/or duration of challenge as birds progress through peak egg production. Maximum challenge feeding should coincide with peak egg output, with lesser quantities given prior to, and after actual peak. On this basis we recommend challenge feeding to be reduced (but not discontinued) once birds are 2% below peak egg production. Following is an example of challenge feeding (Table 5.29).

Table 5.29 Challenge feeding schedule				
Egg production	**Daily base feed allowance**		**Challenge feed**	
35%	162g	(35.6 lb/100)	None	-
60%	162g	(35.6 lb/100	5 g/d, 2x/wk	(1.1 lb/100)
80%	162g	(35.6 lb/100)	8 g/d, 2x/wk	(1.8 lb/100)
-2% from peak	162g	(35.6 lb/100)	5 g/d, 2x/wk	(1.1 lb/100)
79%	162g	(35.6 lb/100)	None	-
<79%	Reduce	-	None	-

Challenge feeding can also be used post peak if there are precipitous declines in egg production related to minor disease challenge or management or environmental stress. Under these conditions, challenges of 10 g/bird/day for two consecutive days are recommended. If no immediate response is seen in egg production, then the challenge should be discontinued. If egg production returns to normal, then the challenge should gradually be reduced over the next 2-3 days.

Challenge feeding allows tailoring of feed allocation to suit individual flock needs. Managers should be flexible in actual allocations, although maximum challenge feed allocation needs to coincide with peak egg production. Breeder hens will respond to a carefully planned challenge program, with sustained peak production and better post peak persistency. On the other hand, the challenge should not usually represent more than 5% of total feed intake, because excessive challenge will invariably result in obesity and related loss in post peak performance. In general, when birds are subjected to such stresses as variable feed quality, mycotoxin challenge and/or fluctuating or extreme environmental temperature, then a high base feed allowance, coupled with aggressive feed challenge is recommended. On the other hand, lower feed inputs are possible where consistent quality high energy feeds are used, and where there is good environmental control.

Once birds have peaked in daily egg mass, it is necessary to reduce feed intake. There is often confusion and concern as to how much and how quickly feed should be removed, and this is somewhat surprising, since the same basic rules used pre-peak also apply at this time. This means that birds should be fed according to egg production, body weight and clean-up time. After peak production feed clean up time often starts to increase and this is an indication of birds being overfed. The main problem is to prevent too heavy a body weight at this time. If feed is not withdrawn after peak, then because egg production is declining, proportionally more feed will be used for growth. Therefore, after peak egg mass, body weight becomes perhaps the most important parameter used in manipulating feed allocation. It is still important for birds to gain some weight, since loss of weight is indicative of too severe a cut back in feed.

Feed allocation and withdrawal for breeder hens has to be based upon needs. The hen needs nutrients for four major reasons, namely for growth, egg production, maintaining normal body functions and for daily activity. Each of these needs varies with the age of hen and environmental temperature, and each need also varies with respect to the type of nutrients utilized. Growth, egg production and maintenance all require protein and energy, while activity is only really demanding on energy needs. Actual estimates for these nutrient needs are shown in Table 5.30. Surprisingly to many people, the maintenance need is by far the largest single factor affecting energy requirements of the breeder. Secondly it is egg production and lastly, growth and activity. In terms of protein needs, egg production and maintenance are the only two meaningful factors. However, as the bird gets older, their actual nutrient needs and the distribution of these needs change (Table 5.30).

TABLE 5.30 Daily protein and energy requirements of breeder hens at 32 and 55 weeks of age

	32 weeks age		55 weeks age	
Nutrient need	**Energy (kcal)**	**Protein (g)**	**Energy (kcal)**	**Protein (g)**
Growth	40	1	5	None
Egg production	80	10	55	8
Maintenance	300	10	320	11
Activity	50	None	30	None
Total	470	21	410	19

At 55, compared to 32 weeks of age, the bird needs less energy and protein for eggs, because egg production has declined (even though egg size has increased) but she needs more of these nutrients for maintenance because over the 23-week period the bird has grown and so needs more feed to maintain herself. At 55 weeks, if all goes well, there will be significantly reduced growth rate, and both protein and energy needs for growth are greatly reduced. The reduction in nutrient needs for lower egg production and less growth outweighs the greater need for maintenance, and the bottom line is overall reduction in daily need of the hen for both energy (410 vs 470 kcal) and protein (19 vs 21 g).

We can best achieve reduced nutrient needs, by simply reducing feed intake, or maintaining feed intake constant but changing the energy and protein levels of the diet. In practice, reducing feed intake after peak production is by far the easiest and most foolproof method of reducing the bird's nutrient intake. Changing to a lower energy, lower protein diet means a change of formulation, which itself can be stressful to the bird. On multi age farms, it is also more hazardous to have numerous different diets being delivered to the farm, which can get placed in the wrong feed tank. Changing diet nutrient density usually occurs only once or at most twice in the life of the flock, whereas in reality the bird's needs are gradually and continually being reduced after peak, a factor that can be accommodated most easily with frequent changes in feed allocation.

The consequences of not reducing nutrient intake of the breeder hen after peak should be fairly obvious. Supplying more protein or energy than is required is not going to force the bird to lay more eggs or become more active. Oversupply of these nutrients goes directly to increased growth which itself quickly results in increased maintenance requirement. This extra growth will be mainly fat, but there will also be some muscle (protein) growth. Obesity quickly leads to reduced egg production, diverting even more nutrients into growth (fat). This vicious circle is often responsible for the very sudden drop in egg production seen with flocks that are overfed after peak egg production. Before proceeding to the discussion of actual reductions in feed allocation, it is pertinent to define "peak production". Peak production is most often used to describe maximum number of eggs being produced, whereas from a feeding point of view, peak output of egg mass is more relevant. For most breeder strains, peak output of egg mass (number x weight) will occur some 4-6 weeks after peak egg numbers. It is this lag in output of egg mass that makes it necessary to temper the withdrawal of feed and the reason why one should not usually react immediately to the first 1-2% decline in production.

Many producers find it difficult to accept that only very small changes in feed intake are necessary at this time. Calculation of the contribution of eggs to total feed intake make this concept more easily understood:

Example: A broiler breeder producing a 65 g egg, and eating 155 g/b/d of a 2850 kcal ME/kg diet.

A 65 g egg contains about 119 kcal gross energy.

This requires the equivalent of 140 kcal feed metabolizable energy.

Therefore, of the 440 kcal consumed each day (155g x 2850 kcal/kg), only 140 kcal (32%) goes towards egg production.

If one wishes to change the feed in response to small changes in egg production, then obviously the overall effect on the bird is quite small. For example, a 3% decline in production from 79→76% means a change in energy requirement for egg production of:

$$3\% \times 140 \text{ kcal}$$
$$= 4.2 \text{ kcal}$$

Therefore in relation to total feed supply of 440 kcal, this change in egg production of 3%, means a $\frac{4.2}{440} \times 100$ or 0.95% change in feed supply.

Therefore a 3% change in egg production means only an approximate 1% change in feed intake.

For a breeder eating 155 g/b/d, it means changing allocation to 153 g/b/d (34 lbs vs 33.7 lbs/100 b/d).

This type of allocation indicates the reasoning behind the caution needed in reducing the feed allocation for breeder hens.

The final questions of course, are how much and how often is feed allocation reduced after peak production? Regardless of how high a peak production is actually realized, we should not start to reduce feed while birds are at ≥80% production. The main reason for this is that peak egg numbers do not usually coincide with peak nutrient needs for eggs, because egg size is increasing through this period. In most flocks, peak nutrient needs for eggs (production x size) will have been reached by the time production has declined to 79-80%, at about 39-40 weeks of age. At this stage of production one can start to gradually reduce feed intake, and in general, the quantity of feed to be removed will depend on peak feed allowance. If birds were peaked on 175 g/bird/day then it is likely that more feed can be removed than for a flock that peaked on 160 g/bird/day. Also, if temperature/seasonal changes are anticipated, then this should be factored into feed allocation - impending warmer weather means that more feed can be removed, while if cooler temperatures are anticipated, very little feed needs to be taken away (because maintenance needs will naturally increase). Assuming that a flock has peaked at 175 g/bird/day, and no major change in environmental temperature is anticipated, then a feed reduction program as shown in Table 5.31 is suggested. With such a low and steady removal of feed, it should be possible to prevent obesity in hens, while at the same time allowing adequate energy and protein for the inevitable slow decline in egg numbers. The reduction in feed intake is necessarily slow and involves small steps because, as shown in Table 5.30, the actual nutrients going into eggs are quite a small proportion of the hen's total needs.

TABLE 5.31 Feed allocation program for heavy breeders after peak production

Egg production (%)	Approx. age (wks)	Daily feed intake (g/day)	(lbs/100/day)
80	39	175	38.5
79	40	174	38.3
78	41	174	38.3
77	42	172	37.8
76	43	172	37.8
74	45	170	37.4
70	50	165	36.3
65	55	160	35.2
60	60	155	34.1
55	65	150	33.0

Responding to a 5% decline in egg production, therefore, requires very small changes to the feed scale. Some producers consider a 1-2 g/bird/day reduction in feed intake hardly worth bothering about, and either make no adjustment, or a few much larger reductions. Sudden large reductions ≥5 g/bird/day can often be very stressful and result in sudden drops in egg production. Making no adjustments and continuing near peak allocation to 64 weeks, will be uneconomical in terms of birds becoming overweight with associated loss of egg production. In the example shown in Table 5.31, a bird fed according to this suggested schedule will eat about 30.8 kg to 65 weeks. Feeding 175 g through to 65 weeks, with no feed withdrawal, will result in an extra 2.3 kg feed intake. This quantity of extra feed will likely result in an additional 0.3-0.4 kg body weight gain, most of which will be fat.

Feeding to body weight **-** It is essential that producers continue to monitor body weight throughout the adult life of the breeder. All too often, the monitoring of body weight stops when birds enter the breeder house and so birds are fed solely according to egg production. The importance of body weight and body reserves of breeders through peak production has already been emphasized and this means continuous monitoring of body weight. It is essential that birds continually gain some weight through peak production. Loss of weight or a stall out in weight usually implies that birds are not getting enough nutrients, and so loss in egg production will occur within 7-10 d. In this context, monitoring of body weight will give an earlier indication of impending problems. From 20-32 weeks of age, pullets should ideally be weighed weekly.

Feeding to body weight assumes that birds are at ideal weight around 22 weeks of age (~2.2 kg). If birds are over weight or under weight, then adjustments to intake must be made. If birds are under weight, then they should obviously be given more feed than the standard recommended allowance in an attempt to stimulate growth. Overweight birds should also be given more feed (Table 5.32).

TABLE 5.32 Example of energy allowance for breeders (kcal ME/day)

Age (wks)	Under weight	Ideal weight	Over weight
18	230	240	250
20	270	250	280
22	310	295	325
24	345	345	380
26	430	430	470

This apparent contradiction of ideas is based on the fact that heavier birds have a larger maintenance requirement and need more feed to meet their overall energy (nutrient) requirement. This is a difficult concept for farm managers to accept, since they are afraid of overweight birds getting even heavier. There is obviously a fine line between overfeeding and feeding to requirement for this overweight bird. Under optimum conditions pullets will not lose weight after 20 weeks of age. Ideally they show continued small increments of weight gain each week and hopefully are around 3.5 kg at the end of their first laying cycle. Environmental temperature will also have a major effect on feed requirements, because as shown in Table 5.33, the largest portion of the feed is used for maintenance needs.

As temperature increases, feed need is reduced. In this example two values are shown for maintenance feed need at 34°C. The value in brackets (130g) represents feed need when the bird is under stress, and panting etc., where it needs energy to drive the cooling mechanisms in the body. In this situation, total feed need becomes 170 g, which is actually greater than that suggested at 24°C. It is often difficult to get breeders to eat more feed under heat stress conditions, yet this increased energy intake is critical if egg production is to be maintained.

TABLE 5.33 Examples of peak feed needs of breeders at various environmental temperatures (g/bird/day)

Feed need	18°C	24°C	34°C
Growth	10	10	10
Maintenance	140	125	110 (130)
Eggs	30	30	30
TOTAL	180	165	150 (170)

Feeding according to feed clean-up time - Feed clean up time should be used as an indication of adequacy of feed allocation. Major changes in clean up time are an indication of over or under feeding, and as such, are an early warning of subsequent changes in body weight and egg production. As a routine management procedure, the time taken to consume most of the feed allocation should be recorded each day, to the nearest 30 minutes. If clean up time varies by more than 60 minutes on a daily basis, then bird weight should be measured immediately. However, major changes in feed allocation should not be made solely on the basis of feed clean-up time, rather these times should be used as a guide to investigate feed needs through more precise monitoring parameters. Feed clean up time with newer high yield strains of breeder is often greater (+1 hr) compared to the more conventional strains and merely reflects a less aggressive feeding behaviour. Clean up time is also going to be affected by environmental temperature (Fig 5.4). In a cool environment, birds consume most of their feed within the first two hours of an egg laying day. Clean up time is slightly delayed for a non-egg laying day, but there is a dramatic decrease in rate of eating when temperature is cycling between 25-35°C compared to 10-25°C.

Clean up time for feed can vary considerably from flock to flock for no apparent reason. For example, one flock may take 4 hr to clean up feed, whereas a sister flock of the same age etc. can take 2 hr. For this reason absolute time taken to clean up feed cannot be used as a management guide. The only useful parameter is change in clean-up time. Sudden changes in clean up time often precede changes in body weight by 2-3 d, and changes in egg production by 10-20 d.

Fig. 5.4. Effect of temperature and oviposition on feed intake of breeder hens.

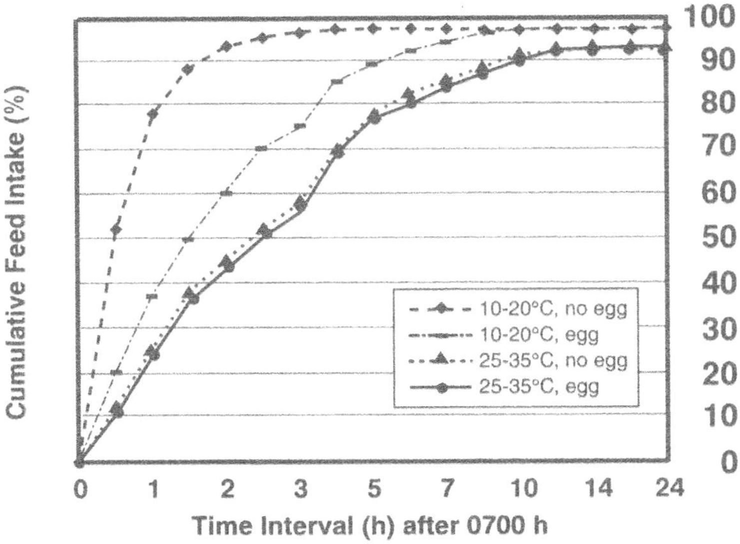

Adapted from Samara et al 1996

Time of feeding **-** Choice of feeding time for adult breeders can influence the production of settable eggs, egg shell quality, fertility and hatch of fertiles. In most instances these factors are a consequence of feeding activity displacing other important daily routines, such as nesting and mating. Breeder hens consume their feed in 2-6 hours each day. This large variation in feed clean up time relates to diet energy level, feed texture and perhaps most importantly, environmental temperature. In hot climates breeders often take much longer to eat feed, and this is especially true of high yield strains. Most managers consider this extended feeding time to be advantageous, because it ensures a more even allocation of feed across the flock where even the most timid birds have time to eat.

If breeders are fed early in the morning, then most intense feeding activity will be over by 9 a.m. Again this is ideal in terms of reducing heat load in the early afternoon period. This timing is also ideal in terms of differentiating the main feeding time from nesting activity. Depending upon when lights are switched on in the morning, most eggs are laid in the 9 a.m.-12 noon period. Feeding at 8 a.m. would, therefore, induce birds to feed at a time when they are usually in the nests. In fact eggs dropped in the area of the feeder are a very good indication of late morning feeding. Obviously some of these eggs will get broken or become too dirty for setting.

A few years ago there was interest in feeding breeders in the late afternoon. The main advantage is claimed to be an improvement in egg shell thickness, and in fact in many field trials this was found to be true. Improved shell thickness is likely a consequence of the bird eating calcium at a time when shell calcification is starting (for the next day's egg) and also the bird having more feed (with calcium) in its crop when lights are switched off. If egg shell quality is a problem, then afternoon feeding seems a viable option. Alternatively, birds could be given a "scratch" feed of large particle limestone or oystershell in the late afternoon. For example, shell thickness is improved by either feeding breeders at 4 p.m. vs 7 a.m. or feeding at 1 p.m. plus a scratch feeding of dicalcium phosphate in the late afternoon.

However, late afternoon feeding has a number of potential disadvantages. Firstly there is an increase in shell thickness. This should not be a problem as long as incubation setter conditions are adjusted so as to maintain normal moisture loss. In most situations this means a reduction in setter humidity to account for less moisture loss through a thicker shell. Because late afternoon feeding is only really useful for improving shell quality, its application is greatest for older breeders. Unfortunately, there seems to be a loss in egg number (up to 10%) when feeding time for older breeders is suddenly changed from early morning to late afternoon.

A greater concern with late afternoon feeding is potential loss of mating activity, and increase in incidence of body checked eggs. Mating activity is usually greatest in late afternoon. If hens are more interested in feeding at this time, then there can be reduced mating activity and also more aggression between males. Body checked eggs are characterized by a distinct band of thickened shell around the middle of the egg (sometimes called belted eggs). This defect is caused by the egg shell breaking during its early manufacture in the bird's uterus. The bird repairs the crack, but does so imperfectly. Such eggs have reduced air and moisture transfer characteristics, and usually fail to hatch. The most common cause of body checked eggs is sudden activity, movement, stress etc. on the bird. This extra activity takes place when feed is given in late afternoon, and so there will likely be fewer settable eggs produced.

Separate sex feeding **-** Almost all breeder flocks today are fed separate sex, which means that the hens and roosters will have separate feeding systems. Although the idea was developed mainly for better control over male feed intake and growth, excluding the males from the hen feeder means that one now has more confidence in all hens receiving the desired allocation. Most equipment relies on the wider head width of the male making it impossible for them to access the "grilled" female feeder. There is obviously variation in head width of both males and females, and so the system is never perfect, especially for young breeders. Feed management of roosters is discussed in section 5.6. For hens, the concern is design of equipment such that roosters are excluded, but that hens do not have to unduly force their head between the grill supports. There are undoubtedly more head and beak lesions and more neck feather loss as a result of this equipment. On average, pullets at 20 weeks will have head widths of around 36 mm, and this increases to about 38 mm by the end of the breeder cycle. Birds with head widths greater than 39 mm almost always have more head lesions.

Hocking (1993) suggests the optimum size of the grill to be 4 mm wider than head width, and that injury is avoided when grill width is 2 mm wider than the head. Fig 5.5 shows the feed intake of young pullets of different weight and head width. The smallest birds were given 53 g feed/day, the intermediate birds 78 g/day while the heaviest birds with 42.6 mm head width were given 135 g/day, which was close to ad lib feeding. There is an obvious correlation between ability to eat, and head width in relation to grill width.

Fig. 5.5 Relationship between head width and grill size as they influence feed intake of caged breeders.

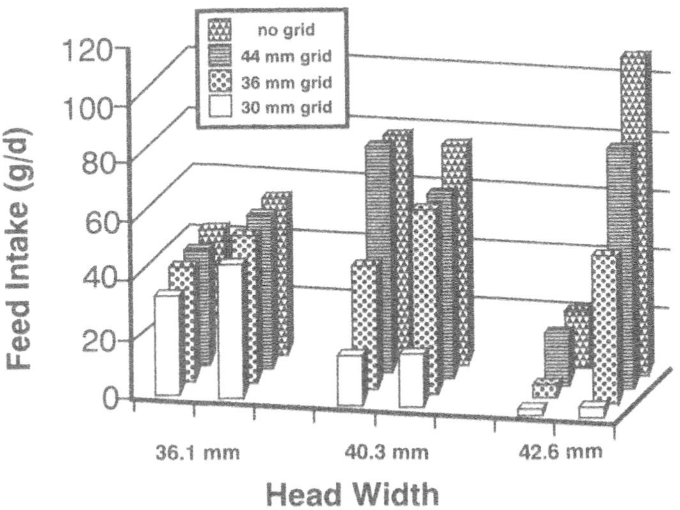

Adapted from Hocking (1993)

Eggshell quality - A distinct disadvantage to high and sustained peak egg production seen today, is associated deterioration in eggshell quality. As occurs with Leghorns, there is frequent loss of shell quality after 25-30 weeks of production. Poor shell quality means potential loss of settable eggs and reduced hatch of fertile due to change in moisture loss from the thinner shelled eggs. Nutritionally, the major nutrients of concern are calcium, available phosphorus, and vitamin D_3. There may be an advantage to phase feeding both calcium and phosphorus, and providing extra vitamin D_3 as a water supplement. Calcium level can be increased over time by adding an extra 5 kg limestone to the diet at 45 and 55 weeks of age. At the same time available phosphorus levels can be reduced by at least 0.05%. If shell quality is problematic, breeders sometimes respond to vitamin D_3 given in the drinking water - 300 IU/bird 2x per week is recommended. While feed is usually the only source of calcium and phosphorus considered in meeting the breeder's needs, it is known that birds eat litter which contains these nutrients. Such litter eating has been suggested as the reason for improved shell quality of floor vs caged birds under experimental conditions. Controlled studies have shown that breeders eating 20 g litter/day, consume an extra 7% calcium and 12% available phosphorus. Unfortunately shell quality is influenced not only by levels of calcium, in the diet, but also feeding time and also particle size. Data for Fig 5.6 was developed with Leghorns, but applies to breeders today at peak production.

Fig. 5.6 Shell mineral deposition over a 24h ovulation cycle.

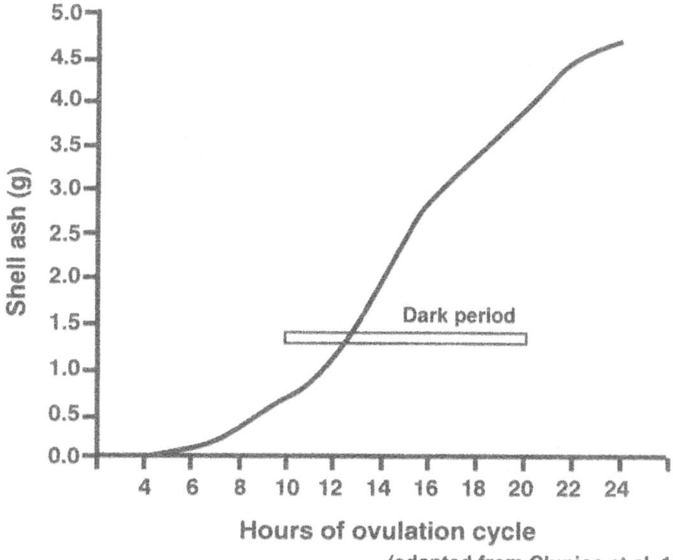

(adapted from Clunies et al, 1993)

Most of the shell material is formed in the daily period of darkness, when the hen is not eating. During this time of rapid shell accretion, the bird relies on the stores of medullary bone (in the long leg bones) for almost 50% of the calcium used to make a shell. Between successive calcifications, this bone must be replenished, in the form of calcium phosphate. One reason for decline in shell quality over time, is gradual loss in efficiency of this deposition and withdrawal of medullary bone. Although the medullary bone reserve is essential to shell formation regardless of diet, its role is somewhat reduced if the bird has some calcium being absorbed from the digestive tract at night. This situation leads to the idea of afternoon feeding of calcium, so as to provide a calcium source in the digestive tract that can slowly be released at night, and so aid shell formation. At the end of the day, the breeder will ideally have a few grains of calcium in the digestive tract, that can slowly be digested and absorbed, and then directed to the shell gland.

Farmer *et al.* (1983) determined the quantity of calcium remaining in various regions of the digestive tract following a 7 a.m. feeding of a diet providing 4.27 g calcium/day (Table 5.34). With lights out at 11 p.m., the breeders had little calcium remaining in the digestive tract overnight. Time of feeding calcium, therefore, seems important. Because most breeders are fed early in the morning and with clean up time of only 2-3 hrs, then there is little potential for calcium reserves remaining in the gut in the evening. When breeders are given experimental diets containing just 0.4% calcium, they are found to be able to maintain shell quality only when an extra 3 g calcium is force fed at around 4 p.m. Such force feeding at 8 a.m. resulted in very poor shell quality.

TABLE 5.34 Calcium remaining in various regions of the digestive tract following 7 a.m. feeding of a diet providing 4.27 g calcium/day (g)

Time	Crop	Gizzard	Upper small intestine	Lower small intestine
11 am	1.64	0.53	0.22	0.32
7 pm	1.36	0.11	0.07	0.14
11 pm	0.86	0.21	0.03	0.07
3 am	0.24	0.20	0.09	0.09
7 am	0.01	0.18	0.09	0.17

Adapted from Farmer *et al.* (1983)

Feeding calcium in the late afternoon therefore seems ideal if shell quality is problematic. This can best be done by simply broadcasting oystershell or large particle limestone directly on to the litter at around 4 p.m. The feeding activity associated with this technique also helps in bringing hens down from the slats, onto the litter, which usually means greater mating activity at this time. This technique raises another concern about calcium source, namely particle size. Usually, the larger the particle size, the slower the rate of digestion, and so the more prolonged the metering out of calcium for shell formation. The reason for poor shell quality following force feeding 3 g of calcium at 8 a.m., as described previously, relates to the fact that the bird cannot utilize this sudden influx of calcium, and has no reserve other than the medullary bone. Large particle limestone and oystershell are usually digested more slowly, and this is the reason suggested for better shell quality with these products. Ideally a mixture of fine and coarse particles should be used because this gives both rapid and slow metering of calcium for metabolic needs. The disadvantage of both oystershell and large particle limestone are that they are very abrasive to mechanical equipment. Table 5.35 is a suggested feeding program aimed at optimizing shell quality.

TABLE 5.35 Diet specification aimed at optimizing shell quality

	Breeder age		
	25 wks	**45 wks**	**55 wks**
Calcium (%)	3.1	3.3	3.5
Available phosphorus (%)	0.40	0.36	0.32
Crude protein (%)	15.5	14.5	14.0
Methionine (%)	0.35	0.32	0.30
Water supplement			
Vitamin D3	-	300 IU/bird/2 consecutive days per week	
Vitamin C	-	20 mg/bird/2 consecutive days per week	

Feed efficiency **-** Most producers in the poultry meat business could give a close approximation of feed efficiency in broilers, but few managers or technicians have comparable values at their fingertips for breeder performance. To some extent this is a fault of breeding companies because virtually no management guides contain this important information.

Table 5.36 shows feed efficiency data for breeders calculated in terms of feed or nutrients per hatching egg or per chick. Data is shown to 64 weeks of age, which is the most common age for flock depletion. Values are also shown for breeder hens alone or hens with 8% males. For hens alone to 64 weeks of age, feed usage is calculated at 300 g during the breeder phase or 370 g including both grower and breeder phases, for each chick produced. Comparable numbers per hatching egg are 260 and 320 g. There is considerable variation in the level of dietary energy fed to breeders worldwide, and so perhaps a more accurate assessment of feed efficiency for comparative purposes, is feed energy usage per egg or per chick. To 64 weeks of age, total energy intake, including the carrying cost of the males, is 980 and 1130 kcal ME per hatching egg and chick respectively. As a simple rule of thumb therefore, we expect an energy cost of about 1000 kcal ME per hatching egg or chick.

TABLE 5.36 Feed efficiency of breeders

	Females only		Females + 8% males	
	0-64 wks	**24-64 wks**	**0-64 wks**	**24-64 wks**
Per hatching egg				
Feed (g)	320	260	345	280
Energy (kcal)	915	750	980	800
Protein (g)	50	40	53	43
Per chick				
Feed (g)	370	300	400	320
Energy (kcal)	1050	860	1130	920
Protein (g)	60	50	62	50

Because there are two values used in calculation of any measure of efficiency, the bottom line can be improved by maximizing one value and/or minimizing the other. This means that in theory efficiency can be improved by increasing egg and chick output and/or by reducing feed intake. Unfortunately these two factors cannot be changed that easily. It is difficult to increase egg output *per se* because hopefully this is already being maximized with the standard on farm management practices. Likewise, we cannot simply reduce feed intake by an arbitrary amount without expecting some loss in performance. However there may be some potential for fine tuning these parameters.

If late cycle increase in egg size can be tempered, then one should be able to improve feed efficiency because feed intake is really a factor of egg mass, rather than just a factor of egg numbers. Once egg size is optimized, there is little advantage to obtaining an ever increasing egg size. Nutritional modification can therefore be considered to limit such egg size increases, and specifically reduce or control the bird's intake of crude protein and/or methionine. Phase feeding of these nutrients will help to temper late cycle egg size and apart from improving feed efficiency, will help maintain hatchability because of better control over shell thickness and shell porosity.

Although feed intake cannot arbitrarily be reduced, the bird's need for feed can be lessened by maintaining optimum environmental temperatures. A major portion of the bird's daily energy intake is used for maintenance of body functions, and in a mature bird this means keeping warm. An ideal temperature for a mature breeder is around 22°C. Much below 20°C, she will start to use more feed to stay warm (about 1% more feed per 1°C change). Similarly above 30°C, depending upon acclimatization, she will use energy to stay cool. Feed efficiency will, therefore, deteriorate (more feed per egg) at either high or low environmental temperatures. At high temperatures feed efficiency falls off even more quickly, because there is often an associated loss in egg numbers.

Feed efficiency will be compromised if there is any degree of feed wastage. This can be due to improper feeder management, especially with pan feeders. Both male and female feeders must be adjusted to the correct height, and the pans adjusted to give the correct depth of feed. Consistency of feed texture is also important - birds often waste more feed (flicking, billing out of feeders) if there is a change in feed texture, especially when suddenly changing from small to large feed particle size.

5.5 FEEDING PROGRAMS FOR ADULT ROOSTERS

Condition and performance of the breeder male are critical for optimum chick yield per breeder hen. Most of our losses in hatchability are due to infertility. If a breeder hen produces an egg, then infertility is usually due to simple absence of sperm in the oviduct, and this itself is directly related to effective mating frequency. In many situations, therefore, loss of hatchability is caused by incorrect body condition of hens and/or roosters, such that mating activity is reduced. For hens this is usually due to overfeeding and associated obesity, and in roosters is caused by overfeeding or underfeeding. Just as care is taken to meet the hen's nutrient requirements with continual adjustments to diet or feed allocation, there is also a need to carefully monitor the male's condition and environment and to feed them accordingly. In many respects it is easy to predict the male's nutrient requirements, because they do not have the complication of egg production as occurs with the hen. The feeding program therefore has to meet just two basic needs namely, growth and maintenance of body functions. The major criteria of male feeding programs, therefore, are monitoring body weight and body condition and controlling frame size and uniformity.

There is much more variation in feeding standards for roosters compared to those used for hens. Diet nutrient density can vary from high nutrient dense diets formulated for hens in hot climates, to low nutrient dense diets formulated specifically for the males. Males have much lower needs for protein/amino acids and calcium compared to hens. Likewise daily feed allocation can vary from as low as 100 g/bird/day to as high as 165 g daily as fed to the hens. Both extremes are undesirable. While extra calcium intake does not seem to be problematic for adult males, high protein intake is correlated with reduced fertility. Energy intake is however probably the critical nutrient for the male, and as such their needs are greatly influenced by environmental temperature. Feeding much less than 350 kcal ME/day to mature males in moderate climates seems to result in reduced fertility. There have also been reports of poorer male broiler offspring performance for chicks hatched from roosters fed 300-340 vs 380 kcal ME/kg.

Bramwell *et al.* (1996) recently correlated energy intake of roosters with both semen production and hatchability (Table 5.37). As energy intake increased there was a greater percentage of males producing semen later in the breeding cycle. This situation was correlated with increased size of the testes (Table 5.37). In addition to more males producing semen, the higher energy intake also resulted in greater sperm penetration of the previtelline membrane, which is a useful measure of potential fertility.

TABLE 5.37 Adult male performance in relation to energy intake

	Males producing semen (%)			**Hatch of set**	**Sperm penetration Day 2**	**Testes wt**
kcal ME/d	**38 wk**	**42wk**	**46 wk**	**%**	**(#)**	**(g)**
290	100	55	36	61	20	9
330	100	73	64	66	100	12
370	100	100	82	65	160	26

Adapted from Bramwell *et al.* (1996)

Young breeder **-** The period during early maturity is probably the most critical in the adult life of the breeder male. Up to about 30 weeks of age the breeder male is still expected to grow quite fast. For example a weight gain of around 1.4 kg is expected between 10 and 20 weeks of age, and this is only slightly reduced to around 1.2 kg weight gain between 20 and 30 weeks. It is very important to maintain this growth potential through to 30 weeks, therefore, continued monitoring of body weight is critical.

The major complication of feeding the breeder male at this time relates to the separate male/female feeding systems now commonly used. Grills on the female feeders are usually around 43 mm in width. Unfortunately 19- 21 week old male breeders, when first moved to the breeder facilities, will have a head width slightly less than this. The males will, therefore, eat from the female feeders while they still have a smaller head size. Different males will grow at different rates, and their head width will reach >43 mm, on average around 26-28 weeks. The larger birds usually have larger heads, and so there is a self limiting system that evolves with gradual exclusion of males from the female feeder lines over time. However one is faced with the problem of trying to estimate the males feed and nutrient intake. One answer to this problem has been the use of so called "nose-bars" which are plastic rods inserted through the nostrils of the bird. This "nose-bar" effectively excludes the male from the female feeder line almost immediately, and the males will only take feed from their own feed line. The effectiveness of "nose-bars" has been reported as quite variable, and like many situations with broiler breeders, there undoubtedly needs to be a desire by the flock supervisors to make the system work. Another potential solution to the problem of male access to the hen feeders, is to delay placement of the males in the breeder house until 22-23 weeks, when the male's head width will naturally be wider. This management decision should not affect fertility, because eggs are rarely saved for hatching until 27-28 weeks of age, and by this time there will be normal male activity in the breeder house. If males are held in the growing facilities until 22-23 weeks, it is important to light stimulate them according to the hen lighting schedule. This will ensure that roosters are as mature as the hens when introduced at this later date.

Leaving males un-dubbed also helps in earlier exclusion of males from the female line. Sometimes this causes problems of roosters getting their combs caught in mechanical equipment. Dubbing the back 20% of the comb seems beneficial in these situations. Consideration of comb size raises another important consideration of feeder design. Much emphasis has been placed on grill width ($\simeq$ 43 mm) although too often grills provide too much height, such that roosters will force their way into the hen feeders. If roosters are not dubbed, then grill height should be no more than 70 mm, and ideally closer to 65 mm. If roosters are dubbed, then grill height should be no more than 60 mm.

The other major variable affecting breeder male feed intake, is environmental temperature. Because maintenance plays such a major role in nutrient needs, then environmental temperature can greatly influence the amount of energy needed to maintain body temperature. Birds will need more energy in cooler environments, and less energy under warmer conditions. Unfortunately it is difficult to differentiate energy from the other nutrients in a diet, and meeting fluctuating energy needs can only practically be accommodated by varying overall feed intake.

Table 5.38 gives examples of feed intake for breeder males, with emphasis on the critical period up to 36 weeks of age. Because in most cases males will have some access to the female feeders, this system has been emphasized in Table 5.38, and suggested intakes are shown under various environmental conditions. Table 5.38 also shows suggested feed intake for males excluded from female feeders, using techniques such as "nose-bars". Under comparable environmental conditions, these birds should be given more feed, because this allocation is their only source of feed.

TABLE 5.38 Examples of feeding schedules for male breeders consuming a diet with 2900 kcal ME/kg (grams/bird/day)

	Assuming males have access to hen feeders until approximately 28 weeks age				Assuming males totally excluded from hen feeders	
Age (weeks)	>35°C	20-28°C	(kcal ME/day)	<15°C	20-28°C	(kcal ME/day)
20	108	110	319	120	115	334
22	110	115	334	125	118	342
24	112	118	342	130	120	348
26	120	125	363	135	130	377
28	124	130	377	140	135	392
30	130	135	392	150	135	392
32	135	140	406	155	130	377
34	130	135	392	152	130	377
36	125	130	377	148	128	371
40	125	128	370	145	128	371
50	120	126	365	140	126	365
60	120	126	365	140	126	365

When roosters have access to hen feeders, we have a major feeding management decision to make at around 28-30 weeks of age. At this time almost all roosters will be unable to get into the hen feeder, and they are suddenly faced with a potential major reduction in feed intake. At this time the roosters can start to lose weight and/or start to become very aggressive. One management decision, as shown in Table 5.38, is to increase the rooster feed at this time, and then more gradually wean them off of this extra allowance over the next few weeks. Roosters that previously had access to the hen feeder line are given more feed, especially from 30-36 weeks, compared to those birds with "nose-bars" etc. By 40 weeks of age, all roosters should be fed about the same amount of feed, regardless of whether or not they previously had access to the hen feeders. The feed intake numbers shown in Table 5.38 correspond to diets of 2900 kcal ME/kg. If diet energy level is much different from 2900 kcal, then daily feed intake should be adjusted so as to maintain these energy intake values. Corresponding daily energy intake values can be calculated for birds kept at <15°C or >35°C. The data shown in Table 5.38 are only guidelines and again it must be stressed that any pre set feeding schedule must be flexible based on actual growth achieved by the breeder males.

Older breeder - After 30-35 weeks of age, a slow down in the male's growth is expected, and so there can be a corresponding reduction in feed intake. Because maintenance requirement assumes almost the entire nutrient needs of this slower growing older bird, the mature male's feeding needs are greatly affected by environmental temperature. After 30 weeks of age the temperature effects on feed intake as shown in Table 5.38 are accentuated relative to that occurring prior to this time. As at other times in the production cycle, it is critical to weigh sample birds in order to determine actual growth and development.

The usual problem encountered in this period is roosters becoming overweight, and especially overly fat. The simple reason for this is excessive nutrient intake in relation to needs for maintenance. Extra growth will only occur if extra nutrients are available. The most important nutrients at this time are energy and protein. After 35 weeks of age, the rooster needs only the equivalent of around 10% crude protein, albeit well-balanced in the important amino acids. Energy needs are shown in Table 5.38, although sample weighing of birds will quickly tell if the allocation is correct. If roosters become excessively overweight/obese, there should be an attempt at reducing their nutrient intake. If roosters are 200-400 g overweight, then body weight control can be achieved by reducing daily feed allowance by 5 g/bird/day each week until desired weight and condition are achieved. If roosters are >500 g overweight, it may be essential to use a low nutrient dense feed (see next section) as well as reducing allocation over time. The reason for using a low nutrient dense feed is to maintain weight uniformity because proportionally more feed can be given daily (albeit at reducing quantities weekly). Any manager facing these problems should seriously evaluate the feeding management strategy of birds in the critical 19-30 week period.

Separate male feeds - Male and female breeders will usually be fed the same diets up to maturity. In the breeder facilities there is the choice of using the breeder hen diet for all birds, or a separate diet specifically formulated for males. Such male diets will usually be much lower in crude protein, amino acids and calcium compared to the breeder hen diet (Table 5.39).

TABLE 5.39 Separate male breeder diet	
Metabolizable energy (kcal/kg)	2650-2750
Crude Protein (%)	10.0 - 12.0
Calcium (%)	0.75
Available Phosphorus (%)	0.30
Sodium (%)	0.18
Methionine (%)	0.24
Methionine + Cystine (%)	0.44
Lysine (%)	0.50
Tryptophan	0.13
Mineral-Vitamin Premix	As per breeder hens

The advantage of a separate male diet is that it more closely meets the male's nutrient requirements and allows for a slightly more generous feeding allowance. The protein and amino acid needs of the mature male are very low, being in the range of 10% CP. Such low protein diets are often difficult and expensive to formulate, but body weight control, and subsequent fertility, will usually be improved. A practical compromise formulation is around 12% crude protein or to use a 14-15% pullet grower diet. When low protein diets are used it must be remembered that protein quality is still very important. For these low protein diets, methionine should be maintained at 2% of the protein, and lysine at around 5%. Using a lower energy level, such as 2650 kcal/kg, together with the lower protein, means that we can give males more feed. This extra feed prolongs feeding time, helps maintain weight uniformity within the group and helps reduce aggressiveness. The calcium present in the hen breeder diet is also excessively high for the male. Because it is not producing eggshells, the male needs only a low level of calcium in the diet. Any extra calcium intake may pose additional stress on the kidney, although under most farm conditions, the roosters can handle this extra calcium load. However, when combined with other stressors to the kidney, such as high intakes of protein or mineral, infectious bronchitis, or mycotoxins such as ochratoxin, there can be problems with the general function of the bird's kidney.

While there are distinct advantages to using a separate male diet, the major disadvantage is the practical problem of handling relatively small quantities of feed, often in bags. The potential advantages for a separate male diet can be quickly lost if male feed is stored on-farm for extended periods. If male feed is stored for more than 6 weeks, especially in hot humid weather, then any advantages may be counterbalanced by potential loss of nutrients and/or mold growth.

5.6 NUTRITION AND HATCHABILITY

Successful hatching of an egg depends upon a fertile egg having adequate nutrients and environmental conditions such that the embryo can develop into a viable chick. From a nutritional point of view, hatchability can be influenced by fertility of both male and female breeders, the nutrients deposited in the egg for the embryo, and certain physical egg characteristics that can affect gas and water exchange during incubation. Traditionally, vitamin status of breeders is often considered the major nutritional factor influencing hatchability, although we now know that imbalance or excess of a number of nutrients can affect embryo viability. In the following discussion it is assumed that incubation conditions are ideal, and also that eggs are stored and transported under appropriate environmental and sanitary conditions.

Fertility - There is surprisingly little information available on the effect of nutrition on fertility, especially for the hen. With hens it is assumed that if she is capable of producing eggs, and if viable sperm are available, fertility will occur. Nutritional effects on female fertility are, therefore, assumed to be quite minor in relation to nutritional effects on egg formation *per se*. While this is true for nutrients such as vitamins and minerals, it may not be true for nutrients affecting general body size and body composition, such as diet protein and diet energy. In a recent study, Lopez and Leeson (1995) indicated that protein level of the diet of breeder hens had a significant effect on fertility (Table 5.40).

TABLE 5.40 Diet protein and female fertility to 64 weeks of age

Diet protein (%)	Fertility (%)
16	91.6[b]
14	93.3[a]
12	95.1[a]
10	95.4[a]

In these diets, methionine and lysine levels were kept constant, as was energy level, and only diet crude protein varied. All roosters were fed a separate male diet at 12% CP, so the data shown in Table 5.40 is a true female effect. Lopez and Leeson (1995) concluded that this apparent crude protein effect was simply due to body weight, because hens on the lower protein diets were smaller throughout the experiment. Birds fed 10% CP were some 500 g smaller than birds fed 16% CP at 64 weeks, even though feed and energy intake were similar for all treatment groups. Limiting excess body weight after peak production is, therefore, important in maintaining greater mating activity of these smaller more active birds. In this respect, overfeeding both protein and energy is expected to reduce fertility, simply by making birds obese, and less willing to mate with the roosters. This same concept also applies to roosters, where overfeeding of protein and/or energy is likely to result in reduced fertility. Overfeeding of male Leghorn breeders results in a dramatic decline in total sperm production with associated increase in production of dead spermatozoa. The introduction of separate male feeding systems has also resulted in better fertility, simply because of better control over feed intake of the rooster. However, even with separate male feeding, it seems advantageous to use low protein diets as described previously (McDaniel, 1986, Fig. 5.7).

Fig. 5.7 Diet protein level and percentage of roosters producing semen (from McDaniel, 1986).

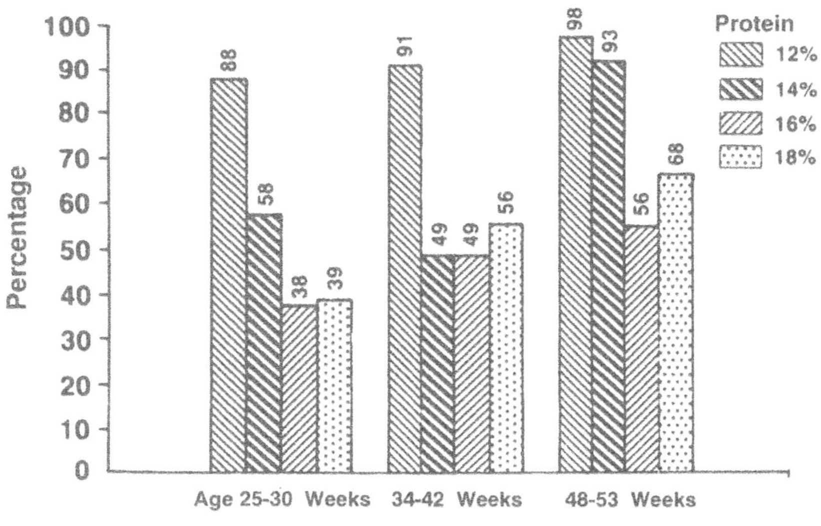

Hatchability - Nutritional effects on hatchability of fertile eggs are not easily quantified, apart from the effect of gross deficiencies of vitamins and some other nutrients. Table 5.41 provides a summary of common embryo deficiency symptoms for selected vitamins and minerals. It should be emphasized that classical deficiency symptoms of individual vitamins are rarely seen. More often, multiple vitamin deficiencies occur when vitamin premixes are inadvertently omitted from the diet, or more commonly, deficiencies are induced by some other nutrient or toxin.

TABLE 5.41 Common embryo deficiency symptoms for vitamins and minerals

Nutrient	Deficiency symptoms
Vitamin A	Early embryo mortality (48 hours) with failure to develop circulatory system.
Vitamin D3	Depending on reserves in hens, stunted chicks and soft bones. Usually associated with shell defects and hence changes in porosity of the shell. Symptoms seen within 12d in diets devoid of synthetic D3.
Vitamin E	Usually see early embryo mortality at 1-3d. Encephalomalacia may be seen in the embryo and exudative diathesis is common.
Riboflavin	Excessive embryo mortality 9-14 or 17-21d. Embryos show edema and/or clubbed down. Chicks may show a curling of the toes. Symptoms occur within 3-5d.
Pantothenic acid	Subcutaneous hemorrhages in unhatched embryos.
Biotin	Reduced hatch without reduced egg production. Peak in embryo mortality during first week and last 3 days of incubation. May see skeletal deformities and crooked beaks.
Vitamin B_{12}	Embryo mortality around 8-14 days, with possibly edema, curled toes and shortening of the beak.
Thiamine	There are two stages of embryo mortality - one very early and the other at 19-21d. Many dead chicks appear on the trays although there are few, if any, deformed chicks. Mortality can be high for 10-14 days for those chickens that do hatch. Injecting the chicks with thiamine results in an almost instantaneous recovery. Certain types of disinfectants, anticoccidials and poor quality fish meal have been implemented in thiamine deficiencies. There is also recent evidence to suggest that thiamine requirements are increased in the presence of some Fusarium molds.
Niacin	Embryo mortality in the 8-17d period, depending upon tryptophan level of the breeder diet. Some skeletal abnormalities and retarded feathering.
Calcium and phosphorus	As maternal deficiency progresses, embryo mortality shifts from later to earlier stages of incubation. Shortened and thickened legs are seen with shortened lower mandible, bulging forehead, edema of neck and protruding abdomen. Shell quality is usually affected.
Zinc	Numerous skeletal deficiencies, and feather down may appear to be “tufted”.
Manganese	Late embryo mortality (18 to 21 days). Embryos show shortened wings and legs with abnormal head and beak shape. Edema is common and feather down is usually abnormal.

These latter effects are obviously difficult to diagnose, because diet analysis reveals a correct vitamin level, even though a deficiency of that vitamin is evident metabolically.

In situations of complex vitamin deficiency, caused for example by accidentally failing to add the vitamin premix, then riboflavin deficiency is often the first to appear, and this has the most dramatic effect on breeders with hatchability reaching very low levels within 3-4 weeks (Table 5.42). In this study, breeder hens were fed corn-soy diets where the premix was formulated without individual vitamins as detailed. For some vitamins, corn and soybean meal will provide some base level, and this may be the reason for differential results. The response to riboflavin is most severe, with hatchability down to zero in seven weeks. After 15 weeks, a regular fortified diet was reintroduced, and as shown in Table 5.42, for all treatments hatchability returned to normal within 4 weeks. Hatchability problems related to vitamin deficiencies therefore appear to be reversible once adequate diets are fed, and there seems to be no long lasting effect. A practical problem with on farm nutritional deficiencies is that hatchability declines are not seen until three weeks after deficient diets are consumed. For this reason, weekly checks on embryo survival will give a much quicker indication of potential problems. This type of data is shown in Table 5.43, which relates to the same study detailed in Table 5.42.

TABLE 5.42 Hatchability of eggs produced by caged breeders fed corn-soybean diets devoid of supplemental vitamins (% fertile eggs)

	Vitamin omitted from control diet							
Week on diet	None (control)	Biotin	B_{12}	E	Folacin	Niacin	Panto-thenate	Ribo-flavin
1	95	86	97	97	97	96	94	95
3	97	83	95	84	89	87	81	55
5	98	63*	84	67	30*	61*	74*	19*
7	92	54*	61*	62*	19*	69	26*	1*
13	88	52	27*	95	38*	50	54	0*
15[x]	90	96	21*	75	70	38*	56	0*
17	95	90	50*	58*	85	61	40*	57*
19	97	99	99	92	99	98	97	96

* Significantly different from control (P < .05).
[X] Vitamins reintroduced.

TABLE 5.43 Incidence and age of dead germs from eggs produced by breeder hens fed diets devoid of supplemental vitamins (% fertile eggs)

Week on diet	Vitamin omitted from control diet																	
	None (control)			Biotin			B_{12}			E			Pantothenate			Riboflavin		
	E	M	L[1]	E	M	L	E	M	L	E	M	L	E	M	L	E	M	L
1	5	0	0	11	0	2	3	0	0	0	1	0	6	0	0	4	0	1
3	2	0	0	11	0	5	3	0	1	6	0	6	18*	0	0	10	7*	24*
5	0	0	0	23*	1	5	10*	1	1	7	15*	6	19*	0	4	34*	31*	5
7	2	0	2	15*	6*	5	4	21*	1	10	14*	4	16*	36*	6	70*	24*	1
13	9	0	2	33	1	3	0	39*	18	2	2	0	28	3	3	47*	36*	0
15[2]	0	0	10	0	0	4	0	0	79*	0	0	25	12*	3	4	28*	16*	39
17	1	3	0	7	2	0	0	50*	0	0	3	35	39*	4	0	7	5	16*
19	2	0	1	0	0	1	1	0	0	1	0	7	1	0	0	1	0	1

*Significantly different from control within each age group ($P < 0.05$)

[1]E, 1-7 days; M, 8-14 days; L, 15-21 days of incubation

[2]Vitamins reintroduced

The pattern of embryo mortality in the treatment groups should be compared with that occurring in the control fed birds. Within 3 weeks, in the case of riboflavin, and within 5 weeks for most other vitamins, there is a dramatic increase in incidence of dead embryos which coincides with the loss in hatchability shown in Table 5.42. The most characteristic feature of this study is embryo mortality occurring in the mid, 8-14 day, period of incubation. For the control birds there is virtually no mortality in this period. Likewise for the treatment birds in the first week of the study, or in the last week of the study 4 weeks after reintroduction of the control diet, there is again no 8-14 d embryo mortality. These data suggest that 8-14 d embryo mortality can be used as a diagnostic tool for establishing hatchability problems related to inadequate breeder vitamin nutrition. Vitamin deficiencies, of course, should not occur under commercial conditions, because all requirement needs should be met by synthetic sources in the premix. In fact breeder diets often contain the highest levels of supplemental vitamins of any class of poultry, and this is sometimes questioned as being too costly. In feeding breeders we not only want to prevent signs of deficiency as detailed previously, but also to ensure optimum production and hatchability. The superior performance of breeders routinely seen today, with peaks of 85-88%, will only be achieved by feeding relatively high levels of vitamins as part of a balanced nutritional program.

One reason for higher vitamin fortifications relative to standards, such as NRC (1994), is the loss in potency of vitamins that can occur between feed manufacture and consumption by the bird. Different vitamins are susceptible to various stresses by varying degrees, but as a generalization it can be stated that the major causes of loss of vitamin potency are storage time, storage temperature, and storage humidity of the premix before mixing, and of the feed after mixing. Another major loss of vitamins occurs if they are premixed with minerals and stored for any length of time prior to incorporation in feed. Also conditions within the premix and feed can cause loss of potency. For example, some vitamins are acidic whereas others break-down under acidic conditions. Finally, breeder feed is sometimes pelleted, and here the temperature and humidity involved can cause vitamin breakdown.

An obvious question is the cost effectiveness of adding relatively high levels of vitamins so as to ensure good egg production and optimum hatchability. A major producer of pure vitamins, recently conducted a survey of commercial breeder operations in the USA and, as anticipated, found a range of vitamin levels being used. This industry data covered 62 broiler companies and represents about 90% of the industry. Table 5.44 shows the highest and lowest vitamin levels being used, compared to NRC (1994). There is about a 100% difference between the top 25% and bottom 25% of reported levels for vitamin fortification. Table 5.44 also shows the cost of obtaining these individual vitamin levels, and the total cost per tonne of mixed feed.

TABLE 5.44 Breeder vitamin levels and costs						
	Industry High (Top 25%)[1]		Industry Low (Bottom 25%)[1]		NRC (1994)	
Vitamin	Level	$/t feed	Level	$/t feed	Level	$/t feed
Vit. A (IU/kg)	12,800	0.68	8,100	0.43	3,000	0.16
Vit. D_3 (IU/kg)	3,500	0.08	2,100	0.05	300	0.01
Vit. E (IU/kg)	36	0.70	14.3	0.30	10	0.19
Vit. K_3 (mg/kg)	3.1	0.13	0.74	0.03	1.0	0.04
Thiamine (mg/kg)	3.2	0.11	1.0	0.04	0.7	0.03
Riboflavin (mg/kg)	9.9	0.53	5.6	0.29	3.6	0.19
Pantothenic acid (mg/kg)	17.3	0.38	9.3	0.20	7.0	0.15
Niacin (mg/kg)	43	0.27	23	0.14	10	0.06
Pyridoxine (mg/kg)	6.0	0.31	1.4	0.07	4.5	0.23
Folic acid (mg/kg)	1.3	0.13	0.63	0.06	0.35	0.03
Biotin (µg/kg)	220	0.77	88.0	0.31	100	0.35
Vit. B_{12} (µg/kg)	17.5	0.09	10	0.05	8	0.04
Total		$4.18/t		$1.97/t		$1.47/t
Cost/breeder 20-64 weeks		17.5		8.24		6.14

[1]BASF Technical Bulletin #KC9305

Obviously the bottom line is how well breeders perform based on high vs low industry values. Such data is unavailable, but it can be noted that the higher vitamin levels cost about 10¢ more per breeder, which in most markets is equivalent to 0.5 chicks per breeder. Considering that a number of the low industry vitamin levels (Table 5.44) are even less than NRC (1994), it is assumed that this will affect hatchability, and this will be much more than 0.5 chicks per breeder. Marginal vitamin levels can easily result in loss of 2-5 chicks per breeder, which is 4-10 times the cost of the extra vitamins in the feed. With these extra levels of vitamins in the feed, there should be no need to use supplemental vitamins in the water, except in situations of environmental or disease stress when feed intake is not optimal, or where there is evidence of enteritis.

If vitamin levels are to be adjusted according to local conditions, then which ones are most likely to influence feed cost? Vitamin E, biotin and vitamin A are usually the most expensive, and together make up over 50% of the cost of the vitamin premix. These three vitamins should, therefore, receive most attention when additions to, or deletions from premixes are contemplated, based upon knowledge of specific needs within a feeding program.

Vitamins are expensive, with the premix representing about 2-3% of the cost of breeder feed. However the effects of deficient or marginal levels in breeder feed can be far greater than the 10¢ per breeder potentially saved by feeding at the low vs high end of current industry standards.

While vitamin deficiencies should only occur under unusual circumstances, there is an indication that lower hatchability, related to vitamin metabolism, may occur when high protein diets are fed. Although there has been no definitive research to implicate high protein intakes with induced vitamin deficiencies, there is substantial circumstantial evidence from a number of studies showing that with high crude protein diets, there is often reduced hatchability and embryo mortality which suggest problems with vitamin adequacy of the egg. It is possible that deamination and transamination involved in "excretion" of excess nitrogen could impose a very high metabolic demand for B vitamins. Work out of the UK and more recent work with both Leghorn and broiler breeders shows a consistently reduced hatchability for birds fed high vs low protein diets.

In relation to industry practice, "high protein" levels as discussed here are really not too high compared to normal feeding practice. In our work "high protein" refers to 25 g protein/bird/day. In order to achieve a "high" protein intake of 25 g/b/d, a flock of breeders consuming 160 g/b/d would achieve this intake with a diet of only 15.7% CP. A comparable protein intake by Leghorns consuming 100 g/b/d would be achieved with a diet level of 25% CP. Obviously the breeder hen requires more protein than does the Leghorn for maintenance, although with a 1 kg body weight difference this should amount to only 3 g/b/d. If these calculations are correct, then breeders are being overfed by some 5 g CP/d.

Breeder nutrition and broiler growth **-** There are a few reports of breeder nutrition having a direct effect on broiler growth. Perhaps the most direct effect is via egg size, because this is correlated with broiler market weight-for-age. In general a 1 g difference in egg size results in a 10-15 g difference in ≥40 d broiler weight, and especially for males. Nutritionally, egg size is controlled by protein intake, or more specifically, the intake of methionine and also linoleic acid. Because most breeders world-wide are fed corn-based diets today, linoleic acid deficiency is not usually encountered. However with wheat or sorghum based diets, it may be necessary to add at least 1% fat to the diet to ensure a minimum 1% linoleic acid level in the diet.

Protein:energy ratio of the diet has also been shown to influence chick weight (Fig 5.8).

Fig. 5.8 Effect of diet protein: energy ratios on chick weight for 28 week old broiler breeders (adapted from Spratt and Leeson, 1987)

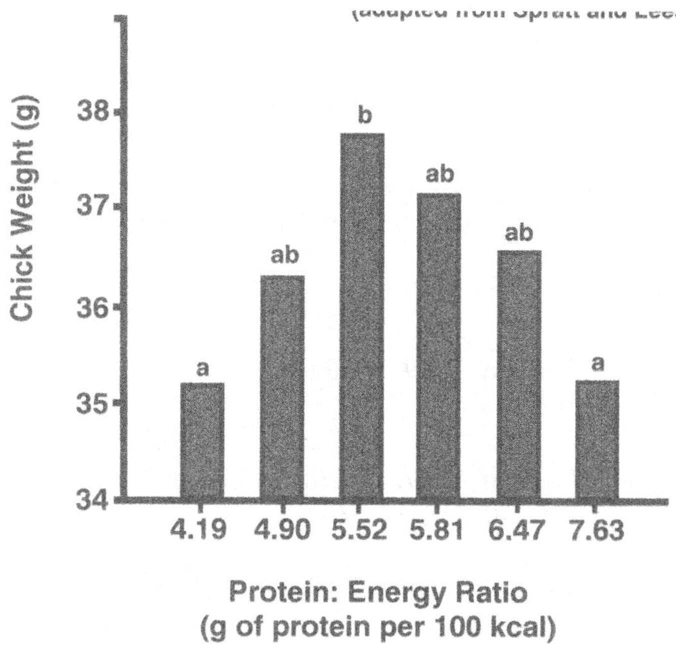

Chick size is reduced when energy:protein is low, which is usually a consequence of high protein, used in conjunction with low energy. Although less frequently seen in industry, small chick size can also occur as a result of a very high energy:protein ratio which is usually a consequence of low protein used in conjunction with high energy.

These results are generally in agreement with the earlier research findings from the UK suggesting that high protein levels are detrimental to breeder performance especially when used in association with lower energy intakes. In our studies, breeders fed the highest energy allowance produced significantly heavier male offspring at 20 d, with the effect being +4% in weight at 41d (Table 5.45).

TABLE 5.45 Effect of breeder diet on growth of male broiler offspring

	Breeder protein		Breeder energy intake		
	High	**Low**	**High**	**Medium**	**Low**
0-20d weight gain (g)	549	548	562a	547ab	537b
0-41d weight gain (g)	1808	1850	1856	1840	1790

Adapted from Spratt and Leeson (1987)

These findings indicate the importance of adequate energy intake by the breeder, not only in terms of breeder performance, but also of early growth rate of offspring.

BIBLIOGRAPHY

Bennett, C.D. and S. Leeson, 1989. Water usage of broiler breeders. Poult. Sci. 68:617-621.

Bennett, C.D. and S. Leeson, 1989. Growth of broiler breeder pullets with skip-a-day vs daily feeding. Poult. Sci. 68:836-838.

Bennett, C.D., S. Leeson and H.S. Bayley, 1990. Heat production of skip-a-day and daily fed broiler breeder pullets. Can. J. Anim. Sci. 70:667-671.

Bramwell, R.K., C.D. McDaniel, W.H. Burke, J.L. Wilson and B. Howarth, 1996. Influence of male broiler breeder dietary energy intake on reproduction and progeny growth. Poult. Sci. 75:767-775.

Burke, W. and L.S. Jensen, 1994. Energy restriction of breeder hens affects performance. Arbor Acres Review 37(1).

Clunies, M., R.J. Etches, C. Fair and S. Leeson, 1993. Blood, intestinal and skeletal calcium dynamics during egg formation. Can. J. Anim. Sci. 73:517-532.

Combs, G.F., 1968. Amino acid requirements of broiler and laying hens. Proc. Maryland Nutr. Conf. P. 86-96.

Farmer, M., D.A. Roland and J. Brake, 1983. Calcium metabolism in broiler breeder hens. Poult. Sci. 62:459-464.

Hocking, P.M., 1993. Optimum size of feeder grids in relation to the welfare of broiler breeder females on a separate sex basis. Br. Poult. Sci. 34:848-855.

Hurwitz, S. and S. Bornstein, 1973. The protein and amino acid requirements of laying hens. Poult. Sci. 52:1124-1134.

Leeson, S. and J.D. Summers, 1983. Consequences of increased feed allowance of growing broiler breeder pullets as a means of stimulating early maturity. Poult. Sci. 62:6-11.

Leville, G.A., R. Shapiro and H. Fisher, 1960. Amino acid requirements for maintenance in the adult rooster. J. Nutr. 72:8-15.

Lilburn, M.S. and D.J. Myers-Miller, 1990. Effect of body weight, feed allowance and dietary protein intake during the prebreeder period on early reproductive performance of broiler breeder hens. Poult. Sci. 69:1118-1125.

Lopez, G. and S. Leeson, 1995. Response of broiler breeders to low-protein diets. 1. Adult breeder performance. Poult. Sci. 74:685-695.

McDaniel, G.R., 1986. Feeding systems found to improve broiler performance. Feedstuffs 58 (49).

Samara, M.H., K.R. Robbins, and M.O. Smith, 1996. Interaction of feeding time and temperature and their relationship to performance of the broiler breeder hen. Poult. Sci. 75:34-41.

Spratt, R.S. and S. Leeson, 1987. Determination of ME of various diets using leghorn, dwarf and regular broiler breeder hens. Poult. Sci. 66:314-317.

Spratt, R.S. and S. Leeson, 1987. Effect of protein and energy intake of broiler breeder hens on performance of broiler chicken offspring. Poult. Sci. 66:1489-1494.

Vaughters, P.D., G.M. Pesti and B. Howarth, 1987. Effects of feed consumption and feeding schedule on growth and development of broiler breeder males. Poult. Sci. 66:134-146.

Waldroup, P.W.A., Z. Johnson and W. Bussell, 1976. Estimating daily nutrient requirements for broiler breeder hens. Feedstuffs 48 (28).

Wilson, H.R., D.R. Ingram, F.B. Mather and R.H. Harms, 1989. Effect of daily restriction and age of initiation of a skip-a-day program for young broiler breeders. Poult. Sci. 68:1442-1446.

CHAPTER 6. ENVIRONMENTAL CONTROL

PAGE NO.

Breeders rarely achieve their genetic potential today if any aspect of the environment is stressful to the bird or is poorly managed. As discussed in Chapter 3, one must have absolute control over the lighting schedule regardless of house design or other environmental factors. There is now a trend towards greater control over the environment, especially in the grow-out period, and so black-out housing is becoming more popular. It is assumed that these more costly building designs are economically advantageous in terms of improved control over sexual development. For breeders, black-out housing is the standard in cooler climates and this technology is now being considered in warmer regions, in order to reduce fluctuations in lighting and environmental temperature. When outside temperature is much above 28°C, then there should be consideration for some form of cooling system, such as foggers or evaporative cool cells.

This chapter centres around control of house temperature and humidity since the critical aspects of light control are covered separately in Chapter 3. However, when designing new facilities or retrofitting established buildings, any attempts at modifying environmental systems must not be at the expense of the lighting program. This latter concern is very important with fan and air inlet design for black-out houses.

6.1 BODY TEMPERATURE CONTROL

After brooding, the bird must maintain a body temperature close to 41°C. Being homeothermic, the bird is continually losing heat to its surroundings although the mechanisms involved change as both temperature and humidity change within the environment. Table 6.1 shows normal heat balance in an adult breeder with the need to remove about 325 kcal heat daily.

TABLE 6.1 Heat balance of adult breeder at 22°C		
ME Intake		450 kcal
ME output:	Egg	100 kcal
	Growth	25 kcal
	Heat production	325 kcal

Depending upon acclimatization, birds will die when temperatures reach 40°C, while few birds can survive for very long at temperatures below -10°C. At -2°C, the comb and wattles will freeze. In most commercial houses today there is concern with bird comfort in the range of 0°C to 38°C depending upon the degree of environmental control. Breeder performance will be optimized at around 22-24°C and apart from changes in egg production, there is an incentive in optimizing feed efficiency by maintaining this ideal temperature. While most discussion on environmental control of breeders focuses on temperature, it must be remembered that the prevailing relative humidity is often the factor causing distress to the bird. Conditions of high temperature and low humidity (eg. 32°C, 40% RH) are quite well tolerated by the bird, while high temperature and high humidity (eg. 32°C, 90% RH) are problematic. Figure 6.1 shows the general relationship between temperature and humidity. The bird loses or gains heat by means of radiation, conduction, convection and evaporation and these various systems assume more importance as environmental conditions change.

Fig. 6.1 Generalized bird response to changes in temperature and humidity.

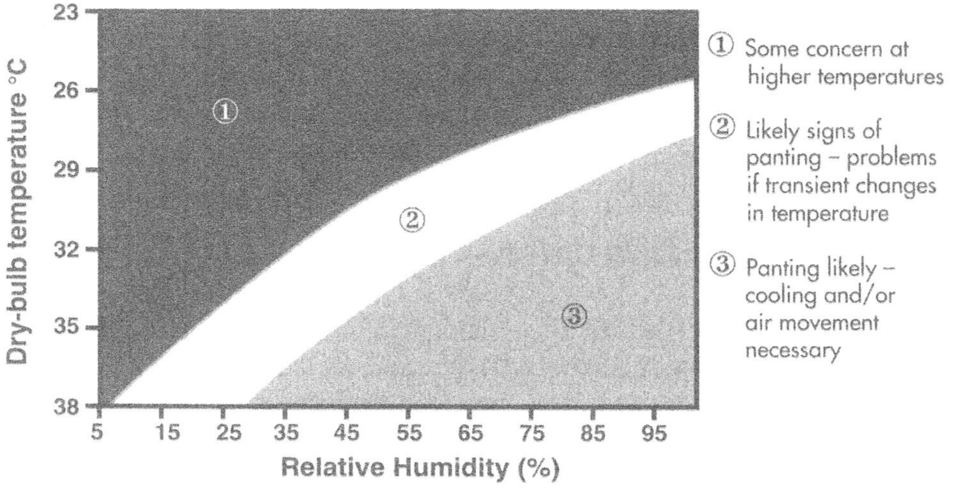

Radiation: Heat is usually radiated away from the bird's body to the surrounding environment, however, there can be a heat load onto the bird in direct intense sunlight. Of more importance, perhaps, is the potential of radiant heat warming up the bird from a heated steel roof. On a sunny day an uninsulated, unpainted steel roof can contribute the equivalent of 5-10°C to the ambient pen temperature. White surfaces reflect solar radiation, and hence the common practice of painting roofs white. At the other extreme, a rusted steel roof provides the worst possible scenario for the birds. As will be discussed later, the radiant heat transfer from the roof can be reduced by applying an insulating layer between the roof and the birds. Layout of the house, in relation to movement of the sun, can also help minimize the effects of solar radiation. Having breeder houses run east-west tends to minimize heat load (Fig. 6.2). When buildings are aligned north-south, then even at sunrise, the east side of the roof is perfectly angled to receive heat from the sun. With an east-west aligned building, the effects of the sun are not maximized until later in the morning, and again more quickly recedes in the late afternoon. With north-south orientation there is also the problem of having different sides of the house heated at different times. In the morning, the east side of the roof is going to be much warmer than the west side, and vice-versa in the afternoon.

Fig. 6.2 Effect of solar radiation on houses aligned East-West and North-South.

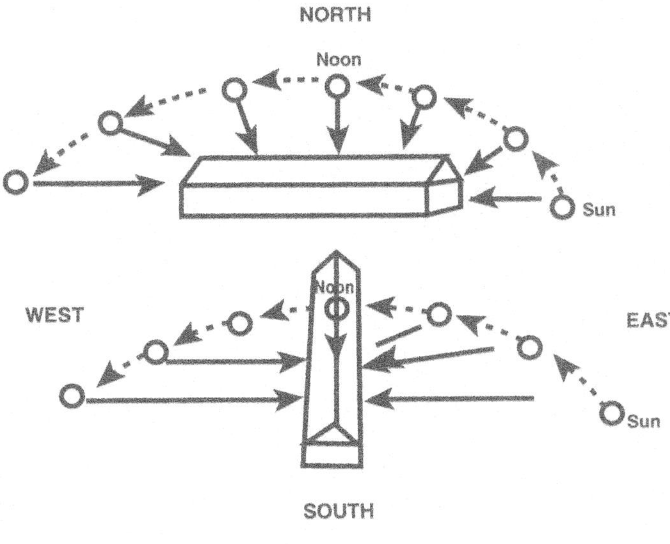

This change in heat load is radiated down to the birds and can cause their migration to the cooler side of the building. Orienting buildings east-west also minimizes the entry of direct sunlight onto the birds and the litter.

Conduction **-** Heat is usually conducted away from the bird to any object that it touches. This situation assumes that such objects are <41°C. In extreme heat stress situations, and especially where litter is wetter than ideal, then heat can be conducted to the bird from litter that is essentially fermenting. It is always useful to measure litter temperature under such conditions, because this may be contributing to the "effective" temperature of the bird.

Convection **-** The air immediately (within 1-2mm) around the bird is trapped in a boundary layer that will be much closer to body temperature than ambient environmental temperature. For example, with air temperature at 30°C, the boundary layer of air may be at 39°C. This situation occurs with all animals, and is complicated somewhat in the bird by the presence of feathers. As the bird moves, the boundary layer is disturbed, and heat is lost from the body. We can make use of this system to mechanically cool birds. At high temperatures, we can disrupt the boundary layer by moving the air around the bird. In fact, during heat stress the bird is less reluctant to move itself, and so sudden air movement reverses the normal situation but has the same cooling effect. This wind-chill effect will only be useful at temperatures up to about 39°C, and obviously becomes less effective as ambient temperature approaches the temperature of the boundary layer. In general, heat loss by convection is proportional to (air speed)^2. For example an air speed of 10 vs 5 meters/min creates a 4-fold increase in cooling.

Evaporation **-** Birds do not sweat and so this important cooling mechanism is unavailable to them. As an alternative, birds lose heat by evaporation through panting and loss of moisture in respired air. Evaporation is a very efficient means of heat-loss. For each 1 g of water vaporized, about 600 calories of energy are utilized. Much above 28°C, evaporation becomes the most important route of heat loss for the bird. Table 6.2 shows water balance of breeders at 22 vs 35°C where increased respiratory loss relates to cooling.

TABLE 6.2 Water balance in breeders at 22 vs 35°C (ml)

	22°C	35°C
Water intake	300	500
Excreta loss	120	200
Egg water	55	55
Respiratory loss	125	245

Under moderate environmental conditions, all routes of heat exchange are important and help to maintain a normal balance. Feather cover will influence conductive and convective heat exchange, and at high temperatures, heavy feather cover becomes a disadvantage. Birds carrying a gene for "naked neck", where there is no feather cover of the head or neck region, seem to be at an advantage under high environmental temperatures. Likewise bird posture can influence heat exchange and we see behavioral changes of birds as they attempt to reduce or increase heat loss from the body. For example, by simply holding their head under the wing, adult birds can reduce their heat loss by 10%, while huddling into groups also reduces loss by up to 10%. During heat distress, birds can increase their heat loss by up to 8% by dropping their wings and by not being in contact with other birds in the flock. When bell drinkers are used, birds are often seen wetting their combs and wattles in an attempt to increase evaporative cooling.

During panting, there is increased air flow through the lungs and air sacs. The air sacs in fact represent about 80% of the tidal volume of air moved during respiration (250 ml vs about 35 ml in the lungs), and so this means that obese birds are more prone to stress because of reduced effective air sac volume.

As environmental temperature increases, then evaporative cooling becomes more important, but in many instances will not be adequate to maintain normal equilibrium. The balance of heat input and output must always equal zero, and so the easiest solution for the bird housed under these extreme environmental conditions, is simply to reduce its heat load. This means reduced feed intake. In essence, the basic aim of our housing systems is to ensure optimum feed intake regardless of fluctuations in the effective environment.

6.2 FEEDING TIME AND HEAT PRODUCTION

Most of the bird's heat load comes from the feed, as consequences of digestion, absorption and nutrient assimilation or excretion. Because there are few nutrient reserves in the body, then these activities occur at fairly predictable times following feed intake. This situation is made even more precise in breeders because of our restricted feeding programs which result in a very predictable time of feed intake. Figure 5.1 (Chapter 5) shows the heat production of growing 12 week old pullets fed 74 g of feed either daily or skip-a-day. As shown in Fig. 5.1, there is a major difference in heat production on feed vs non-feed days for the skip-a-day fed birds. On the feed day, heat production peaks 3-5 hrs after feeding and represents almost 100% increase in heat production compared to unfed birds. While heat production peaks 3-5 hrs after feeding, it is significant over the period from 2-6 hrs following feeding. Increase in heat production is associated with about +1°C rise in body temperature.

This mechanism of heat production associated with feeding is the basis for early morning feeding of breeders. If birds are fed at 6 a.m., then peak heat load will be at 9-11 a.m. which is usually prior to the natural peak heat load in the building. Most problematic for the bird would be feeding at around 10-11 a.m., when heat of feed utilization coincides with the warmest part of the day.

6.3 LIGHTING

The basic principles of lighting programs have been described in Chapter 3. Implementation of a lighting program involves simply manipulating daylength and light intensity within controlled environment buildings or manipulating artificial daylength to augment natural light within open-sided houses. The quantity of light emitted by a lamp is measured in lumens, and efficiency of artificial light is rated in watts per lumen. In this latter respect, the conventional incandescent light provides less lumens per watt of power input than do fluorescent lamps, and these are less efficient than are sodium vapor lamps. Light intensity in the building is measured in lux, which is simply 1 lumen/m^2. The imperial equivalent is the foot candle, which is 1 lumen/ft^2. One lux therefore approximates 10 foot candles.

Incandescent lamps - Conventional light bulbs are referred to as incandescent, where the light source is generated by heating a tungsten filament to about 600°C. Most bulbs are coated inside with a white metal film in order to give a more diffuse light, although this does reduce efficiency somewhat. The main advantage of incandescent lamps is that they are inexpensive. However their disadvantages are a low efficiency of around just 20 lumens per watt and a low life expectancy. Bulbs are rated at so many hours of life, which means the time over which 50% of the bulbs are expected to have burned out. Incandescent lamps are usually rated at 1,000 hours, and so a considerable number of lamps will have burned out by this time. Most bulbs produce a full even spectrum of light, which mimics natural light.

Fluorescent: These bulbs have been used extensively in offices and industrial applications for many years, although they have had little use in poultry buildings until the recent introduction of compact fluorescent fixtures. Fluorescent bulbs produce light from ultra violet radiation resulting from a controlled gas discharge. The inside white lining of these tubes, which is a phosphorus coating, then converts the ultraviolet into visible radiation. These fixtures usually give about 70 lumens per watt of energy input, and are rated for about 10,000 hrs of use. Until quite recently, fluorescent fixtures had the major disadvantage of not being dimmable, so as to change light intensity. Another disadvantage is that light output is affected by temperature, with intensity declining dramatically at temperatures approaching 0°C. Most regular fixtures also fail to "start" at 0°C, although this situation can be overcome by installing more expensive (3-4x) cold start ballasts. All fluorescent fixtures need a ballast to supply the correct voltage to start the gas discharge and then maintain operation. In conventional long tube fixtures, the ballast is large and heavy and this limits application. Compact fluorescent fixtures have a small ballast fitted into the base and these simply screw into the conventional socket. Ballasts are rated A-F, with A being the quietest, and most expensive. F rating ballasts are usually appropriate for use in the poultry house, where noise is of little importance. As previously discussed, "electronic" ballasts are available, at 3-4x the cost, which operate effectively at low temperatures.

Some types of reflectors increase effective light output down to the birds by up to 80%. As a rule-of-thumb, when using reflectors, incandescent wattage) 8 = fluorescent wattage *ie.* a 60 w incandescent = 8 w fluorescent. Without reflectors, the relationship is to divide by a factor of 4. This increased efficiency is realized at an increased capital cost of 8-10x the incandescent bulb.

Gas discharge **-** While fluorescent is a type of gas discharge, this description is usually applied to sodium and mercury vapor lamps. Sodium lamps are usually low pressure (at vacuum) or high pressure (1-2 atmospheres) that produce light by emitting radiation when an electric current is passed through the vaporized sodium. Low pressure sodium lamps are probably the most efficient light sources available today, producing about 140 lumens/watt - this is 7x incandescent and 2x fluorescent. Bulbs are rated for extremely long life at 20,000 hr, but are another magnitude of cost above fluorescent fixtures.

6.4 GAS AND DUST LEVELS

Respirable gas and dust have become an issue in recent years in terms of how they influence humans as well as poultry. European standards are as follows for birds subjected to continuous exposure:

Ammonia 20 ppm
Carbon dioxide 3,000 ppm
Carbon monoxide 10 ppm
Inhalable dust 3.4 mg/m^3
Respirable dust 1.7 mg/m^3
Bacterial toxins 500 ng/m^3

For most people working in breeder houses, ammonia is the most common irritant. Ammonia becomes noticeable at around 20 ppm whereas 40-50 ppm will cause eye irritation within 2-3 minutes. Ammonia levels much above 30 ppm can cause chronic respiratory distress in birds and predispose them to other respiratory infections. Virtually all the ammonia will come from the litter or beneath the slats and is most noticeable in warm humid conditions. However little ammonia is given off from really wet litter or manure. Various feed additives and litter treatments are available with claims of reducing ammonia release from the decomposing litter, which is often a factor of pH change.

In breeder houses, most of the airborne dust will come from the birds themselves, being feather or skin material. This dust is very high in protein and can cause allergic reaction in humans. Dust particles less than 0.5 microns in size rarely settle out unless they join with other particles, or come in contact with vertical surfaces. It is these very small particles that can reach the lung of the birds or humans, and so extra care must be taken when dusting such vertical surfaces. As a generalization, dust that can be seen is called inhalable dust and is usually 2-5 microns in size. Most of these larger dust particles settle out quickly and if inhaled are captured by the epithelial lining of the trachea. It is the respirable dust that is usually invisible to the human eye that can reach the lung and cause chronic respiratory problems.

Dust production will be much higher in situations of low humidity. At 40% relative humidity, dust production per bird has been measured at close to 100 mg/day, while at 70% humidity, production is halved at 50 mg/day. An average dust value in adult breeder houses, at bird level, is around 2-5 mg/m^3, which is a level that likely contributes to respiratory problems in the breeders and attendants. Dust also carries odor compounds, and so filtering air as it leaves a house dramatically reduces odor exhaust from a building. Ammonia can also be absorbed by dust particles which can carry this irritant into the lung. Free ammonia rarely reaches the lung, because it is so soluble in water that it is taken out by the mucous lining of the trachea.

Many bacteria are also carried by dust particles. The most commonly found bacteria are streptococci or staphylococci, although, E. coli has also been isolated from dust. Viruses can also survive attached to dust particles, the classic situation being the realization that Marek's virus can be transmitted by this route. Total microbial counts in breeder houses can be as high as 100 million/m^3. This compares to about 5,000/m^3 in a ventilated egg room and 100/m^3 in fresh outside air.

6.5 BUILDING DESIGN

Breeder houses are of two basic designs, namely total control environment (black-out) and curtain-sided. The majority of birds world-wide are housed in curtain-sided buildings, although there is a trend to black-out housing, even in warmer climates. The main advantage of black-out housing is absolute control over the lighting program together with moderate saving in feed intake. On the other hand, black-out housing costs 3-5x as much as comparable sized curtain houses, although with newer sophisticated curtain mechanism and cool cell additions, the price differential is less.

The actual design and construction of buildings is the responsibility of architects and engineers who are familiar with local laws and restrictions governing farm constructions. As a generalization, houses today are from 10-20m wide and up to 100m long depending upon the need for mechanical ventilation. There is no alternative to concrete floors and steel roofs are becoming universal. Most managers are likely to consider some form of mechanical ventilation in new breeder houses, and so material selection of the walls becomes more critical. Because of the need for relatively long runs of mechanical equipment, there is little alternative to using pressure-treated wood or steel studs for wall construction. Walls constructed from untreated wood or raw poles will invariably warp to some degree, and this compromises most mechanical ventilation systems that rely on inlets managed along the walls.

a) Insulation: Insulation material will be used during construction in order to slow down heat flow through the roof, walls and foundation. Such heat flow can be from the birds to the outside air in cool weather, or from the outside to the birds in warmer climates. In the latter situation, roof insulation is the most critical.

Insulating materials are rated by their "R" value or by the RSI, which relates to resistance to heat transfer. Dense materials such as wood, steel and concrete are poor insulators because they conduct heat very quickly. Good insulators contain trapped air, and so by definition, are very light weight. Table 6.3 shows relative value for 25 mm thicknesses of various construction materials.

Fibreglass and mineral wool have both been used extensively for insulating breeder houses. In N. America, products are usually 40 cm (16") wide so as to fit between wooden studs. Friction-fit, rather than paper wrapped are now preferred, because this product is more elastic and is less prone to sagging over time within the wall.

TABLE 6.3 Insulating values for 25 mm thickness of construction materials		
	RSI[1]	**R value**
Fibreglass	0.60	3.4
Polystyrene	0.65	3.7
Polyurethane	1.00	5.7
Wood	0.30	1.7
Concrete	0.00	0.01
Window-single	0.15	0.85
Window-thermal	0.33	1.87
[1]R x .176 = RSI		

Polystyrene foam is also used to insulate new buildings, but tends to be more expensive than fibreglass. Polystyrene is perhaps the best floor insulator when placed under poured concrete. Most heat loss that occurs from the floor actually takes place at the perimeter through the foundation wall. Insulating the outside of the foundation wall is therefore critical in cooler environments. Polyurethane foam is an ideal material for retrofit insulation. The foam can be sprayed onto existing surfaces, and is particularly useful in insulating roofs. If foam is applied to the outside of the roof, then it usually needs some protective cover, such as plastic resin so as to make it impervious to insects and wild birds. Regardless of the type used, insulating material is very attractive to rodents and insects, and so it should be protected within practical limits. Many insulators, and especially polystyrene and polyurethane are fire hazards, although the problem can be limited by the incorporation of fire retardants during manufacture. Following are guidelines for insulating values suggested for breeder houses:

TABLE 6.4 Insulating values for breeder houses				
	Wall		**Roof**	
	R	**RSI**	**R**	**RSI**
Hot climate	2	0.35	8	1.40
Cold climate	20	3.50	30	5.30

Table 6.5 shows the quantitative effect of insulating a breeder house. In scenario A, the building is uninsulated, and the heat loss is greater than the heat gain from the birds. In scenario B, with insulation, the heat loss is less than the heat gain.

TABLE 6.5 Effect of insulation on heat balance of a breeder house (kcals/hour)	
Scenario A (uninsulated)	
Heat produced by birds =	**60,000**
Heat needed to remove moisture via ventilation =	47,000
Heat loss through building	
- Ceiling	8,000
- Walls	6,000
- Floor	4,000
∴ **Total heat loss =**	**65,000**
Scenario B (insulated)	
Heat produced by birds =	**60,000**
Heat needed to remove moisture via ventilation =	47,000
Heat loss through building	
Ceiling	3,000
Walls	3,000
Floor	2,000
∴ **Total heat loss =**	**53,000**

In reality, heat loss must always equal heat gain. In scenario A, therefore, the ventilation rate must be reduced because the heat loss through the building cannot be controlled. This results in inadequate air movement in the building. Alternatively, if the ventilation rate is maintained, the building will cool down, and birds will have to eat more feed in order to increase heat output. In scenario B, where the building is insulated, we actually have an increased heat load. This latter situation can be accommodated by either increasing the ventilation rate or by reducing feed intake. In such situations, adjustments to the feed intake can only be quite small (4-5%), and so the major resolution to these changing situations will be to move more or less air through the building.

In poorly insulated buildings, the lower limit to ventilation rate is often what is needed to remove moisture from the building. Table 6.6 shows the moisture holding capacity of air at different temperatures. As air temperature rises, it is able to hold much more water. The example shown at the bottom of Table 6.6 indicates the importance of having warm air in the breeder house. In this extreme example, outside air is at -10°C and 90% RH. This air is virtually saturated with water, but because it is cold, it can only hold 40 g of moisture. On entering the breeder house, the air is warmed to 15°C where the original 40 g of moisture now represents only 10% RH. This volume of air can be saturated to 80% RH before it is taken out by the fans, and in this process, the warm air can pick up an extra 260 g of moisture. In cooler, uninsulated buildings, the air cannot be warmed and so it cannot pick up and exhaust as much moisture coming from the birds and litter. Cooler houses will therefore always have wetter litter. In an uninsulated building, the water in the house can also condense out on the walls. This situation happens when the air temperature is below the dew point of the air, or the temperature at which it physically cannot hold more water. Because there is a boundary layer of still air immediately adjacent to the walls, this air will be 4-6°C less than ambient room temperature, and so the dew point can be reached even with ambient house temperatures of 8-12°C.

TABLE 6.6 Moisture holding capacity of air

°C	kg water/450 kg dry air
-20	0.4
-15	0.6
-10	0.8
0	1.7
10	3.2
20	6.0
30	12.0

Eg. 30 m3 air @ -10°C @ 90% RH holds 40 g moisture
30 m3 air @ 15°C @ 10% RH holds 40 g moisture
30 m3 air @ 15°C @ 80% RH holds 300 g moisture

b) Vapor barriers: Insulation used in moderately moist environments is always prone to damage from migration of water through the wall or roof structure. Water vapor in the air exerts a pressure, and so when there is more vapor on one side of the wall than the other side, moisture will migrate - this usually means from inside to outside of the house. Air cools as it passes through the wall and condenses at the dew point as already described. Wet insulation loses up to 80% of its value. This transfer of moisture can be greatly reduced by placing a vapor barrier, usually plastic film, between the inside wall sheathing and the insulation. A plastic vapor barrier must never be placed between the outside wall cladding and the insulation, because this prevents any trapped moisture from eventually moving out of the wall.

6.6 CONTROLLED ENVIRONMENT OR BLACK-OUT HOUSING

Windowless solid-sided buildings, rely totally on mechanical ventilation to remove heat and moisture from the building, and to provide air exchange. For these buildings, the most critical piece of equipment is an alternate source of electricity, because with power disruption birds usually start dying within 1-4 hours depending upon the age and stocking density. Black-out housing is ideally suited to regions where environmental temperature rarely exceeds 32°C, although the incorporation of fogging or evaporative cooling systems can extend this upper range. Well insulated houses are necessary when winter temperatures are consistently below 10-12°C.

Air movement in the breeder house will be controlled by fan numbers, speed and size and more importantly by the design of the air inlets. For adult breeders, air movement needs to be around 10 m^3/bird/hr. However, the ventilation system also needs to have the added flexibility of providing from 5 m^3/bird/hr at the slowest rate and up to as high as 60 m^3/bird/hr for heat stress situations. This assumption is based on a stocking density of 0.3 m^2 per bird, and a ceiling height of 3 m *ie.* a breeder occupies around 1 m^3 of air space in the building.

Actual ventilation rate may be accommodated by fans of different sizes or variable speed fans. The rate of 10 m^3/bird/hr is equivalent to 2.8 litres air/hen/second or 14,000 litres/second for a flock of 5,000 breeders. This capacity could be accommodated by, for example, 3 small fans with capacity of 1,000 litres/second and 3 larger fans rated at 5,000 litres/second. The combination of fans, or regulation of their speed, therefore has to accommodate background continuous ventilation (minimum rate) through to temperature control during hot weather (maximum rate). Fans rarely run unimpeded by wind. Fan rating should be based on a minimum of 31 Pa static pressure (0.125" static pressure). For example; a 25 km/hr wind blowing against the fan is equivalent to 30 Pa static pressure while a 50 km/hr wind increases this loading to 125 Pa.

Air will be brought into the house through inlets that usually run continuously down the angle of the roof and wall of the building. Inlet size needs to be about 65 cm^2/m^3

air moved/minute. In the previous example of 5,000 breeders needing 10m^3/bird/hour, this equates to the need for 54,000 cm^2 of inlet area. If the building is 100 meters long, then inlet capacity can be accommodated by a continuous inlet of 5 cm height running the length of the building. Because inlets tend to become moist, when incoming cold air condenses, inlets can become warped and so a continuous 100 m inlet becomes impractical. Inlet sections of 7-10 m are more manageable. In addition to balancing inlet area with fan capacity, the most important characteristic of the inlet design is the directional flow of air into the building. It is this initial flow of incoming air that dictates air movement throughout the house (Figures 6.3 and 6.4)

Fig. 6.3 Air flow with inlet discharge across the ceiling.

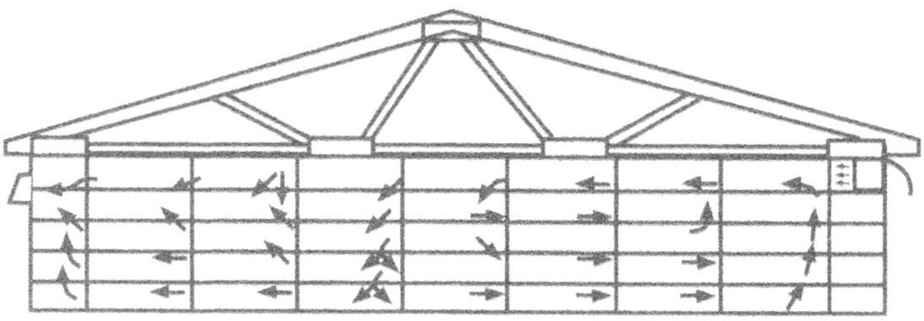

Fig. 6.4 Air flow with inlet discharge vertically onto the litter.

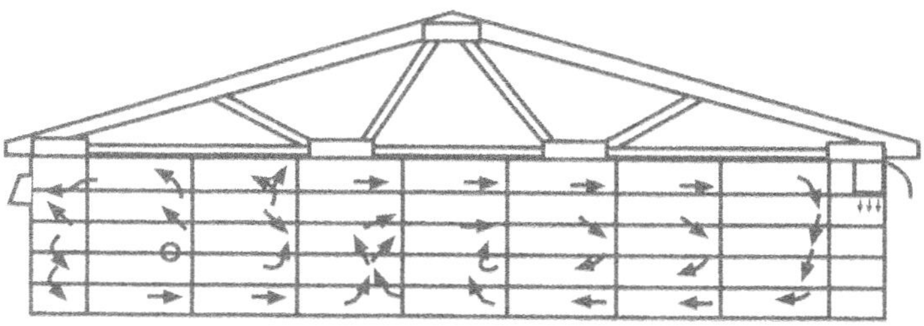

Figure 6.3 shows air movement at various locations in the house when air is initially directed across the ceiling. In Fig. 6.4, the initial air flow is 90^0 different to that of Fig. 6.3, being directly onto the birds. Changing this initial air flow changes air movement by 180° in any section of the house studied *ie.* air flow is reversed. This effect is independent of position in relation to the fan. Inlet design therefore dictates air flow, and such air flow is little affected by fan positioning, or fan speed. Ideally, air will always be vented across the ceiling, rather than directly on to the

birds (*ie.* Fig. 6.3 vs 6.4) since this gives cooler air a longer time to mix with the heated air, prior to its falling on to the birds. Venting cool air directly on to the birds, immediately below the inlet, causes drafts and birds are usually reluctant to stay in this area of the building.

Fans can be positioned on the side wall opposite the inlets to create simple cross ventilation, where air has a minimum distance to travel before being exhausted. Tunnel ventilation can be created by having fans at one end of the house, and the inlets at the opposite end, so that the air has to travel the whole length of the building before being extracted. Such tunnel ventilation usually involves higher air speeds, and so this can be beneficial as a cooling mechanism (see section 6.7). Operation of the fans can either be by thermostats that are reactive to temperature, or to changes in static pressure. Thermostats should be at bird level, or if set at 1.5-2 m height then calculations made for the assumption of a higher temperature at this point than at bird level.

There needs to be a minimum ventilation rate regardless of the environmental temperature. Low temperature sensed by the thermostat should be connected to an alarm system. At higher temperatures, fans can be made to operate sequentially until the maximum ventilation rate is achieved. A high set point temperature can again be connected to an alarm system. Specialized control systems can also use changes in static pressure to control ventilation. Such systems usually involve a powered inlet that can be opened or closed so as to maintain a given level of static pressure in the building. In most situations, the inside of the house will be at a negative static pressure, meaning that slightly more air is removed than is being drawn into the building. Such systems are noticeable by the slight force needed to open the door. Table 6.7 outlines potential ventilation problems that can arise in controlled environment buildings, together with corresponding solutions.

6.7 OPEN OR CURTAIN-SIDED HOUSING

Open or curtain-sided buildings are more suited to warmer climates because even with insulated curtains, it is difficult to maintain house temperature when outside air is <8-10°C.

Without any system of power ventilation, then 13 m is about the maximum width possible because wider buildings will tend to have poorer air movement towards the central locations. Height from the floor to eaves should be at least 2.4 m, and ideally 3 m in very hot climates so as to ensure good air movement. Length of the building, if not ventilated, is usually dictated by the physical terrain. Houses up to 100 m length are standard, but not essential if this means extensive landscaping. As

TABLE 6.7 Ventilation troubleshooting		
Problem	**Potential Causes**	**Potential Solutions**
Building is too cold	Thermostats are set too low or are out of calibration.	Raise thermostat setting. Check thermostat against accurate thermometer.
	Building is not properly insulated.	Properly insulate building.
	Air is being exhausted at ceiling level - the coldest air is at floor level. Removing air from ceiling level removes heat, even at lowest ventilation rates.	Remove air from as low in the building as possible. Air circulation is dictated by air inlets, not fan positioning or size.
	Inlets may be opened too wide - at very low ventilation rates, inlets must almost be closed in order that sufficient pressure differences inside versus outside building are maintained.	Reduce air inlet opening. Implement winter ventilation program.
	Extensive air leaks.	Tighten building by plugging air leaks.
	Insulation may be wet.	Replace wet damaged insulation.
	Too high ventilation rates.	Decrease fan capacity or increase air inlet opening.
Building is too warm	Thermostats are set too high or are out of calibration.	Decrease thermostat setting. Check against accurate thermometer.
	Thermostats located on outside wall.	Relocate thermostats to the middle of house at bird level.
	Thermostat is improperly located - if the thermostat is located in the path of incoming cool air, it gives false reading that is too low.	Relocate thermostats to the interior of the building, which accurately reflects conditions to which chickens are exposed.
	Some fans may not be operating or some fan louvres may be stuck shut.	Check all fans and louvers. Silicone should be used to lubricate fan louvers rather than oil.
	Fans may actually deliver less air velocity than their rated capacity.	Check that all fans are cleaned.
	Air inlets may be partially clogged- suspect this if door slams too hard, indicating too much air pressure difference inside versus outside building.	Clean air inlets
	Inlets closed too tightly.	Open air inlets slightly.
Adapted from Summers 1997. Ventilation Factsheet #88. Poultry Industry Centre, R. R. #2 Guelph, Ontario.		

TABLE 6.7 Ventilation troubleshooting

Problem	Potential Causes	Potential Solutions
Extensive dead air pockets or draftiness	Poorly adjusted inlets.	Close inlets enough to keep air moving at 300 m per minute.
	Air inlets may be partially clogged with dust or feathers.	Clean air inlets.
	Fans may be too few or too small.	Clean fans or increase air volume by increasing fan capacity.
	Building may have air leaks preventing adequate static pressure difference inside versus outside building	Eliminate air leaks.
Extensive moisture in building	Inadequate ventilation if building is too warm.	Reduce air inlet opening slightly while running fans at same or at increased capacity.
	Too much ventilation if building is too cool.	If air is not allowed to warm as it passes through the building, it cannot carry much moisture. Reduce air volume by running fewer fans or reduce air velocity by maintaining fan capacity and opening air inlets slightly.
	Leaky waterers - 1 dripping waterer can add 80 litres of water per day per house.	Stop leaky waterers.
	Unvented gas heaters in work areas - a by-product of combustion is water vapour.	Vent gas heaters directly outside house.
Extensive condensation on walls and ceilings	Building not properly insulated.	Insulate building properly.
	Wet insulation-if insulation gets wet, it is not effective.	Replace wet damaged insulation.
	Inadequate ventilation.	Add heat to building.
	Leaky waterers.	Increase ventilation by increasing fan capacity while maintaining air inlet openings.
		Repair leaky waterers.
Ammonia buildup or wet manure	Ventilation rate too low.	Increase air velocity by reducing air inlet opening or by increasing air volume by increasing fan capacity.
	Thermostat set too high.	Reduce thermostat setting to generate more fan capacity at lower temperatures.
	Leaky waterers.	Repair leaky waterers.
	Watery, loose droppings.	Check for enteritis; check salt content of feed.

Adapted from Summers 1997. Ventilation Factsheet #88. Poultry Industry Centre, R. R. #2 Guelph, Ontario.

with black-out housing there is no substitute for concrete floors and up to 2 m of crushed stone to 0.5 m depth around the perimeter to ensure good drainage. Roof overhang at the eaves should be at least 1m, and designed to prevent direct sunlight hitting the litter between 8 a.m. - 4 p.m. Trees or shrubs planted around buildings are a controversial topic. Most trees are planted for shade. If trees are to be planted, varieties with a large canopy are ideal. The trees should be pruned such that only the trunk is visible up to 2 m in height, such that air flow is not disturbed (Fig 6.5). Thick shrubs at ground level can reduce air flow by up to 30%.

Fig 6.5 Shading from trees, with minimal disturbance to air flow (Avicola Villalobos, Guatemala)

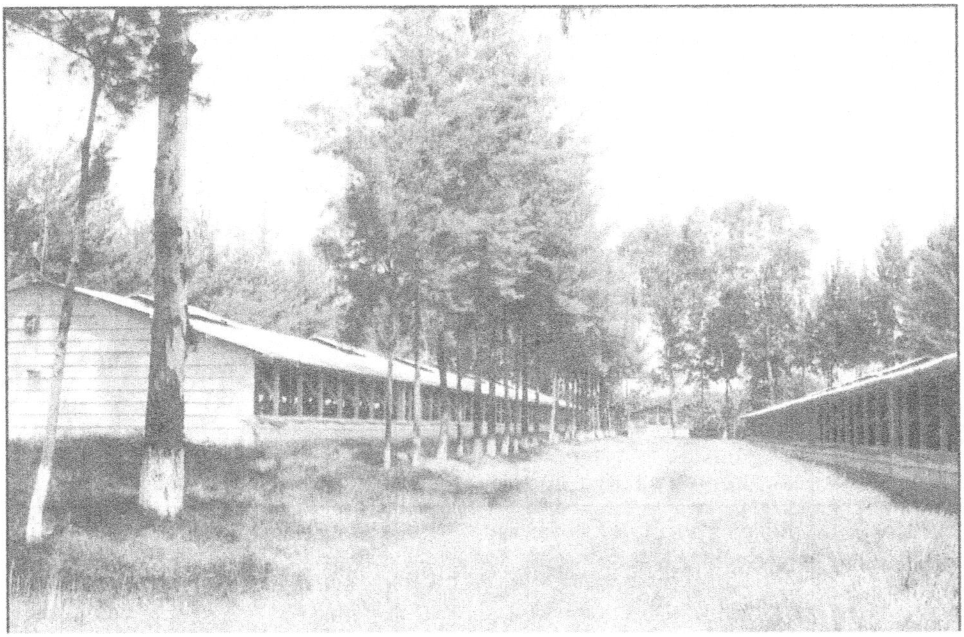

In open-sided buildings there will likely be an advantage to moving air over the birds maintained at high temperatures. As previously discussed, there is a boundary layer of air around birds which will be closer to body temperature than to ambient temperature, and so moving this air will have a cooling effect on the bird. Obviously the closer that ambient air temperature is to body temperature, the less effective is evaporative cooling. Recirculating fans can be arranged so as to direct air across the birds, and when arranged in a pattern such that they are aligned, this is commonly called a "raceway". Table 6.8 shows mean cooling effect of air movement at 29°C. Although the effect is real, it is difficult to measure. Ambient air temperature is not changing, and so there will be no change in temperature recordings in the breeder houses. Because the birds themselves greatly disrupt the air flow, the air speed about 1 m above the birds (where it is usually measured) is around 25% greater than at bird level - air speed has to be adjusted accordingly.

TABLE 6.8 Cooling effect of air movement at 29°C for adult breeders	
Air speed (meters/min)	**Cooling effect (°C)**
15	0.5
30	1.0
45	2.0
60	3.0
75	4.0
90	5.0
105	6.0

Curtain-sided houses, and black-out houses can be ventilated by tunnel ventilation. Black-out houses have conventionally been ventilated by having inlets on one side of the building and fans on the opposite wall as shown in Fig. 6.4. With tunnel ventilation, all fans are located at one end of the building, with inlets at the other end.

The direction of air flow is down the length of the building, and so this tunnel effect usually involves higher air speed (100 m/min 1 meter above the birds) with the associated cooling effect. Tunnel ventilation implies some type of ceiling structure, and in curtain-sided houses, the curtains must be relatively air tight. With tunnel ventilation, and associated use of cool cells, then stocking density can be increased by up to 30% *eg.* 7 birds/m^2 utilizing a b slat system is now common. Tunnel ventilation also usually implies better light control. Balanced against these advantages are increased capital cost, the need for superior management and most importantly the need for reliable electrical supply.

Another system used for reducing the heat load is evaporative cooling. If air is passed over a fine stream of water, then it heats and evaporates some of the water, which takes substantial quantities of heat from the air. The system obviously works best in conditions of moderate humidity because the air must pick up moisture, and so at the extreme of 100% humidity in outside air, evaporative cooling is ineffective. With incoming air at 20% RH, a 15-20°C reduction in temperature by evaporative cooling is theoretically possible. At more normal levels of 60-70% RH, an 8-10°C cooling effect is possible, while at >75% RH the cooling potential is about 5°C. Each 1°C of cooling is associated with about a 5% increase in RH.

Evaporative cool cells are usually located at one end of the house and fans at the opposite end pull air through the saturated cell and down the length of the building. Water usage can vary greatly with the system used. The ideal situation is to have the pad wetted evenly by fogger nozzles or continuous drip systems. With fogger nozzles, working at about 4 litres/hour, then three rows are usually used, spaced at 450 mm centres. About 6.0 m^2 of pad surface area is required for each 1.2 m fan. As a rule of thumb, one 1.2 m fan is required for each 12 m length of housing. For a 100 m long house, with a 3 m ceiling, 8 fans would be needed with about 48 m^2 of pad area (*ie.* 24 m x 2 m pad). Cool cells can also be used with cross ventilation, having the cell on one wall, and fans on the opposite side. If the building is >80 m long, it may be beneficial to split the cool cell area into two, locating each unit at opposite ends of the building. Alternatively, the cell can be positioned in the centre of one side, and exhaust fans located on each end wall.

An alternative system of evaporative cooling often used in curtain-sided houses, is some type of fogging system involving overhead sprinklers. Fogging nozzles should be designed to provide a minimum of water so as not to saturate the birds or litter. In this regard, high pressure foggers (33 atmospheres or 500 PSI) producing fine water droplets (10F diameter) help to minimise water usage and the wetting effect within the house. For example, foggers at 6 atmospheres (100 PSI) characteristically produce droplets of 30F diameter, and while using the same volume of water, will have a noticeable wetting effect on the birds, equipment and litter.

Roof sprinklers can also be used to cool birds during hot weather, where again the concept of evaporative cooling is utilized. Roof sprinklers can reduce inside house temperature by up to 5°C, but tend to use a high volume of water (1 litre/bird/hour) compared to in-house foggers. In order to reduce heat load from the roof, then the surface should ideally be reflective and a light color rather than a dark color. Roofs can be painted with a "paint" made up of 10kg lime and 1 litre of PVA acetate (binder) added to 20 litres of water.

There have been attempts at constructing naturally ventilated breeder houses. If such houses are managed and designed adequately then they seem to work in temperate climates. Air movement relies on natural convection currents to carry air over the birds, and as it becomes warmed, it rises to the roof vents situated down the ridge of the building. The roof needs to be quite high with at least a 30° pitch and with a minimum of obstruction to the air flow. Because of the slower air movement, the inlets need to be proportionally larger and this imposes some limitations if light control is desired. The slower moving air is more easily disrupted by winds, and so both inlets and ridge vents need protection. The roof vents must also be designed so as not to allow rain to fall on the litter.

SUGGESTED READING

Curtis, S.E., 1987. Environmental Management in Animal Agriculture.
Publ. Iowa State Press.

CHAPTER 7. BROODING AND MANAGEMENT OF THE GROWING PULLET AND ROOSTER

PAGE NO.

7.1 INTRODUCTION

The goals of the brooding and grow-out systems are to provide pullets and roosters of ideal weight, condition and stage of sexual maturity as they enter the breeder facilities. Such management requires knowledge and understanding of the growth and development of the birds and how these factors are influenced by husbandry decisions. The major factors influencing development of breeder birds are:

Nutrition and feeding management

Environmental control

Health status

Behavioral and social interactions

Strain specific development

Table 7.1 outlines major production goals for breeders in the growing period as well as the breeder cycle. All too often in integrated companies, the goals of the grow out manager are separated from those of the breeder manager. It must be remembered that the simple criterion for adequate grow-out management is optimum adult breeder performance, and so it is necessary for all managers to consider themselves as essential components of the production of hatching eggs and chicks - regardless of how distant they may be in time or geography from the actual production of hatching eggs. Expressed another way, the egg production goals shown in Table 7.1 are as much dependent on the skills of the pullet grower manager, as they are on the skills of the breeder manager.

TABLE 7.1 Major production goals

Hen Body wt.	6 wk	600g
	12 wk	1150g
	22 wk	2300g
	64 wk	3700g
Rooster Body wt.	6 wk	850g
	12 wk	1650g
	22 wk	3000g
	64 wk	4600g
Egg production	Start	24 wk
	50%	26 wk
	Peak (85%)	29 wk
	#wks >80%	8 wk
	#wks >70%	20 wk
Hatchability	24-64 wks	Av 85%
Hatching eggs/hen	24-64 wks	175
Chicks/hen	24-64 wks	150
Mortality	0-22 wks	4%
	22-64 wks	7%
Feed consumption	0-22 wks	10 kg
	22-64 wks	45 kg

General management guidelines are shown in Table 7.2 outlining the basic space requirements and needs for various types of feeding and watering equipment. If birds are raised in the same facilities through to maturity, then obviously the guidelines for 7-20 weeks apply in terms of the number of birds that can be housed and basic needs for feed and water supply.

TABLE 7.2 General management guidelines			
	0-6 wks	**7-20 wks**	**21-64 wks**
Floor space	8/m2	4/m2	3.5/m2
Feeder space - Trough - Tube	7.5 cm/bird 4/100 birds 5 cm/bird	15 cm/bird 7/100 birds 12 cm/bird	15 cm/bird 10/100 birds 14 cm/bird
Water space - Bell - Nipple	1/150 birds 1/15 birds	1/80 birds 1/10 birds	1/70 birds 1/10 birds

The key to successful breeder management is conscientious record keeping. Most breeder companies collect and maintain copious quantities of records on their breeders. Unfortunately, few companies use these records to their full potential in terms of analyzing performance against all the variables influencing profitability in the grow-out and breeder houses. Table 7.3 is an example of a summary of important records that should be maintained on all flocks. Grow-out and adult breeder data are combined on this summary report.

While most breeder managers now work in metric units, the influence of the industry in the USA means that imperial systems of measure are still used as guidelines by a number of organizations. Table 7.4 shows some common conversion figures, metric: imperial, that may be of use to breeder managers.

7.2 BROODING

Preparation for brooding starts with depopulation of the previous flock. A major requirement for successful early chick development is minimal challenge from bacteria, viruses, mycoplasma, molds and parasites. Consequently the building must be thoroughly washed and disinfected following clean out of litter. Periodically the brooding area should be fumigated. Once the feeding equipment has been reinstalled then ideally 200-300 kg feed + 30 kg propionic acid, should be loaded into the feed tank and flushed through the feeder system. Water lines will need to be flushed, disinfected and then sanitized with 10 ppm chlorine, followed by a final flushing with clean water.

TABLE 7.3 Flock Summary

Farm #	**House #**	**Breed: M**	**Supplier:**
Date placed:	**Date 24 wks:**	**Date depleted:**	
Comments:			

Growing:
Birds placed including extras
Mortality (%)
Culls (%)
Feed consumption (kg)Starter
Grower
Prelay
Total

Observations:

Breeder:	**Comments:**
Age at 1st egg (days) 50% production (days) Peak production: % Weeks over: 80% 70% Mortality(%) ♀ ♂ Culls (%) ♀ ♂	
Feed consumption (kg) Breeder 1 Breeder 2 Male feed Total Total eggs collected Total hatching eggs shipped Hatchability Saleable chicks	**Comments:**

TABLE 7.4 Conversions

Temperature		Stocking density	
°C	°F	Birds per m^2	Sq. Ft. per bird
-5	23	14.3	0.75
0	32	10.8	1.00
2	36	8.6	1.25
4	39	7.2	1.50
6	43	6.1	1.75
8	46	5.5	2.00
10	50	4.8	2.25
12	54	4.3	2.50
14	57	3.9	2.75
16	61	3.6	3.00
18	64	3.3	3.25
20	68	3.1	3.50
22	72	2.9	3.75
24	75	2.7	4.00
26	79	2.5	4.25
28	82		
30	86		
32	90		
34	93		
36	97		
38	100		
40	104		
Weights		**Egg size**	
		Grams per egg	**Ounces per dozen**
1 gram.	0.0353 oz.	42.5	18
1 oz.	28.4g	44.9	19
1 kg	2.2 lbs	47.3	20
l pound wt	0.454 kg	49.6	21
1 tonne	1000 kg	52.0	22
1 ton	2000 lbs	54.3	23
1 tonne	1.1 ton	56.7	24
1 ton	0.9 tonne	59.1	25
		61.4	26
		63.8	27
		66.2	28
		68.5	29
		70.9	30

There are two basic types of systems used to supply heat, and maintain the brooding area at 34-35°C in the first few days. The conventional system relies on spot heating under brooders, which are usually propane fueled systems. With curtain-sided buildings or controlled environment houses, whole or partial house heating is more common. In this latter system, all or part of the brooder house is heated, usually fueled by propane. The whole room heating provides a more uniform environment for the chicks which are usually easier to observe because brooder surrounds are rarely used. There is no need to confine the chicks because the whole environment is heated. Partial room brooding is usually accomplished by means of temporary plastic walls used to partition off 25-30% of the brooder house. With this brooding system the initial space requirement up to about 14 days of age, is 20-25 chicks/m^2. With spot brooders, it is usual to use brooder surrounds or brooder guards that are 20-30 cm high and confine the chicks to the immediate area of the heat source. Disposable cardboard surrounds are ideal, and as the chicks grow, the confinement area should be gradually increased. The surrounds can be taken down completely after 10-14 d depending upon general house temperature and the potential for cool air currents to adversely affect the birds. In very hot, humid environments, wire mesh rather than cardboard brooder guards are preferred because they allow for more air movement. However these wire mesh surrounds are notoriously difficult to clean prior to re-use. The general concept of brooding is to gradually reduce the air temperature corresponding to the lower critical temperature of the chick. At day of age the chick's lower critical temperature is around 30°C, which means that at temperatures below this, the chick will have to start using feed as a source of body heat in order to stay warm. However, feathers quickly develop, and as the chick grows, its surface area relative to body mass quickly declines, and so it can function well at ever decreasing temperatures as it gets older. In fact there is a tendency for chicks to be overheated, rather than underheated, after the first 3-4 d of brooding. The main advantage of whole room brooding is that it provides the chick with a greater range of ambient temperature within the building, and so the chick can move in and out of "warm" to "warmer" areas as needed. With spot brooders and confining brooder surrounds, the manager has to be much more careful about overheating or underheating chicks. Table 7.5 shows ideal mean brooding temperatures and humidity, together with corresponding ideal room temperatures.

While thermometers can give a general indication of the quality of the brooding environment, chick behaviour is perhaps the best guideline. The young chick has a very narrow band of heat tolerance, meaning that it can become overheated or chilled within very narrow limits. At day of age, the chick will likely be chilled at constant temperatures much below 29°C and become overheated at temperatures above 34°C. This is not to say that the chick cannot tolerate these temperatures for a short period of time, and in fact this happens (quite successfully) with chicks in whole or partial room brooding, where chicks move in and out of heat zones established within the building.

TABLE 7.5 Suggested brooding and room temperatures and humidity

	Temperature °C		
Days of age	Brooding[1]	Room[2]	Relative Humidity (%)
1	32	30	85
2	32	29	85
3	31	28	85
4	31	27	82
5	30	26	82
6	30	26	82
7	29	25	80
8	29	25	80
9	29	24	80
10	28	24	80
11	28	23	80
12	27	23	80
14	26	22	75
16	25	22	75
18	24	22	75
20	23	22	70

[1]2-5 cm above the litter, at edge of heat source
[2]1 m above the litter

If chicks become overheated, then much like adult birds, they will try and move away from the heat source, and away from other chicks. If it is too cold, then chicks move as close as possible to the heat source, and as close as possible to other chicks. This simple change in behavior and distribution of chicks therefore is usually the best guideline for adequacy of the brooding environment. Figures 7.1 and 7.2 show representations of chick distribution for spot brooding within brooder guards, and whole room brooding respectively.

To some extent the chicks exhibiting huddling behavior related to overheating as shown in Figures 7.1 and 7.2 are stressed, and so there will likely be other related signs. Chicks can be listless and reluctant to move and often are more noisy, displaying an increased chirping sound that can be almost continuous in large flocks. Feed and water intake will be affected, because chicks are reluctant to move, and then growth rate and feathering will subsequently deteriorate. Early heat distress can often lead to irreversible cannibalism and feather pecking.

Fig. 7.1 Chick distribution within brooder guards using a central heating source.

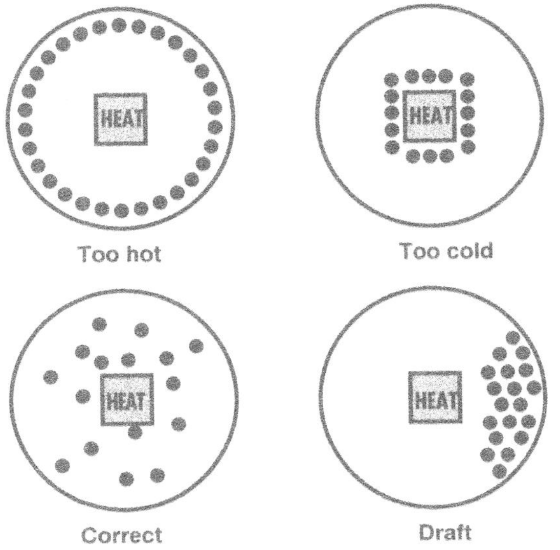

Perhaps the most characteristic sign of overheated or chilled chicks is pasting of the vent. Manure becomes more viscous and adheres to the feather down around the vents. Pasted vents can also be caused by bacterial infection, such as E. coli, but in most instances a 15-20% incidence of this condition is the result of inappropriate environmental temperature.

As in any environment, relative humidity is a factor influencing “effective” conditions for the bird. Relative humidity of 80-85% is ideal at bird level, and this is more difficult to achieve with whole room rather than spot-brooding systems. In order to maintain ideal humidity it is sometimes necessary to use open pans of water inaccessible to the chicks. This situation becomes more critical where coccidiosis vaccines are used because successful cycling of oocysts through the litter is essential for resistance to develop. Such oocyst cycling is less efficient with very dry litter.

Even though maintaining an ideal temperature range is the major factor for environmental management in the first 7-10 d, it is also necessary to think about air movement and ventilation patterns. Adequate air movement is needed in order to maintain the balance

Fig. 7.2 Chick distribution with whole-room brooding.

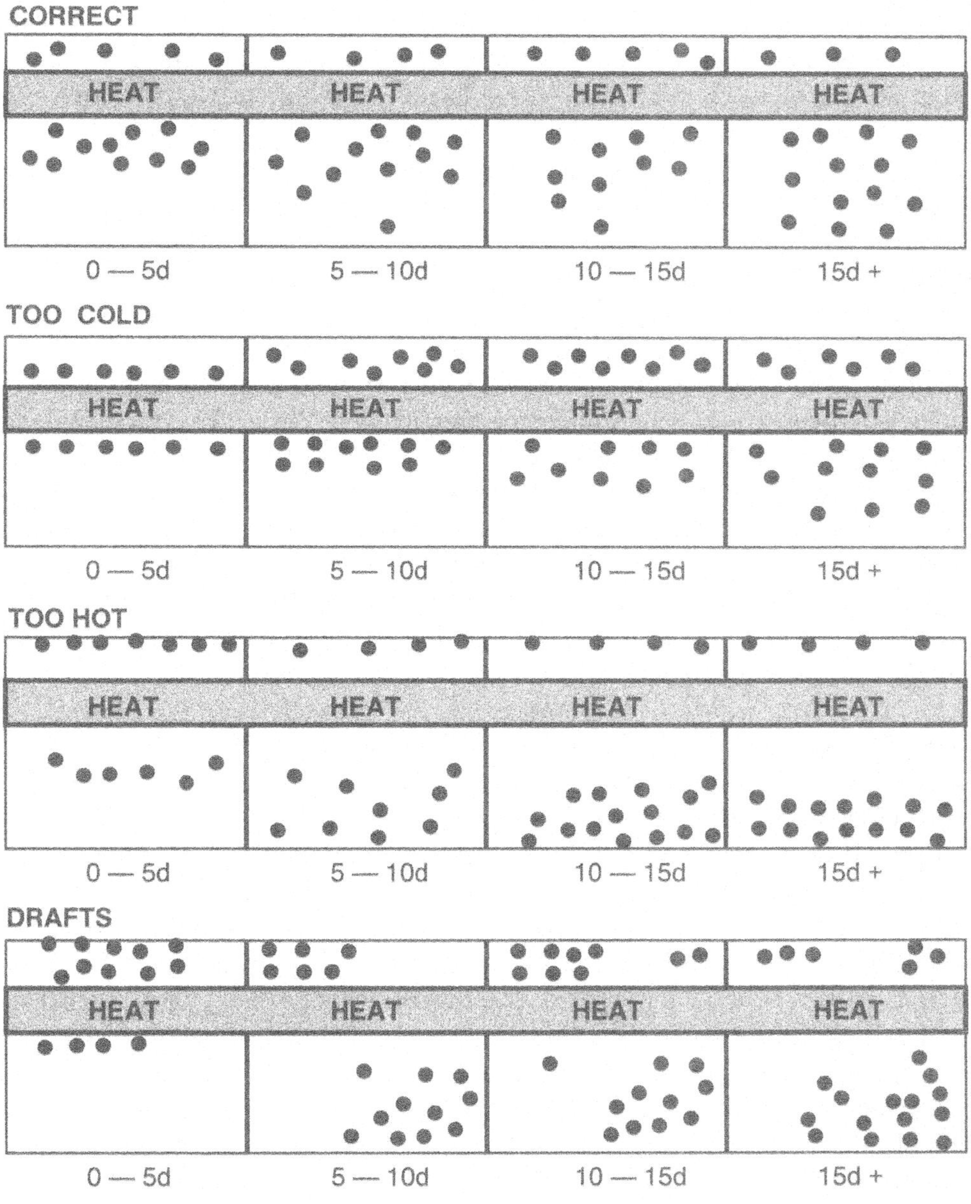

of oxygen, carbon dioxide, moisture, and under extreme cases, to limit build up of carbon monoxide from propane brooders. Very little air movement is usually necessary up to 5 d of age, and a general guideline is 2 m^3/second/tonne feed consumed, up to a maximum of 20 m^3second. This value can be applied up to about 17 d of age, at which time, the normal ventilation rates necessary to maintain house temperature will apply. It is obviously very important to have incoming air well mixed with ambient inside air before it falls on to the chicks. With these types of ventilation rates, air speed should be quite minimal, because even at 30°C, chicks can be chilled if air speed is too high (eg. 2 m/second).

Chicks should be provided with light regardless of the brooding system used. Even with open-sided houses, the brooding area should receive up to 50 lux light intensity, at least for the first 5-7 d of age. In controlled environment brooder houses, it is ideal to have the immediate brooding area under relatively high light intensity (60-70 lux) while the remainder of the floor area is at around 15-20 lux. Adequate light intensity at day-of-age can be provided by one 60 watt bulb per 4 m^2 of floor space, suspended 2.5 m above the litter. This graduation of light intensity helps to confine the chicks closer to the heat source for the first few days. Effective daylength should be 23 hrs for the first day regardless of the housing system. In open-sided buildings, lighting should be reduced to natural daylength (maximum prevailing up to maturity, see Chapter 6, Section 3) by 10 days of age. With curtain-sided or controlled environment houses, daylength can be reduced to 10 hr at 10 days and then to 8 hrs by 14 days of age. If there are any undue stresses on the chicks, such as disease challenge, mycotoxin contamination of the feed etc., it is advisable to delay the reduction in daylength so as to ensure greater feed intake.

When chicks first arrive, their immediate need is usually for water, rather than feed. To stimulate early water intake, some managers will not provide feed in the first 6 hr after placement. Water should obviously be clean and ideally at around 20°C. The water should not contain any additives, unless an antibiotic is required for a specific disease situation. A new innovation to prevent dehydration and ensure good early nutrition is to provide hatchling supplements, such as Oasis™, either at the hatchery or immediately upon placement in the brooder house. Depending upon drinker design, it is often beneficial to provide satellite drinkers to ensure that all chicks are drinking as soon as possible. Satellite drinkers also help to reduce the distance that chicks have to move to find water, because in most brooder houses the nipple or bell drinker lines are essentially designed for the larger pullets. There should be at least 10 nipples per 100 chicks or 1 bell drinker per 100 chicks, and water intake will be stimulated by providing 2-3 small satellite drinkers per 100 chicks for the first 4-5 d. Satellite drinkers can be gradually removed starting at 5 d of age, since this encourages regular use of the permanent water system. A water meter is an essential tool for the breeder manager because deviations from the normal pattern of intake are an early warning of health or management problems. Water consumption will increase from 50 to 200 litres/10,000 chicks/day over the 1 to 14 d period.

There are many different techniques used to supply feed in the first 5-7 d of the brooding period. It is inadvisable to have the large pan or trough feeders available at day of age, because most are designed for larger birds, and so chicks can physically get into the feeders and often become trapped or damaged. Feed can be provided in specially designed chick feeders, in lids from the chick boxes, or on paper spread evenly throughout the brooding area. Feed wastage should not be a concern at this time, because it is important to ensure easy access to the feed, even by the smallest chicks in the flock. Such floor feeding can gradually be discontinued after 5-7 d of age. Feed should be continually available, and ideally female chicks will consume about 0.5 kg starter and roosters 0.7 kg starter in the brooding period. If insoluble grit is part of the management system, then chick-size grit should be introduced around 7-10 d of age, using initially 1 kg/1000 chicks.

Chicks should not have to walk more than 2 m to find either feed or water, and ideally they will find some feed and water within 1 m of the major heat source.

7.3 SEXING ERRORS, TOE CLIPPING AND COMB DUBBING

Regardless of whether chicks are vent sexed or the sexes identified by traditional feather sexing or feather color, no system is 100% accurate and sexing errors must be removed. This is especially important for the males, because a male from the female line will have inferior genetic growth potential, and his offspring will not perform well in the broiler house. A single male can produce up to 1,000 broiler offspring, and so it is very important to remove any males from the female lines that have been sexed incorrectly. Many breeding companies will dubb male chicks, which involves trimming the comb at day-of-age. As the bird grows, its comb remains small and has a rounded top surface (Fig 7.3). Male chicks may also be toe clipped, removing the nail of the inside one or two toes - this is to prevent damage to the hen during mating. If male chicks are dubbed, then any undubbed male is likely a male from the female line, and so should be culled from the flock, as soon as possible during the rearing period. Such suspect males will not be toe clipped, which is further confirmation for culling. Likewise any females that are dubbed or toe clipped should also be culled, because they will likely be mis-sexed birds from the male line, and so have inferior egg production potential.

In very hot weather, it may be inadvisable to use dubbed males, because the comb is an important system for heat loss by the bird. It is also more difficult to subsequently keep dubbed males out of the female feeder grills. However, while it is easier to exclude undubbed males from the female grills, they do have a tendency to catch the back edge of the comb in the grill system, and other equipment, and in extreme cases this can lead to severe injury. Under these conditions, it may be preferable to merely "back-dubb" the bird as shown in Fig 7.3. In this situation there is no leading back edge to the comb, and so the rooster is less likely to become trapped in mechanical equipment.

Fig. 7.3 Dubbing and toe clipping of breeder males.

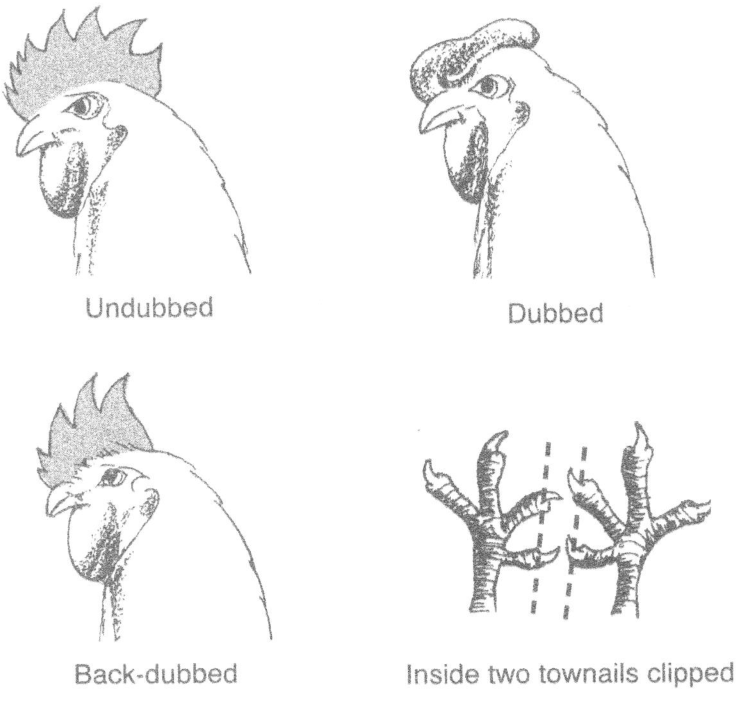

7.4 FEEDING MANAGEMENT

Most aspects of feeding management and nutrition have been covered in Chapter 5, and especially sections 5.1 and 5.2. Pullets and roosters are usually fed on a two or three stage program through to 19-20 weeks of age. In summary, the major nutrient specifications would be as shown in Table 7.6.

Some type of feed restriction program as shown previously in Table 5.8, will have to be started anywhere from 14-28 d of age depending upon the feeding behavior and growth characteristics of the breed. It is usual to ensure that pullets consume a minimum of 0.5 kg starter that provides at least 90 g crude protein and 1450 kcal ME before changing over to grower, regardless of age or climatic conditions. Ideally, roosters should consume at least 0.7 kg of the same feed before changing to the lower nutrient dense grower feed. Starting roosters on lower protein starters or changing to a lower protein grower diet too early often results in poorer feather development.

TABLE 7.6 Major nutrient specifications for growing birds

	Starter	Grower	Developer
Protein (%)	18.0	16.0	14.0
Metabolizable energy (kcal/kg)	2950	2900	2850
Calcium (%)	0.95	0.90	0.87
Av. Phosphorus (%)	0.44	0.40	0.38
Sodium (%)	0.19	0.19	0.19
Methionine (%)	0.36	0.33	0.30
Methionine+cystine(%)	0.72	0.64	0.60
Lysine (%)	0.95	0.80	0.70
Feeding schedule			
2-diet program	0-6 wk	6-19 wk	
3-diet program	0-4 wk	4-12 wk	12-19 wk

There are many variations of the programs used to gradually change birds from a full feeding to a restricted feeding program. Changing when feed clean up time reaches 5-6 hr is one system, although this is notoriously variable from flock to flock even in the same pullet house from year to year. Another option is to introduce restricted feeding at a set age, which is usually around 15 or 20 d, again depending upon the breed chosen. If accurate scales are available, then the ideal system is to change feeding strategy when birds are eating a predetermined quantity of feed, usually around 35 kg/1000/day (6-7 lbs/100). Table 5.8 outlines controlled daily feeding starting at 25 g/bird/day and moving to skip-a-day at 4 weeks of age.

Birds should be fed early in the morning, so as not to impose undue heat load during the day. However feeding should never occur too early in the morning, when attendants may not be present to observe feeding behavior with mechanical feeding systems. A key to uniform pullet growth is even distribution of feed such that all birds have access to feed. Even though theoretically adequate feeder space is provided, the effective space may be less, especially if feed delivery is slow or there are problems with the system. These problems can only be resolved by daily observation, where the attendant is looking for uniform distribution of birds throughout the feeding system within 15 minutes of the delivery system being switched off. In order to maintain or improve uniformity of growth, it may be necessary to change from skip-a-day to alternate restriction programs as suggested in Table 5.15. Up to 20 weeks of age the pullet should consume about 8 kg feed that provides 1.2 kg protein and 22 Mcal energy (Table 5.16).

7.5 WATER MANAGEMENT

The watering system is often used to supply other nutrients, antibiotics and vaccines, as well as provide the water needed for daily growth and development. Daily water intake values are shown in Table 5.21. A typical watering system is shown in Fig. 7.4. In this situation bell drinkers are shown, although the same type of equipment is needed for nipple drinkers.

Fig. 7.4 Water supply system.

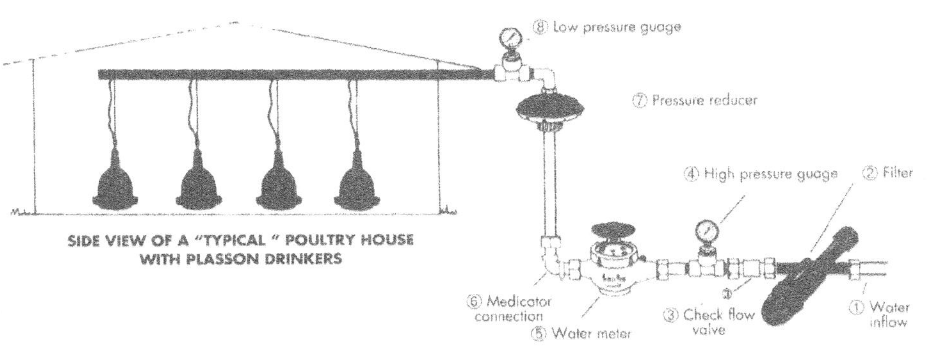

The major management decisions for water supply, are number of drinkers, the level of water in bell drinkers, and the height of bell or nipple drinkers. During brooding, a minimum of one bell drinker per 150 chicks is recommended, although ideally this will be supplemented with satellite drinkers or manually filled chick founts. For the remainder of the growing period, one bell drinker for each 80 birds is recommended. During brooding it is common to supply one nipple per 15 chicks, supplemented with satellite drinkers or water fonts. For older pullets, and roosters, one nipple per 10 birds is acceptable. Birds should not have to travel more than 2 m in order to find water. With nipple drinkers, the height should be adjusted such that birds just have to reach for the bottom of the nipple. If nipples are set too low, then birds have greater difficulty in drinking, and there is also more chance of birds physically moving the nipple as they walk around, and this increases leakage. Setting nipple drinkers too high quickly leads to loss of uniformity since smaller birds have difficulty reaching the nipple. For the first few days it may be necessary to reduce water pressure by 10-15%, such that a large water droplet is clearly visible on the end of each nipple. As the birds grow, it will be necessary to raise nipples at least on a weekly basis.

With bell drinkers, the lip of the drinker should be at back height. This means continual adjustment to drinker height throughout rearing. During brooding, it is common to place bell drinkers on a plywood base, and to fill to the lip for the first 24-36 hrs. Once birds are familiar with the drinkers, then water depth should be adjusted so as to minimize spillage. This usually means no more than 1.5 cm depth of water which is about one-third the depth of the trough around the drinker. Depending upon the level of biosecurity desired, bell drinkers should be cleaned daily, or at least every third day. Most bell drinkers will contain a ballast which prevents excessive movement of the drinker as birds drink or accidentally move the drinker as they walk around the area. Water is usually used as ballast, and antifreeze can be added to this ballast if there is a chance of temperature below 0°C. On most breeder farms, the water supply to each building will be from an overhead storage tank. Ideally these tanks will be white plastic in order to reflect heat from the sun. All too often one sees rusted galvanized tanks, or even tanks painted black, that obviously conduct radiant heat to the water supply very quickly. In heat stress conditions, there is ample evidence to show that water should be kept as cool as possible. White tanks, with a heat deflecting roof are therefore acceptable although the ideal situation is to encase the tank in insulation. Fig. 7.5 shows a schematic diagram outlining the main features of an overhead water tank.

Fig. 7.5 Water tank design.

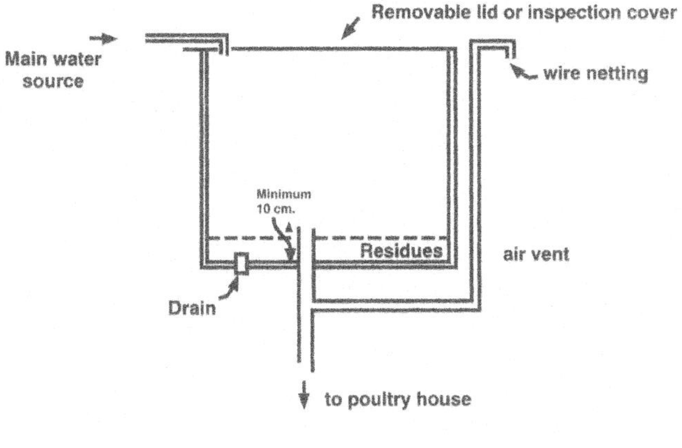

Both the inlet main water supply and the air vent must be protected with wire netting in order to prevent rodents and large insects from entering the tank. The outlet leading to the poultry house should not start at the bottom of the tank, rather this outlet should extend a minimum of 10 cm into the tank in order to prevent residues from entering the system. This type of outlet design reduces up to 50% the labor involved in cleaning filters and blocked nipples.

As discussed in Chapter 5, there will likely be a need to implement some type of water restriction program in order to maintain litter quality. With skip-a-day feeding it is common to give water for at least 1 hr before feeding and continue until 1 hr after the feed is cleaned up, and then to give another hour sometime in late afternoon. On the off-feed day, water availability is usually confined to one hour in the morning and one hour in the afternoon. While these are merely guidelines, it is very important to emphasize to farm staff the need for flexibility according to environmental temperature. Bird behavior is perhaps the best guideline, although at temperatures much above 28°C, it may be necessary to increase water availability. As a generalization, water intake will be 1.5-2.0 x feed intake at 22°C, and this increases to 2.5-3.0 x feed intake at 28°C depending upon acclimatization.

Water quality is variable in different locations depending upon depth of water source and soil composition. Table 7.7 outlines general guidelines for the major potential contaminants of water. Sanitizing the water system is an essential part of the health management program. Before chicks arrive the water system must be thoroughly cleaned and sanitized, and then on an on going basis it is advisable to periodically sanitize the water lines. Between flocks it is essential to first clean the filter, and then increase pressure at the reducer valve and flush the system. The lines should then be flushed with sanitizer, which is allowed to sit in the water lines for at least 3 hours. The lines should then be re-flushed with clean water and the filter replaced. Concentration of sanitizer should be varied commensurate with health management goals.

Whatever system is used, it is essential to remove sanitizers at least 48 hours prior to administering any vaccines via the water system. Table 7.8 and 7.9 provide general guidelines for use of sanitizers.

TABLE 7.7 Water quality standards			
Contaminant	**Ideal level**	**Upper acceptable limit**	**Potential problems**
Total bacteria	0/ml	100/ml	Low levels of bacteria may be present without causing problems.
Coliforms	0/ml	50/ml	The presence of Coliforms usually indicates fecal contamination of the water supply.
Nitrates(ppm)	10	25	Levels greater than 20 may result in performance problems.
Calcium (ppm)	600	---	
Magnesium (ppm)	14	125	Laxative effect.
Manganese (ppm)	0.01	1.0	May leave black deposits on valves causing leaky waterers. Discolors bell drinkers.
Iron (ppm)	2	10	Higher levels may be safe but the water has a metallic taste and causes staining of drinkers.
Sodium (ppm)	32	50	Laxative effect.
Hardness (ppm)	60	180	Interferes with the effectiveness of soap, many disinfectants and some water medications.
pH	7	6.8-75	pH lower than 6.0 may cause performance problems.
Chloride (ppm)	14	250	Laxative effect.
Copper (ppm)	0.002	0.06	Liver toxicity.
Sulphate (ppm)	125	250	Laxative effect.
Adapted from Gillingham (1997)			

TABLE 7.8 Cleaning and sanitizing water lines				
	Between flocks		While birds present	
	Proportioner	**Bulk tank**	**Proportioner**	**Bulk tank**
Citric Acid	200g/litre	2kg/1000 litres	50g/litre	500g/ 1000 litres
Vinegar	No dilution	8litres/ 1000 litres	50cc/litre	4 litres /1000 litres
Concentrated Ammonia Solutions	100cc/litre	200cc/ 1000 litres	25cc/litre	100cc/ 1000 litres
Concentrated Chlorine Solutions	100cc/litre	200cc/ 1000 litres	25cc/litre	100cc/ 1000 litres
Hydrogen Peroxide	-	-	5cc/litre	50cc/ 1000 litres
Iodine	-	-	100cc/litre	500cc/ 1000 litres

TABLE 7.9 Comments on choice of water sanitizers	
Product	**Comments**
Chlorine	Inexpensive, but quickly inactivated by organic matter. Corrosive at 75 ppm, even to stainless steel.
Iodine	Corrosive at >5 ppm.
Hydrogen peroxide	Very corrosive and explosive at full concentration when contacted by metals.
Ammonia	Quickly inactivated by organic material. At low concentrations helps maintain the stability of sulfur drugs
Citric Acid	Helps maintain stability of tetracycline antibiotics. Ideal product to replace sugar as a carrier in vitamin-electrolyte packs. Corrosive to galvanized steel.
Note* - Never mix sanitzers because of potential violent reactions and gas production	

The choice of sanitizers depends on microbial load in the water, design of the watering system and compatibility with other drugs and medications. Table 7.9 discusses some of the issues to consider in selecting sanitizers.

7.6 BEAK TRIMMING

Most breeder pullets will be beak trimmed during the growing period. The advantages to beak trimming are reduced picking of the feathers, vent and toes of other birds, together with reduced feed wastage and improved uniformity of growth. The disadvantages are that it is a stressful procedure, and if carried out much later than 4 weeks of age, it will result in 1-2 week's loss of normal growth. Usually the older the bird that is beak trimmed, the greater the problems of loss of growth rate and uniformity. It is not advisable to beak trim birds if they are under any stress, such as heat, cold or disease challenge. Likewise some sulfur drugs if used at this time can cause prolonged bleeding time, and especially in 5-7 d old chicks hatched from breeders fed marginal levels of vitamin K (<2 mg/kg diet). Most breeding companies now recommend precision beak trimming at 5-8 d of age (Fig. 7.6).

Fig. 7.6 Appearance of correctly beak trimmed chick at 5-8d, and adult at 23 weeks.

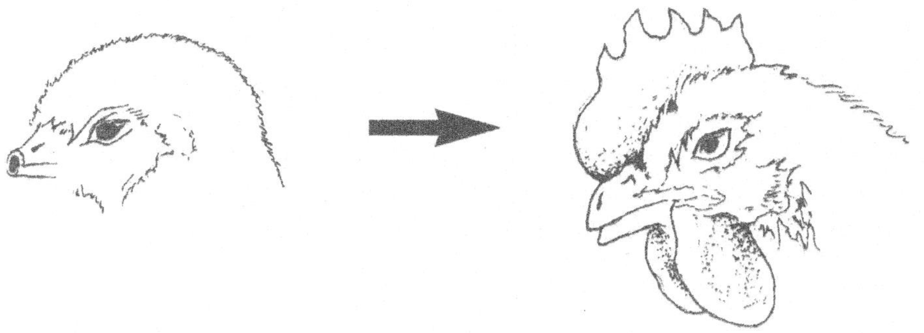

Beak trimming at 5-8d.

Adult hen without further trimming.

When beak trimming is carried out correctly, as shown in Fig. 7.6, there should be no need to re-trim as birds get older. Beak trimming procedures should be re-evaluated if more than 5% of pullets need further work when they are moved to the breeder facilities. For effective precision beak trimming at 5-8 d of age, the operator must be in a comfortable position in order to realize the goal of 750-800 chicks/hr. The beak trimmer should be at chest height, and the operator seated adequately, with easy access to the chicks provided by the catching crew. The blade should be cherry red in color which indicates a temperature of around 700oC. If there is no color, the blade is too cold and there will be tearing of the beak. A yellow-red blade that is too hot can distort and cut the beaks unevenly. The blade should be used for no more than 5,000 chicks (1 day). It can then be turned over or sharpened. The operator holds the chick in one hand with the thumb behind the head and the first (index) finger under the beak. Slight pressure under the beak causes the bird to withdraw the tongue. Depending upon age of chick, the upper and lower beak will be trimmed through the 0.4 cm opening. The cut will then be about 2 mm in front of the nostrils. The cut surfaces of the beak can then be held on the hot blade for 2-3 seconds to cauterize and prevent bleeding. The processed chick should not be dropped on to the litter, rather it should be placed on a chute (PVC piping) angled at no more than 45o to the horizontal. Operators should continually be re-evaluated for efficiency of their beak trimming skills. This is most easily accomplished when individual operators are responsible for specific pens of birds.

7.7 MONITORING BODY WEIGHT

The major criterion used in assessing the progress of pullets and roosters is the average flock body weight and the uniformity of this weight. Each breeding company publishes guidelines for the weekly growth and body weight of their birds, and achieving this goal is one of the most important management criteria. In large part, the growth of the pullet and rooster is governed by the feed allowance, and monitoring body weight is unquestionably the best system for monitoring adequacy of the controlled feeding system. In fact, body weight of the birds should dictate the feed allocation schedule, and not vice versa. Fluctuations in the digestibility of nutrients in the diet, ingredient quality, and environmental temperature result in daily or weekly fluctuations in effective nutrient supply relative to expectations, and these effects can only be "corrected" by observing bird response and then adjusting nutrient supply accordingly.

After 6 weeks of age, pullets should gain about 100g in weight each week. To be more precise the values are 14 g/d from 6-14 weeks, 17 g/d from 14-20 weeks and 20 g/d in the pre-breeder period from 20-24 weeks. Obviously there will be strain differences in this growth pattern, and the breeder's guide should be the standard used. Tables 7.10 and 7.11 show average guidelines for growing pullets and roosters through to 22 weeks of age.

These values shown in Tables 7.10 and 7.11 have been taken as a mean across values for six commercial strains. Associated with these values are guidelines for feed intake, feed type and expected uniformity.

Birds should be weighed at least weekly, and ideally, at the same time and day each week. With skip-a-day feeding, it is best to weigh on a non-feed day. If birds are weighed on a feed day, then adjustments must be made for the weight of feed and water consumed. If pullets are allotted 100 g of feed, then about 2 hr after starting to feed, they will be about 150 g heavier (feed & water). After this time, they can be expected to lose about 10 g weight/hr as feed is digested and water is metabolized. These feed and water induced changes in apparent body weight must be accounted for as the birds are changed from skip-a-day to every day or alternate feeding systems. Ideally 2% of the flock will be sampled at each weighing, with a minimum of 50 birds regardless of flock size.

TABLE 7.10 Guidelines for weekly body weight and feed intake of growing pullets

Weeks of age	Body weight		Feed intake*		Feed type	Weight Uniformity
	g	lbs	g/bird	lbs/100		“15%
1	120	0.26	25	5.5	Starter	75
2	230	0.51	27	5.9	↓	75
3	330	0.73	29	6.4		75
4	420	0.93	31	6.8	Grower	80
5	510	1.12	34	7.5	↓	80
6	610	1.34	36	7.9		80
7	680	1.50	40	8.8		80
8	760	1.67	43	9.5		80
9	860	1.89	46	10.1		80
10	960	2.11	49	10.7		80
11	1050	2.31	53	11.7		80
12	1150	2.53	58	12.7		80
13	1250	2.75	62	13.7		80
14	1350	2.97	66	14.5		85
15	1450	3.19	70	15.4		85
16	1550	3.42	75	16.5		85
17	1670	3.67	80	17.6		85
18	1790	3.94	85	18.7		85
19	1900	4.18	92	20.3		90
20	2040	4.49	97	21.4		90
21	2200	4.85	103	22.7	Breeder	90
22	2320	5.11	110	24.2	↓	90

*Mean diet ME 2900 kcal/kg

TABLE 7.11 Guidelines for weekly body weight and feed intake of growing roosters

	Body weight		Feed intake*		Feed type	Weight Uniformity
Weeks of age	g	lbs	g/bird	lbs/100		“15%
1	125	0.28	27	6.0	Starter	70
2	280	0.62	30	6.6	↓	70
3	440	0.97	32	7.0		70
4	610	1.34	34	7.5		75
5	720	1.59	36	7.8	Grower	75
6	840	1.85	39	8.5	↓	75
7	930	2.05	42	9.2		75
8	1040	2.29	46	10.1		80
9	1180	2.60	50	11.0		80
10	1300	2.86	53	11.6		80
11	1420	3.13	57	12.5		80
12	1550	3.41	61	13.4		80
13	1700	3.74	66	14.5		80
14	1880	4.14	71	15.6		82
15	2060	4.53	76	16.7		82
16	2200	4.85	81	17.8		82
17	2320	5.11	90	19.8		85
18	2450	5.39	100	22.0		85
19	2600	5.72	105	23.1		85
20	2830	6.23	110	24.2	Breeder	85
21	2970	6.54	115	25.3	or	85
22	3100	6.82	120	26.4	Male diet	85

*Mean diet ME 2900 kcal/kg

There is often discussion about the need to sample at different locations in the building or within individual pens of birds. Certainly sampling from 3 locations may improve accuracy, but test results suggest that this improvement is quite minimal and the extra time involved is best spent in conducting a slower, more thorough, weighing at one location, which is less stressful to the birds. In this same regard, there seems little advantage to weighing more than 2% of the flock as a sample, because accuracy is little improved, and the process is more stressful to a larger number of birds.

Automated scales are sometimes used to record bird weights, the most common being platforms about 25 cm square and 6-8 cm high. The birds voluntarily stand on the scale and weight is recorded automatically. The system is much less stressful to the birds because there is no handling. The associated software can be programmed not to record weights that are > or <50% from the daily mean weight. This ensures no recording of a bird standing on the scale with just one foot on the scale and the other on the litter, or two birds standing on the scale at one time. Behavioural studies have shown that individual birds tend to use the scales more frequently than others, and so this can bias the mean accordingly. This problem can be resolved to some extent by having multiple scales located throughout the building. As a move towards greater mechanization of management systems, the automated weighing system can be connected to the feed scale, and so daily feed allocation will be driven by the previous day's weight. If such recorded body weight is below standard, then proportionally more feed can be given and vice versa. With manual weighing, there is sometimes discussion about weighing birds in groups of 5 or 6, rather than individually. This usually means weighing birds in crates. The mean weight recorded is often similar to that obtained by individual bird weighing, and the advantage being less stress on the bird (hanging from a conventional scale by the legs) and less time involved. However the weight of the crate must be accurately accounted for, especially after multiple weighings where manure can build-up in the crate can bias the recordings. The obvious disadvantage to group weighing is loss of accuracy in recording uniformity.

Recording of weights is most often done manually, although data can be entered directly into hand-held computers. With a manual recording, one of the simplest methods is to record observations according to pre-assigned weight categories. In the example shown in Table 7.12, body weight categories are in units of 50 g, assuming this is the degree of accuracy on the scale. A bird weighing 500 g is therefore recorded as an "x" on the record sheet. The person reading the scale is trained to categorize birds to the nearest 50 g. In Table 7.12, there were two birds at 500 g, 5 birds at 550 g etc. The advantage of this type of recording is less error in transposing numerical data, and more importantly there is an associated visual output of the variance or uniformity of the flock.

Simply looking at the "x" weight recordings in Table 7.12 suggests a mean weight of around 700 g. In fact subsequent calculations provide a mean of 703 g. In this example the accepted uniformity range is “15%. With a mean of 703 g for the flock, our acceptable range becomes 703”15% = 597 to 808 g. This is rounded off to the nearest category of weights, which in this example becomes 600 to 800 g. There are 36 birds in this acceptable range, and so uniformity is (36÷50)x100 = 72%. All of this information is recorded on the production sheet and provides a quickly assessed overview of the status of the flock for attendants, managers and supervisors. As previously discussed, the intent of the weighing and uniformity calculation is to assess flock performance, and to provide a basis for decisions on feed allocation. For this reason it is essential to use this data for such purposes, and so the 'comments' section of the record sheet (Table 7.12) is perhaps the most important information. In the example shown, flock mean weight at 703 g, is about 3% over standard, and the poorer than accepted uniformity (72% vs 80-85% standard) is due to too many heavy birds. These facts combined suggest overfeeding, and so the decision is made to reduce or at least not to increase feed allocation the following week.

The conclusion of the example weighing procedure depicted in Table 7.12 is that the pullets are overweight and that this needs to be corrected. It is usually inadvisable to attempt too quick a correction of flocks that are either over or underweight. Rather, the return to standard should be more gradual because sudden changes (either more or less) in feed allocation usually cause loss in uniformity. The goal should be a gradual return to standard. This situation is perhaps easiest with underweight flocks, where increased feed allocation causes increased growth. The ideal way to accommodate these changes to growth rate is to specify an alternate weekly weight standard for these problem flocks. Table 7.13 shows four such examples, together with the standard weight-for-age as specified by the breeding company. Flock #1 (Table 7.13) for example is at 0.75 kg body weight at 6 weeks, which is excessively heavy compared to the standard of 0.61kg for this age of bird. The newly devised standard aims to gradually reduce this weight difference, so that by 20 weeks pullets will be 2.09 kg vs 2.04 kg as the ideal standard. In this example we are taking 14 weeks to correct the problem, which will pose little added stress on the bird.

Flock #2 (Table 7.13) is underweight at 6 weeks (0.5 kg vs 0.61 kg standard). In this situation we can correct the problem more quickly, by increasing feed allowance, and the new goal is to have the correct weight by 16 weeks of age (1.55 kg). Where possible, we should have underweight flocks on target by 16 weeks of age, so as not to cause permanent reductions in shank length and skeletal development.

Flocks #3 and #4 pose more of a problem, because the weight discrepancies occur much later during growing. The same concept of gradual correction applies, but in these situations it is often difficult (and inadvisable) to obtain complete correction of growth. For example with Flock #3 which is overweight at 14 weeks, the new standards are imposed so as to prevent even greater variation from standard. This growth is tempered although the actual weight at 20 weeks is still

TABLE 7.12 Flock weight and uniformity record

Farm: Orogrand	Flock: #28	Sex: ♀	Breed Hycross:82
Flock size: 5,700	Hatch date: 28.10.99	Week: #7	
Number weighed:50	Weighing time:8:00 am	Feed day yes ( ) No (✓)	
Target weight: 680g	Actual weight:703g	Uniformity 72%	
Comments: Birds slightly heavy. Uniformity poor because of heavier birds. Suggest hold feed increase next week			

GRAMS		GRAMS
50		1kg 550
100		600
150		650
200		700
250		750
300		800
350		850
400		900
450		950
500	xx	2 kg 000
550	xxxxx	50
600	xxxxxx	100
650	xxxxxxxx	150
700	xxxxxxxxx	200
750	xxxxxxxx	250
800	xxxxx	300
850	xxx	350
900	xx	400
950	x	450
1kg 000		500
050		550
100		600
150		650
200		700
250		750
300		800
350		850
400		900
450		950
500		3 kg 000

Total #Birds weighed:	50		
Total Bird Weight: 35,150g		Uniformity range: 600-800g	
Average Bird Weight:	703g	Birds within range:	36
-15%	597g	% Birds within range:	72
+15%	808g	Uniformity:	72%

TABLE 7.13 Weight adjustment schedule for pullets that become overweight or underweight throughout the growing period

Wks age	1	2	3	4	5	6	7	8	9	10	11	12	13	14	15	16	17	18	19	20
Standard wt. (kg)	.12	.23	.33	.42	.51	.61	.68	.76	.86	.96	1.05	1.15	1.25	1.35	1.45	1.55	1.67	1.79	1.90	2.04
Flock #1 Overweight at 6 wks						.75	.81	.88	.97	1.06	1.15	1.24	1.34	1.43	1.52	1.61	1.73	1.84	1.95	2.09
Flock #2 Underweight at 6 wks						.50	.58	.69	.79	.89	.99	1.10	1.21	1.32	1.44	1.55	1.67	1.79	1.90	2.04
Flock #3 Overweight at 14wks													1.40	1.49	1.58	1.67	1.79	1.90	2.01	2.14
Flock #4 Underweight at 14 wks													1.10	1.21	1.32	1.44	1.59	1.72	1.84	2.00

heavy, because achieving the standard would necessitate severe feed restriction which would impact uniformity at this critical time. Likewise with Flock #4, we accept that the flock will only be partially corrected. It will still be slightly underweight at 20 weeks, because total correction would likely necessitate large increases in feed, leading to obesity. Weight adjustments must therefore be gradual, and not at the expense of uniformity, frame size or obesity.

7.8 UNIFORMITY

Body weight of pullets at 20 weeks of age is highly correlated with age at sexual maturity. This means that on average the heavier pullets in a flock will mature much earlier than the lighter weight birds. Because we will be feeding breeders according to their egg production, then ideally we want all birds at the same stage of production. For example, if we plan to give peak feed allowance when the flock reaches 45% egg production, we assume all birds are at this stage of production. In reality, this does not happen because we can never achieve 100% uniformity of sexual development in birds. However the higher the uniformity, the greater the chance of being correct in feeding all birds in a flock. If for example, we have very poor uniformity, (eg 50%), then when flock mean egg production is 45%, we are likely to have the heaviest birds close to peak, and the smallest birds not yet laying. We will be under feeding the heavy early maturing birds, and grossly overfeeding the smaller immature birds. Certainly black-out growing facilities help to improve uniformity of sexual development, but by far the biggest factor is uniformity of body weight. Within the growing facilities we must strive to obtain the highest uniformity achievable within the limitations of the production facilities. Most managers accept values of 80% (“10%) or 85 (“15%) as standards of uniformity. In reality 90% (“10%) is achievable, even with large flocks, but this is at the expense of additional labor input. It has been suggested that each 1% improvement in uniformity is worth about +1 egg/breeder. When records are reviewed, then we hope to see all individual bird weights as close to the mean as possible (Fig. 7.7). An accepted degree of uniformity at the breeder farm is 80% of the flock being within “10% of the flock mean. Deviation from this normal pattern, as shown in Fig 7.7 is a cause for concern because subsequent egg production will be adversely affected. Loss of uniformity is commonly due to poor or slow feed distribution, feed separation or disease challenge. Uniformity is most often calculated as shown in Table 7.12. Another statistical measure that is sometimes used is coeffecient of variation (CV).

The CV of a flock is obtained from the following equation:

$$\frac{\text{Standard Deviation}}{\text{Mean weight}} \times 100$$

Fig. 7.7 Patterns of uniformity of body weight of growing pullets.

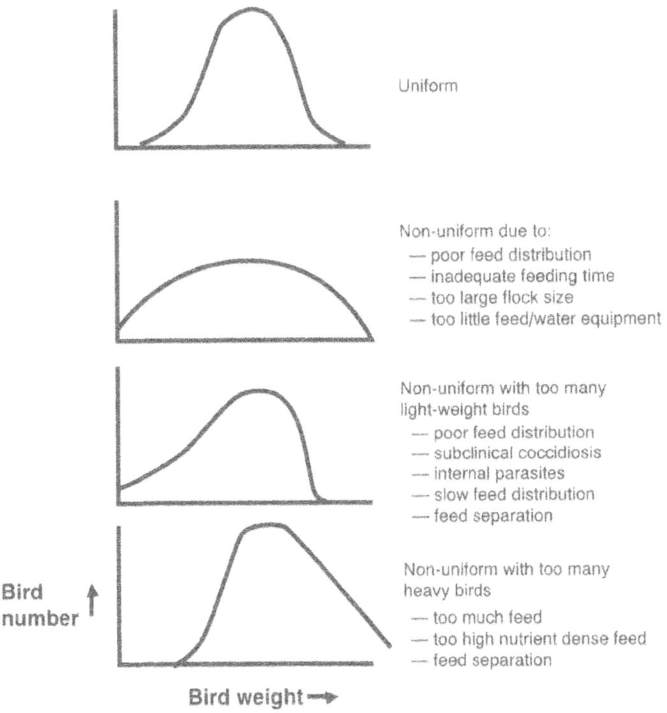

The standard deviation is another statistical measure that assesses the variability within a sample population. Most managers using this system will derive the standard deviation and CV from a computer system or programmable calculator. The values are more difficult to calculate by hand, and so if computing systems are not available, then perhaps derivation of CV should be avoided. The standard for CV is around 8%. Values higher than this indicate poorer uniformity, and vice versa.

Improving the level of uniformity in a flock is quite difficult, and the best solution to the problem is to never allow uniformity to deteriorate. However in the competitive environment of the pullet house, this is often difficult to realize, and so we are faced with both preventative and correctional management techniques. The major factors contributing to a loss of uniformity are detailed in Table 7.14.

TABLE 7.14 Factors causing loss of uniformity of body weight in breeder pullets
1. Too slow feed distribution
2. Inadequate feeder space
3. Feed segregation
4. Inadequate water allocation
5. Inadequate water space
6. Disease challenge, especially coccidiosis and internal parasites
7. Too large a flock size (consider subdividing into pens)
8. Variable effective environmental conditions throughout the house

Correcting problems with uniformity, therefore relates to solving any problems found as described in Table 7.14. Slow feed distribution is one of the major causes of loss in uniformity. For example, chain feeders should run at a minimum 30 meters/min, while tube feeding systems need comparable fast filling. It is unusual to fill feeder lines while they are winched above bird height, and subsequently lowering the filled lines to the birds simultaneously, but this is an excellent way of ensuring even feeding activity throughout the pullet house. This system has become very popular with rooster feed systems. With hand feeding, it is ideal to have at least two people feeding a flock at any one time, and for these two people to start feeding at opposite ends of the house or pen.

Another very effective way to improve flock uniformity is to weight segregate flocks and then to feed them according to their weight status. For example, suppose a flock is weighed at 8 weeks of age and found to have an average weight of 750 g with uniformity of just 60%. The average weight is acceptable, but uniformity is very poor. It is found that 33% of the flock are small, with a mean weight of just 650 g, 33% are heavy with a mean weight of 850 g, while only 34% are of ideal weight at 750 g. If we could separate the different types of bird, then we could re-assign weight standards (Table 7.13) and then feed them separately so as to achieve ideal weight at say, 16 weeks. The goal perhaps would be to have all three subgroups of the flock reach a mean weight of 1600 g at 16 weeks. Without such intervention we will likely have exceptionally heavy and light birds at this critical time.

Success of weight segregation relies on the farm staff being able to manage the logistics of weighing all birds in a flock, and then physically relocating them according to their weight category. This task appears simple in theory, but requires careful planning if it is to be successful with minimum stress placed on the birds. Advocates of this management technique often weight segregated twice, usually at around 8 and 14 weeks of age. In most countries it costs the equivalent of one hatching egg, for the labor involved in weighing and/or relocating an individual bird. One therefore expects at least one extra egg to result from the improved flock uniformity. When carried out under ideal conditions, uniformity of 90+% is seen, and so the technique can be very profitable.

7.9 FLESHING, FEATHERING, AND SHANK AND KEEL LENGTH

While body weight and uniformity are usually the main criteria used to assess the feed management program, the condition and physical appearance of the pullet and rooster can also be taken into consideration. While many breeding companies talk about the importance of fleshing of their birds, there do not seem to be any procedures established for accurate assessment. As with any such characteristic it is difficult to quantitate conformation measurements, and so qualitative observations must be accepted. Both pullets and roosters need to be well fleshed which means that the muscle can easily be felt in the breast and thigh regions. After 12 weeks of age, the breast bone should not be prominent, because the breast muscle is taking on a characteristic rounded appearance. Associated with fleshing is the need for a minimum, but not excessive, fat content in the body. Excess fatness can best be determined around the vent area, although the wing web is also a good indicator of general fat reserves in the body.

All managers want their pullets and roosters to be well feathered, although there is little reliable data to correlate degree of feathering in 16-18 week pullets, with subsequent egg production. As birds grow they can be expected to progress through a predictable pattern of molt, where they will lose their juvenile feathers, to be replaced by adult feathers through successive molts. This is most obvious in the wing primary feathers, where the number of juvenile primaries (first to appear) molt in a fairly predictable pattern over time (Table 7.15). However it is not uncommon to see specific pullet flocks with 8 juvenile primary wing feathers at 20 weeks that subsequently perform well in the breeder house. Feather condition can be affected by nutrition. Inadequate level or balance of amino acids, especially methionine and cystine, can cause abnormal feather growth, while the imbalance of lysine to arginine sometimes causes the feather sheath to not fully open, and so the birds have a juvenile appearance. Deficiencies of most vitamins will also cause slower than normal feather growth, while T-2 mycotoxins cause feathers to be frizzled in appearance.

TABLE 7.15 Molting pattern and average shank and keel length of breeder pullets			
Age (wks)	#Juvenile primary feathers remaining	Keel length (cm)	Shank length (cm)
2	10	5.0	5.0
4	10	6.0	7.0
6	10	7.0	8.0
8	9	8.0	9.0
10	9	9.0	10.0
12	8	10.0	11.0
14	6	11.0	11.5
16	4	11.5	12.0
18	3	12.0	12.2
20	2	12.5	12.4
22	1-2	13.0	12.5

Shank and keel length can also be monitored as a means of assessing pullet development. In most situations, shank and keel length are correlated with body weight, meaning that underweight birds can be expected to have shorter keels and shank bones, and vice versa, especially up to 14-16 weeks of age. In fact, it is difficult to influence shank and keel lengths experimentally, without also affecting body weight. These measurements vary with strain, although some average values are shown in Table 7.15. It is important to remember that most bones in the skeleton lose their active growth plates, and become capped with calcium, when birds reach 14-16 weeks of age. It is therefore impossible to expect changes in skeletal growth, after this time, in response to changes in feed supply or diet nutrient specification. Attempting to correct skeletal inadequacies in older pullets, through diet manipulation, usually leads to obesity and a subsequent increased incidence of prolapse in the breeder house.

7.10 LIGHTING PROGRAMS

The concept and use of lighting programs has been extensively covered in Chapter 3, and examples of life cycle programs for most housing systems are detailed in Table 3.6.

The basic concept that must be remembered is never to increase daylength while birds are immature, and once the mature pullet is given extra light, never to subsequently decrease this amount. In open-sided growing houses, the daylength should be adjusted such that it coincides with the maximum that the birds will be exposed to over the 19-20 week growing period. This extra light can be given in either the morning or the evening, since both are equally effective in controlling sexual development. From a management viewpoint, it is easier to give additional light in the morning, because evening light means that birds are suddenly confronted with darkness when lights are switched off. Morning lights also allow for earlier feeding which is useful in hot weather conditions.

In black-out or fully controlled environment growing houses, daylength can quickly be reduced to 8-10 hours, because this will save feed as birds are less active in the dark and so use less feed energy for maintenance. The intensity of the 8-10 hr light period can also be quite low, usually being around 30-40 lux.

7.11 VACCINATION PROGRAMS

Pullets will be vaccinated against various potential endemic diseases, in order to protect them against infectious agents and also to ensure that adequate maternal antibodies are transferred into the egg for the broiler chick. When eggs or chicks are exported or transferred any great distance, it is important to understand the potential disease challenge likely to be encountered in the customer's region for these broiler chicks, and give initial protection through the breeder health program. It may therefore be necessary to vaccinate for diseases not necessarily endemic at the location of the breeders.

While vaccination programs vary in different countries and at various locations within a given area, a generalized program is outlined in Table 4.3. Vaccination programs will likely involve a combination of live and dead (inactivated) vaccines. Live vaccines are often used as an initial primer to the immune system, and then as birds get older they respond much better to the inactivated vaccines that give much longer lasting protection. Managers therefore have to be skillful in both types of vaccination methods.

With live vaccines, the application system is usually much easier, with many being given as a coarse spray (see Section 4.3, Chapter 4). The main practical points to consider, are cleanliness of equipment used in preparing the vaccine/ water mixtures, spray particle size and the absence of chlorine in the water mix. If the water quality on farm is at all questionable, it may be advisable to purchase distilled water. Application must ensure that all birds receive the vaccine, because any unvaccinated bird will receive a natural infection from their flock mates, usually 3-7 d later when the live vaccine is multiplying in the vaccinated birds. This "rolling" vaccination can continue almost indefinitely, especially with some of the respiratory vaccines, and the flock continually has sub-clinical cases of the disease.

Inactivated vaccines must be injected, which involves handling all birds and giving subcutaneous or intramuscular injection. Although the problem is less obvious, it is important to stress that all birds should be vaccinated, because often groups of birds are missed or even whole pens within a house are forgotten. The vaccine reaction is a stress to the bird, but this is often less than the physical catching and handling of the birds. There should be no bonus for speed of operation, because this often involves rough handling of birds, and leg problems in particular are aggravated by poor handling techniques. Pullets and roosters should never be held by just one leg. The only adequate way to evaluate the vaccination program is periodic ELISA testing of sample birds, and review of the antibody titres. This technique not only indicates the effectiveness of the vaccines, but also shows if the birds are naturally challenged.

7.12 MALE GROWING SYSTEMS

Brooding and management techniques as described in this chapter relate to both pullets and males. The manager has the choice of growing the males together with the pullets, or as is occurring more frequently, the sexes will be grown separately. The major problem of growing the sexes intermingled, is that the feed allowance must be dictated by the needs of the pullets, and so the roosters can become lighter than standard. In order to resolve this problem during the critical first few weeks of growth, it is important to brood the sexes separately and not mix them until the males are at least 140% of the weight of the female chicks - normally this will occur in about the 3rd or 4th week. The males are disadvantaged when the sexes are brooded together because they are usually smaller chicks and have been more stressed because of toe clipping and perhaps dubbing.

When sexes are grown together, the males should be sampled at regular female weighing times, and weight and condition recorded. If roosters are immature in terms of weight and fleshing at 19-20 weeks, because of the mixed-sex growing system, then it may be necessary to move the males to the breeder house 1-2 weeks earlier than scheduled, such that they can be pre-conditioned with extra feed. Alternatively, after 14 weeks, it may be possible to introduce some hanging tube feeders, positioned out of reach of the females, so that again the males can get extra feed. This method is often not too successful however, because it is the underweight males that need extra feed, and often they cannot reach these feeders.

If males are grown separately, then the manager has the ideal situation in feeding to growth requirements as previously described for the pullets. With black-out housing, males can be grown at low light intensity of around 10 lux, in order to prevent fighting and cannibalism. It is very important to ensure adequate frame size in males by 14-15 weeks of age, and as described in section 7.9, this is highly correlated with body weight. Small framed birds have a tendency to subsequent obesity and have problems with mating the larger sized hens. The testes will also start to develop after 16-17 weeks of age, and it is important not to have males on a declining plane of nutrition at this time, ie. undue heavy feed restriction or diets of very low nutrient density. Through the 16-26 week period, the males should be uniformly gaining weight each week. Depending upon the management system, it is usual to move males ahead of females, so that they receive light stimulation earlier and become trained to use the dedicated male feeders.

7.13 GROWING COSTS

Following are average costs for growing breeder pullets and roosters to 20 weeks of age (Table 7.16)

TABLE 7.16 Growing costs (US$)

	PULLETS	ROOSTERS
Chick	2.25	3.40
Feed	1.05	1.25
Labor	0.50	0.50
Vaccine, vaccinations	0.30	0.25
Maintenance, repair	0.10	0.10
Building depreciation	0.10	0.10
Miscellaneous	0.05	0.05
Mortality	0.20	0.20
Total	$4.55	$5.85

7.14 MALE SELECTION

The primary breeders place great emphasis on selecting the largest males from within a population of male-line birds. Because of genetic correlation, the offspring from larger males, on average, will be heavier than offspring from smaller males. This is because the heritability of body weight is reasonably high at 0.3-0.4 (or 30-40%), meaning that larger males produce larger offspring. Commercial breeders very rarely use this technique, since they assume that the primary breeder has done all the genetic selection necessary. Certainly the primary breeder has selected out the fastest growing male-line males, but within these birds, there will still be genetic variation and this can be utilized by selecting out the fastest growing birds. This management technique is rarely used in commercial breeders however, because it is difficult to implement, and initially it looks a very expensive proposition.

The main management problem is that in order to select out the fastest growing males, they must be fed a relatively high nutrient dense diet on a free-choice basis. The primary breeders accomplish this by feeding their potential breeders on broiler type diets. The male-line males will grow even faster than commercial broilers, and they end up with 3 kg males at 6-7 weeks of age. At this broiler age, the males are then selected on the basis of body weight (and other characteristics thought important by the geneticist). However, we now have a 3 kg male at 7 weeks, and need this bird to be around 3 kg as a young mature breeder. Obviously the growing management of this bird has to be very specialized.

For commercial breeder males, if we want to carry out any weight selection, then it has to follow an ad-lib feeding program. Selecting the heaviest males at 18 weeks following the usual restricted feeding program will result in identifying the most aggressive birds that can compete well at the feeder. This characteristic may be important (or not) in the breeder house, but is of no commercial significance to the broiler grower. If we want to select parent males, then it would have to be at about 3-4 weeks of age, or whenever the restricted feeding program normally starts. Genetics will contribute part of the reason why some chicks are heavier than others at this time. If we work out the genetics of heritability of growth and account for variance and the diluting effect of the hens, then we can expect the following improvement in broiler offspring (male and female) to result from various degrees of male selection (Table 7.17).

TABLE 7.17. Percentage improvement expected in growth rate of broiler offspring resulting from selection of the heaviest male breeders at 3-4 weeks of age

Male chicks selected (%)	% Improvement in broiler growth
20	1.9
40	1.3
60	0.9
80	0.5
100	0.0

If we select 100% of the male breeder chicks at 3 weeks, as most commonly occurs in industry, then we cannot expect any improvement in broiler growth. At the other extreme, if we select only the heaviest 20%, then all the broiler offspring will be about 1.9% heavier than if no selection was practiced. The cost of such selection is the extra day-old males that are needed. Suppose we use a 50% selection at 3 weeks, and expect this to give us a 1% improvement in broiler growth. For a flock of 10,000 breeder hens, then we would normally place about 1,200 breeder male chicks, with the expectation of housing 800 adult breeder males.

If we want a 50% selection at 3 weeks, then we need to place 2400 male breeder chicks. Table 7.18 shows the economics of this decision. The extra cost of male selection is calculated at just over $6,000, assuming no salvage value of the 1,200 males selected out as being the 50% smallest chicks. The 1% improvement in weight of the broiler offspring from these "superior" male chicks is calculated to return an extra $28,000 giving an overall improved return of around $22,000 to an integrated poultry company.

BIBLIOGRAPHY

Gillingham, S., 1997. Vaccination - a critical participant in poultry disease prevention in Compendium of Veterinary Products. Publ. Compendium Veterinary Products. Hensall, Ontario, Canada.

TABLE 7.18. Costs and returns associated with 50% selection of male breeder chicks at 3 weeks of age, based on body weight (US$)

Costs	No selection	50% male selection
a) Male chicks	1200 @ $3.40 = $4080	2400 @ $3.40 = $8160
b) Growing costs to 3 wks	$1200	$2400
c) Chick weighing, selection	---	$1000
TOTAL COSTS	**$5280**	**$11,560**
Returns	**No selection**	**50% male selection**
1% improvement in growth of 2 kg broilers @ $1kg/ liveweight. Assume 140 chicks from each of the 10,000 breeder hens.	---	$28,000
TOTAL RETURNS		**$28,000**

CHAPTER 8. MANAGEMENT OF ADULT BREEDERS

PAGE NO.

The major goals in managing the adult breeders are to maintain the health status of the flock, while allowing for continued, but slow increases in body weight. As in the rearing period, some form of controlled feeding is essential in order to maintain ovary function. Under feeding causes failure to attain peak egg numbers, while overfeeding is more commonly associated with very rapid decline in egg numbers following a brief period of peak egg output. Body weight and condition therefore continue to be the major criteria for monitoring the development of the birds. Separate sex feeding of hens and roosters is almost universally accepted, although there has been a trend away from using specialized male diets, with all birds being fed diets formulated to the needs of the breeder hen. This choice of diet for the males is based simply on convenience for the manager. Because the hen diet is of a higher nutrient density than are specialized male diets, lesser quantities are necessarily given, and in part this accounts for the male aggressiveness seen in some flocks. The ultimate profitability of the breeder flock is dictated by the number of eggs produced. However not all eggs are suitable for incubation and measures of hatching success are usually incorporated into egg payments. The main concerns of the breeder manager in this regard are egg size, egg cleanliness, floor egg production, eggshell quality, fertility, hatchability and ultimately, chick quality. In truly integrated operations the growth performance of the broiler offspring becomes the ultimate goal in assessing breeder efficiency.

8.1 PRODUCTION STANDARDS

Breeder hen performance will obviously vary across strains and even between flocks of the same strain due to the many "environmental" factors that can influence egg production and fertility. As a generalization, however, we ideally expect flocks to peak at around 85% egg production and to produce 150 chicks to 64 weeks of age. Average guidelines for breeder hen performance are shown in Table 8.1. The level of daily feed intake will obviously depend upon the environmental temperature and the energy level of the feed. The values for feed intake shown in Table 8.1 assume an energy level of 2850 kcal/kg. Diets as low as 2600 kcal ME/kg are sometimes used in temperate climates where there is an abundance of high fibre cereal by-products. Conversely 3000 kcal ME/kg is sometimes used in warm climates involving corn or milo based diets. Table 8.2 shows the adjustment to feed intake necessary as energy density of the feed varies. This means that if peak allocation is to be 460 kcal/hen/day, and the diet is at 2900 kcal/kg, then daily allowance should be 159 g. Intake would be around 167g if diet energy was changed to 2750 kcal/kg. As will be discussed in a subsequent section, egg size is very important to the hatchery, because it influences chick size and also the incubation conditions necessary for consistent hatchability. Monitoring egg size, and uniformity of egg size is therefore an important management tool. Figure 8.1 shows normal development of egg size.

Fig. 8.1 Egg weight of breeders.

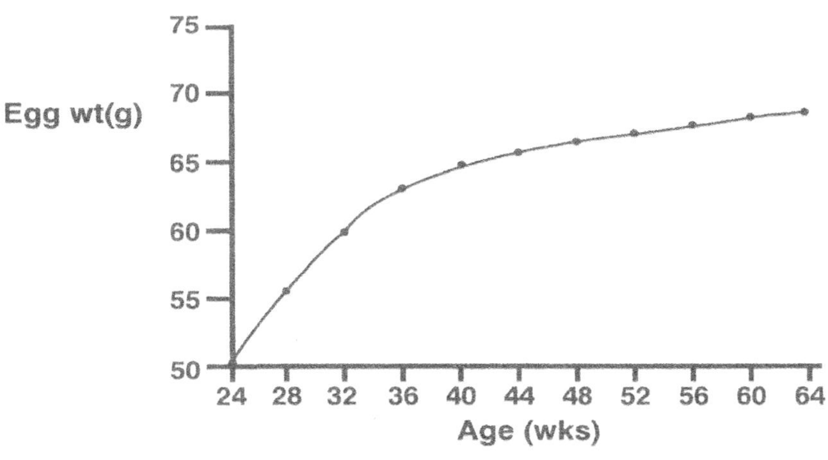

The challenge is to increase egg size, such that a minimum of unsettable small eggs are produced, while later in production it is often necessary to try and limit egg size due to problems with breakage on egg trays during transportation and

TABLE 8.1 Guidelines for mature breeder hens

	Body weight		Feed intake[1]		Egg numbers	Hatchability	Cumulative	
Weeks of age	g	lbs	g/bird	lbs/100	%	%	Hatching eggs	Saleable Chicks
22	2320	5.11	110	24.2	-	-	-	-
24	2550	5.61	130	28.6	5	-	-	
26	2800	6.16	150	33.0	35	80	2	1.6
28	3100	6.83	160	35.2	75	84	10	8.4
30	3250	7.16	160	35.2	85	88	20	17.2
32	3300	7.27	160	35.2	85	90	32	28.0
34	3350	7.38	160	35.2	84	92	42	37.2
36	3400	7.49	158	34.8	82	92	55	49.2
40	3450	7.60	154	33.9	78	90	75	67.2
44	3500	7.70	152	33.4	74	88	95	84.8
48	3550	7.80	150	33.0	70	86	115	102.0
52	3600	7.92	148	32.5	66	85	130	114.8
56	3650	8.00	146	32.0	62	84	145	125.5
60	3700	8.15	144	31.7	58	82	160	137.8
64	3750	8.25	142	31.2	55	80	174	144.0

[1]Diet ME 2850 kcal/kg

TABLE 8.2 Adjusting feed intake according to diet energy level (@22°C)

	g/bird/day					lbs/100/day				
	Diet ME (kcal/kg)					Diet ME (kcal/lb)				
Daily energy need (kcal)	**2600**	**2700**	**2800**	**2900**	**3000**	**1180**	**1225**	**1275**	**1320**	**1360**
300	115	111	107	103	100	25.4	24.5	23.5	22.7	22.0
320	123	119	114	110	107	27.1	26.1	25.0	24.2	23.5
340	130	126	121	117	113	28.8	27.8	26.7	25.8	25.0
360	138	133	129	124	120	30.5	29.4	28.2	27.3	26.5
380	146	141	136	131	127	32.2	31.0	29.8	28.8	27.9
400	153	148	143	138	133	33.9	32.7	31.3	30.3	29.4
420	162	156	150	145	140	35.6	34.3	32.9	31.8	30.9
440	169	163	157	152	147	37.3	35.9	34.5	33.3	32.4
460	177	170	164	159	153	39.0	37.6	36.0	34.8	33.8
480	185	178	171	166	160	40.7	39.2	37.6	36.4	35.3
500	192	185	179	172	166	42.4	40.8	39.2	37.9	36.8
520	200	193	186	179	172	44.1	42.4	40.8	39.4	38.2

handling. Most breeder managers utilize a quick visual reference chart to monitor flock performance, an example of which is shown in Fig 8.2.

Fig. 8.2 Breeder production monitoring chart.

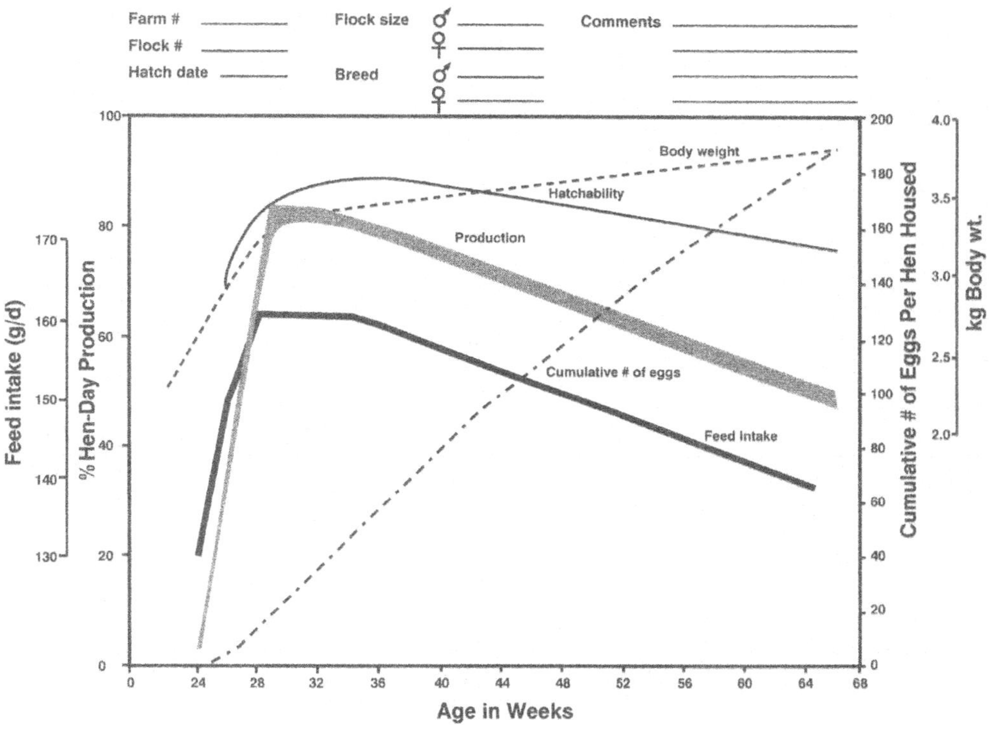

Management guidelines for roosters are less extensive, but still very important to ensure optimum fertility. There is a very good correlation between body weight and fertility, where it seems as though constant, but small increases in weight are important for life time fertility in the rooster. As a generalization, roosters will be about 33% heavier than hens at the start of production, and about 20% heavier after 40 weeks in the breeder house (Table 8.3).

As previously described for the hens, the allocation to the roosters will be influenced by the actual energy level of the diet used. For both hens and roosters, energy and feed needs will also be influenced by environmental temperature as previously described in Table 5.23.

TABLE 8.3 Guidelines for mature roosters (@ 22°C)						
			Daily Feed Intake			
Weeks of age	Body weight		Breeder diet[1]		Separate male diet[2]	
	g	lbs	g/bird	lbs/100	g/bird	lbs/100
22	3100	6.82	120	26.4	123	26.4
24	3270	7.20	123	27.0	126	27.8
26	3500	7.70	125	27.5	126	28.2
28	3650	8.00	128	28.2	131	28.9
30	3820	8.40	130	28.6	133	29.3
32	4000	8.80	130	28.6	131	28.9
34	4100	9.00	132	29.0	134	29.5
36	4200	9.25	132	29.0	134	29.5
40	4250	9.36	132	29.0	134	29.5
44	4300	9.47	134	29.5	136	30.0
48	4350	9.58	134	29.5	136	30.0
52	4400	9.69	134	29.5	138	30.4
56	4450	9.80	136	30.0	138	30.4
60	4500	9.90	136	30.0	140	30.8
64	4550	10.00	136	30.0	140	30.8

[1]Diet ME 2850-2900 kcal ME/kg, CP @ 15.5%

[2]Diet ME 2750 kcal ME/kg, CP @ 12%

8.2 GENERAL HOUSE DESIGNS AND LOCATION

There are three basic breeder house designs that vary with the degree of environmental control. Traditionally there have been totally open-sided houses, designed for warm climates. These allow for maximum natural air movement, but provide no light control and the inside temperature is very much a reflection of outside environmental conditions. Figure 8.3 shows a typical open-sided breeder house - the extensive roof overhang is to prevent rain and direct sunlight from hitting the birds.

Fig. 8.3 Open-sided breeder house (Campi, Merida, Mexico).

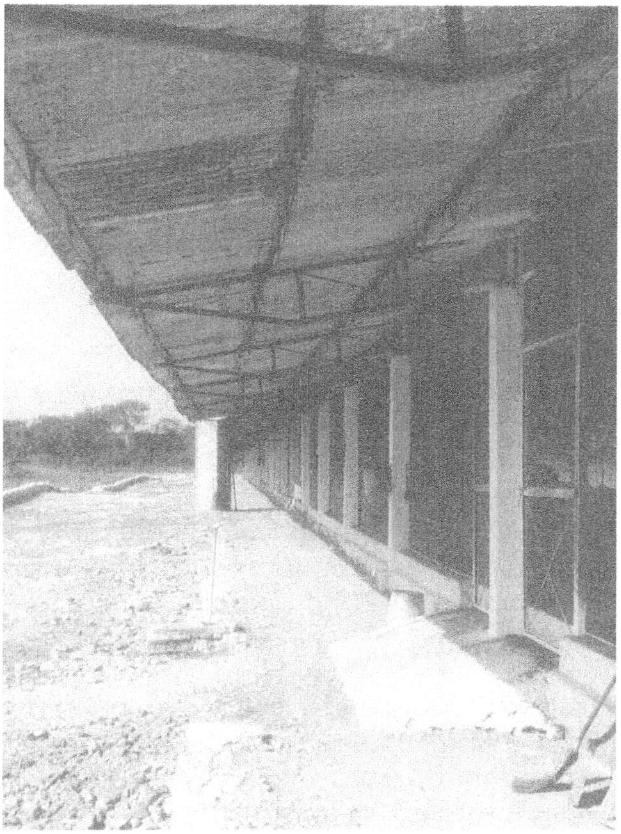

Most open-sided breeder houses will be litter floored. In order to provide some degree of protection against colder environments, the next phase of development was the curtain-sided breeder house. In this design, house construction is similar to that of open-sided buildings, although a movable curtain of plastic or cotton-type material provides greater protection to the birds in winter months and/or at night time (Fig. 8.4). Again most of these houses are total litter floor design.

The latest innovation for breeder houses in warm climates is the evaporative-cooled tunnel ventilated design, that provides much closer control over environmental conditions. As shown in Fig. 8.5, the ventilation is 100% mechanical, being provided by a cluster of fans situated at one end of the building (for building lengths up to 120 meters). Air is drawn in through evaporative cooling cells at the opposite end of the building, and the air is forced down (tunneled) the length of the building. The sidewalls are plastic or laminate that will never be moved except under emergency conditions. In the event of power failure, and where there

Fig. 8.4 Curtain-sided breeder house (Dagranja and PenaBranca, Brazil).

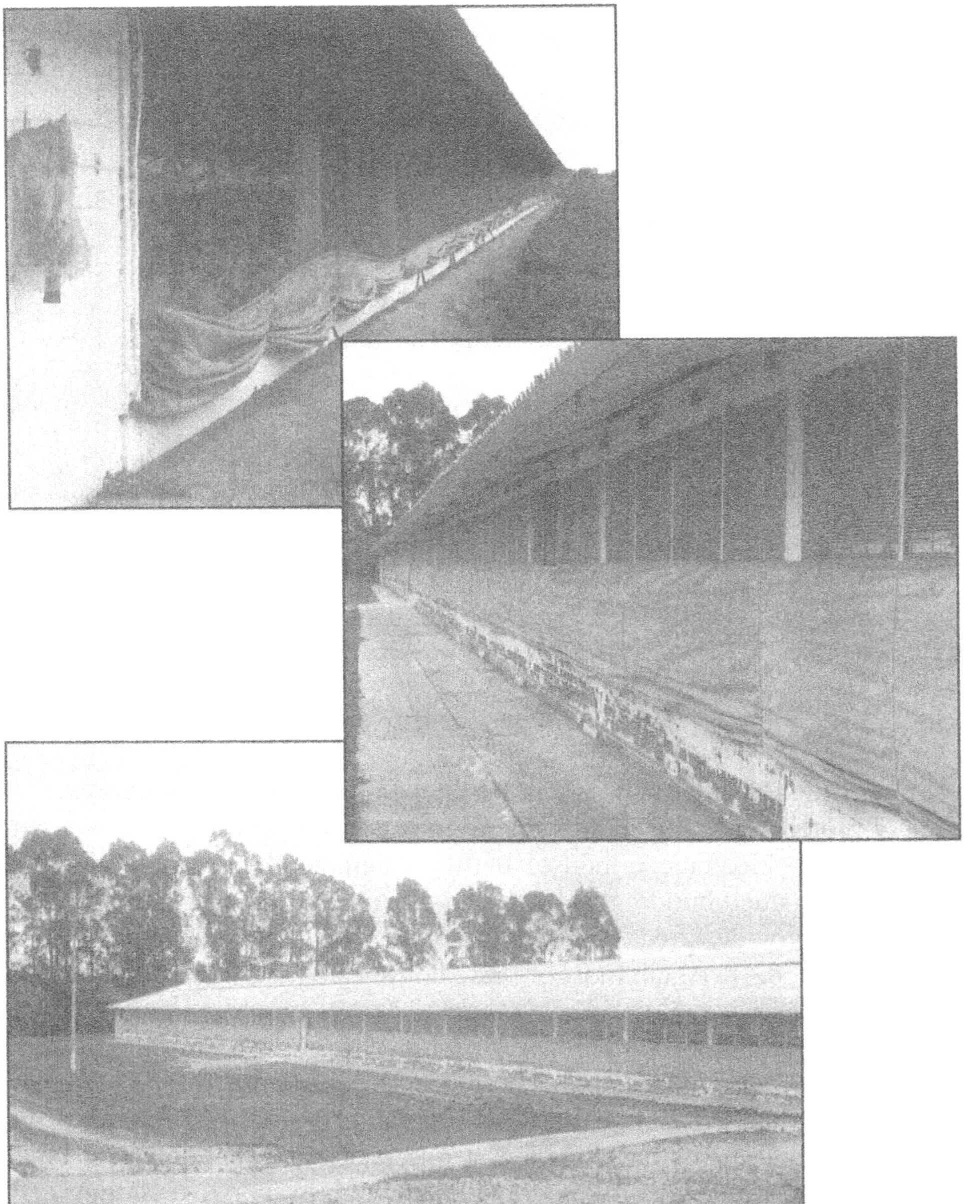

Fig. 8.5 Evaporative cooled tunnel ventilated breeder house. Bottom photo shows safety mechanism used to lower curtain during power loss. (Campi, Merida, Mexico).

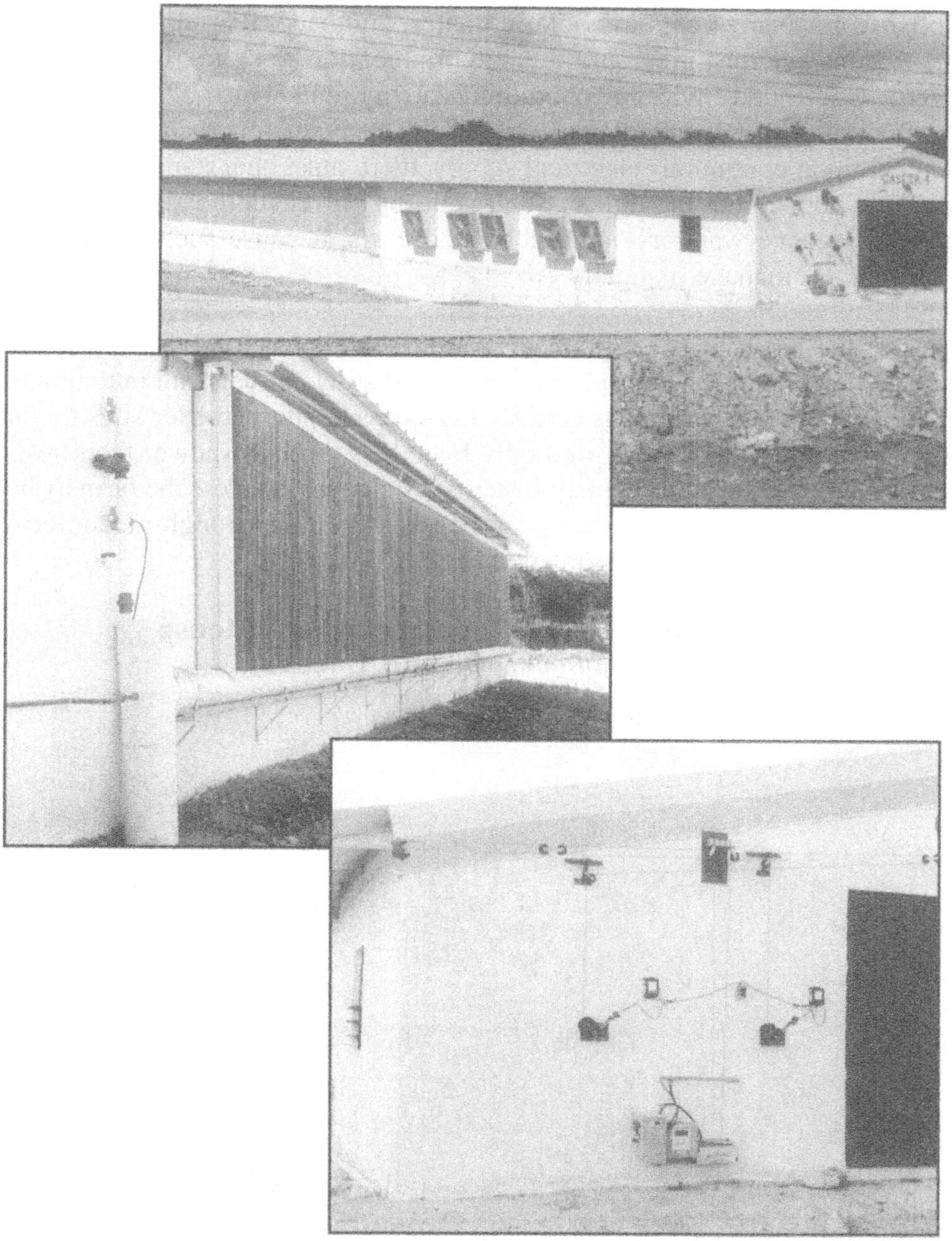

are problems with standby generators, the curtain sides can be lowered. Such a safety mechanism controlled by high temperature thermostats and/or mechanisms responsive to 7-10 minutes of power disruption is shown on the bottom photo of Fig 8.5.

Established for many years in cooler climates, and becoming more common in warm-weather regions, are controlled environment or black-out breeder houses (Fig 8.6). Controlled environment buildings are more likely to have some portion of the floor as a raised slatted area. Because these types of structures are totally dependent upon continuous electrical supply, there must be a stand-by generator available to power fans and lights. Such stand-by power should also be adequate to operate feeders, waterers and mechanical nests, because such equipment is very difficult to manage manually.

As part of the biosecurity program, it is advisable to fence the immediate area around the farm. This ensures protection against stray animals and intentional or unintentional access by humans (Fig 8.7). Access to such breeder sites by farm staff and visitors should be allowed only by access through shower facilities. A major limitation to such biosecurity systems is the need to access the farm by both feed trucks and egg trucks. Trucks can be made to pass through a disinfection tank and sprayed externally as shown in Fig 8.7.

Fig. 8.6 Controlled environment breeder house (Fleming chicks, Ontario, Canada)

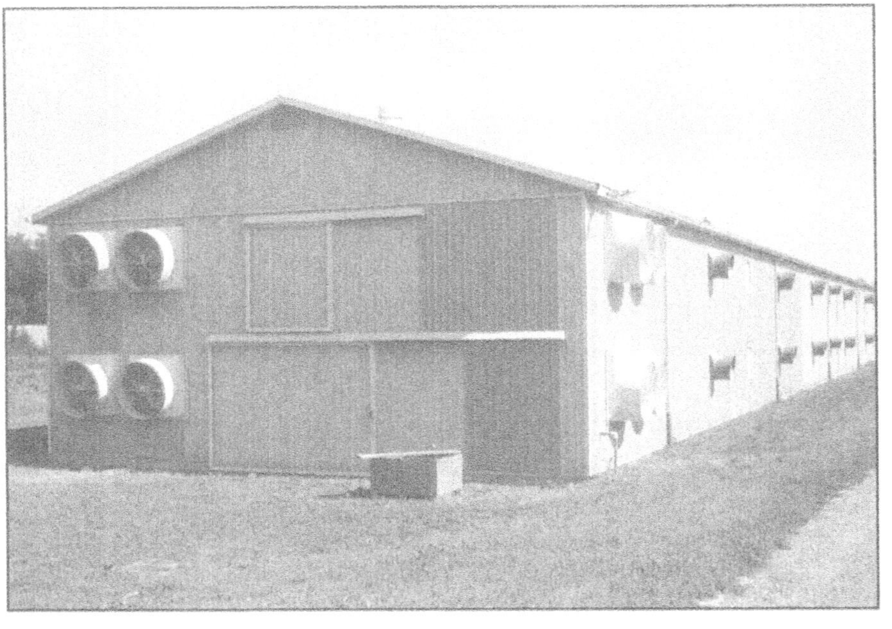

Fig. 8.7 Security fences around breeder facilities. Bottom photo shows vehicle washing facility (Campi, Merida, Mexico)

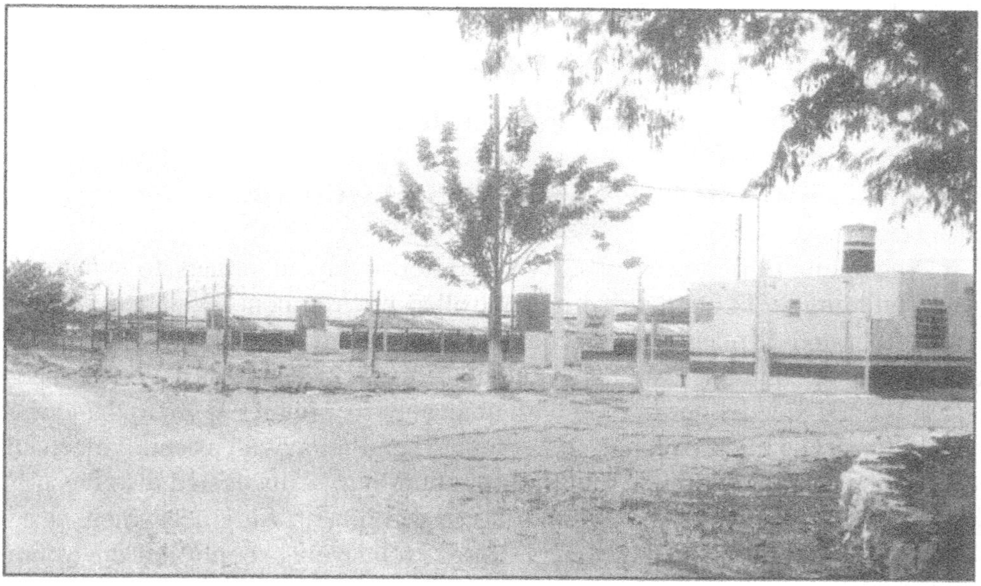

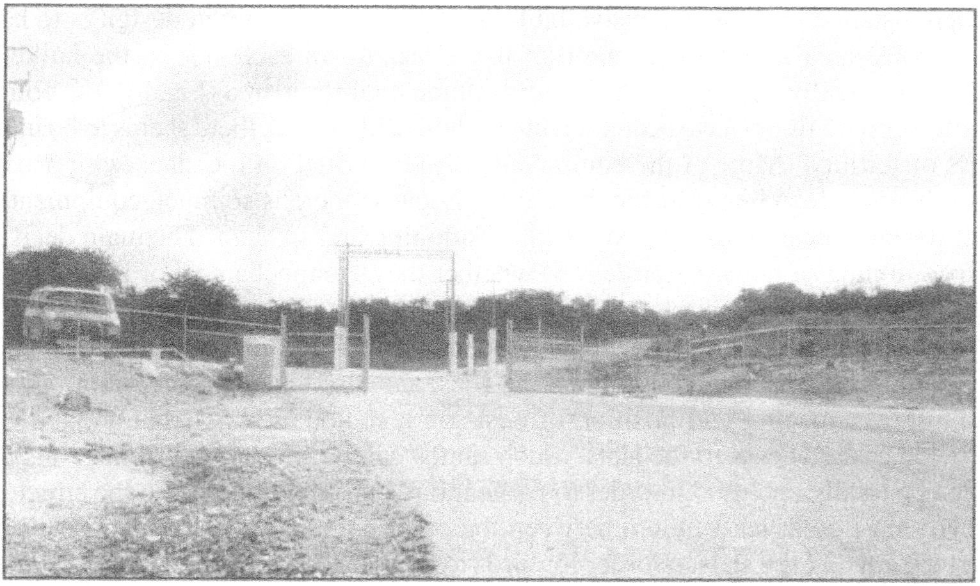

Alternatively, such vehicles can be denied access to the farm, and so delivery of feed and pick up of hatching eggs is from facilities located on the boundary of the farm (Fig 8.8). Figure 8.8 shows (top) access for staff through a "shower-in" facility, (middle) feed delivery to storage silos located on the boundary and (bottom) the central egg room, also with access by hatchery trucks outside the farm boundary fence. Feed and eggs have to be transported within the farm area by use of dedicated vehicles that are solely located on this farm.

8.3 INTERIOR HOUSE LAYOUT AND EQUIPMENT

The major differences observed in interior layout relates to whether the building is **1)** open sided or controlled environment **2)** slatted vs littered floor and **3)** manual vs mechanical nests. Figure 8.9 shows interior layout for an open-sided, tunnel ventilated and controlled environment building. The top design is open-sided, litter floored with manual nests running at 90° to the length of the building. The middle picture shows tunnel ventilation with a central mechanical nest running parallel with the length of the building. This design also has a litter floor. The bottom picture shows controlled environment, with mechanical nest and 2/3 slats, 1/3 litter floor. Slats are used almost exclusively in controlled environment buildings, and are becoming more common in tunnel ventilated houses. Slats allow for up to 20% increased stocking density, and so there is some economic saving when installed in these expensive buildings. The most common design is to have the slatted area running the length of the house, down each side of the building. The slats usually occupy about 2/3 thirds of the total floor area (Fig. 8.10.). Totally slatted or wire floors have been tried but without a litter area, there seems to be major loss of fertility. Most of the equipment will be located on the slats, with usually just the male feed line over the litter area. Because there is so much equipment on the slats, then care must be taken with positioning and spacing. The main decision is positioning of nests, regardless of whether they are mechanical or traditional in design. Traditional nests are usually aligned at 90° to the slats, with just the first 1m on the slats, and the remainder suspended over the litter area. Mechanical nests must be positioned entirely on the slats, and also take up more room. Figure 8.11 shows spacing and position of nests on a slatted area ngled at about 45° to provide easier access to the slats. Such ramps can be spaced at 5 m intervals and must be totally enclosed in order to prevent birds nesting underneath the structure. There must be at least 38 cm between the outer edge of the nest facing the litter and the edge of the slats, in order for birds to be able to get into and out of the nests easily, and not be disturbed by other birds jumping up to the slats. If this distance is much less, then there will be greater competition for nests on the alternate side, and also more floor eggs. There will usually be two hen feeder lines and two rows of drinkers running down each slatted area, and none of these should be positioned closer than 60 cm to the interior face of the nest. The equipment layout and design shown in Fig 8.11 will be duplicated on both slatted areas.

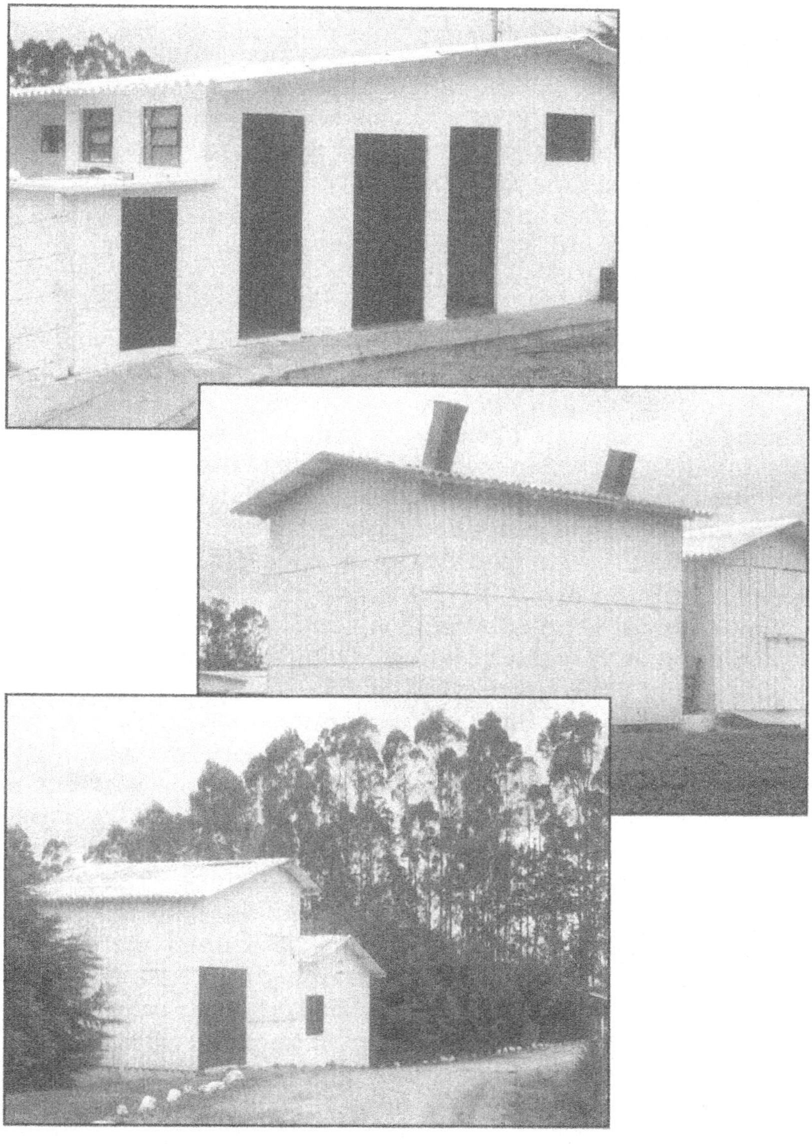

Fig. 8.8 Biosecurity showing perimeter access only. (Top) people showers (Middle) feed and (Bottom) egg pick-up. (Dagranja, Brazil).

Fig. 8.9 Interior design for (Top) open-sided curtain (Middle) tunnel ventilated and (Bottom) fully controlled environment breeder houses. (Campi, Mexico; Fleming chicks, Ontario)

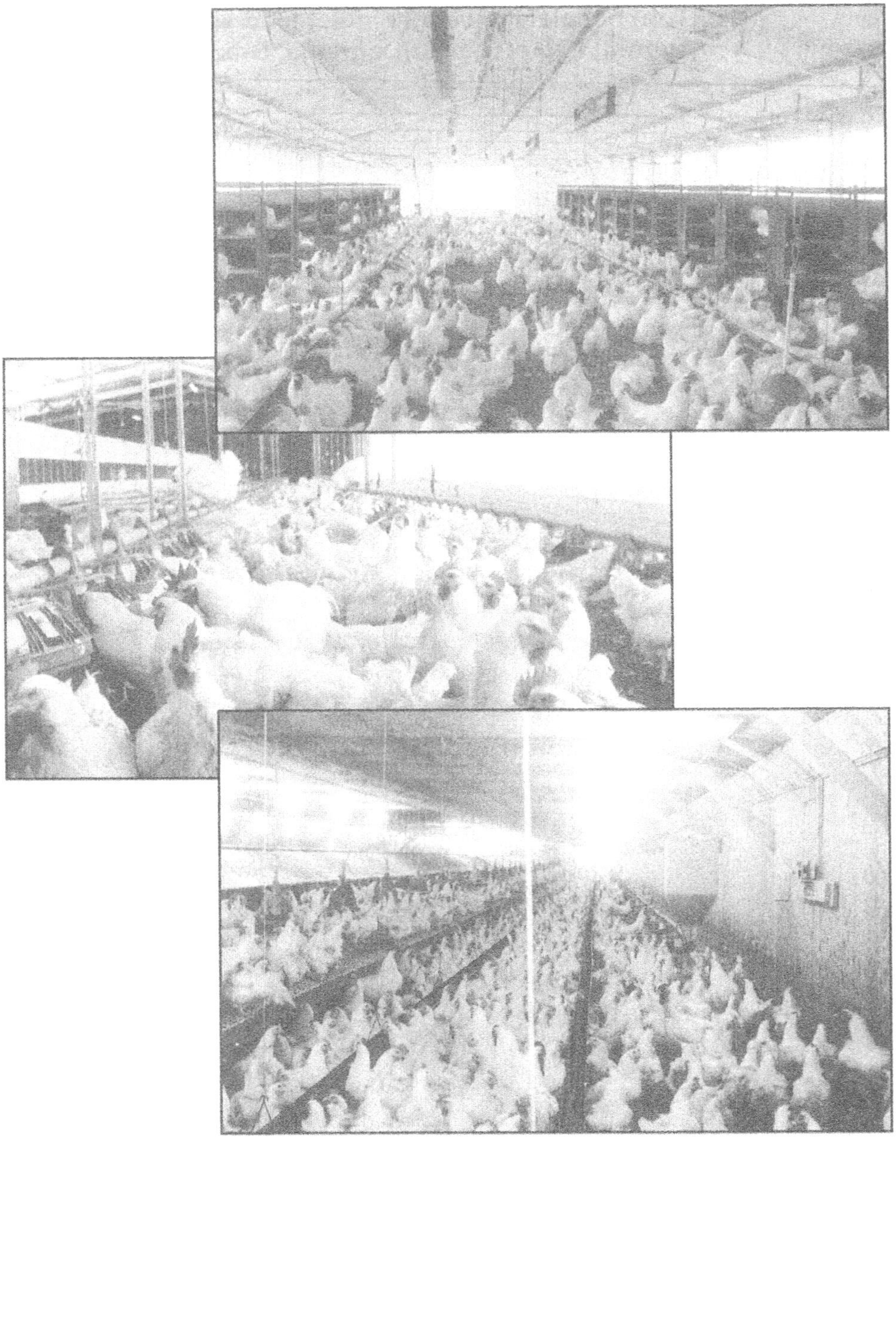

Fig. 8.10 Interior of slatted floor breeder house.

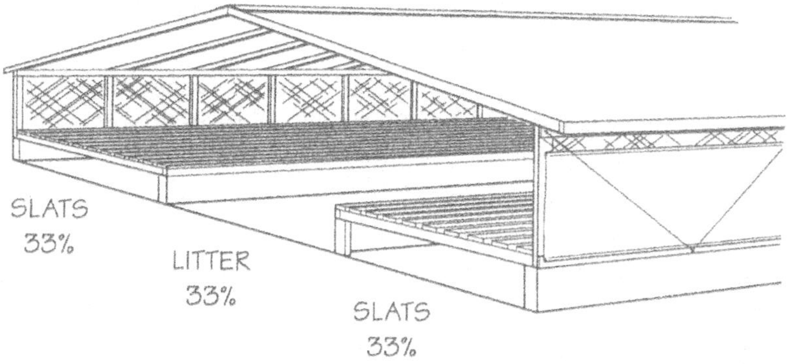

Source: Big Dutchman (1998)

Fig. 8.11 Positioning of equipment on one side of 2/3rd slat breeder house.

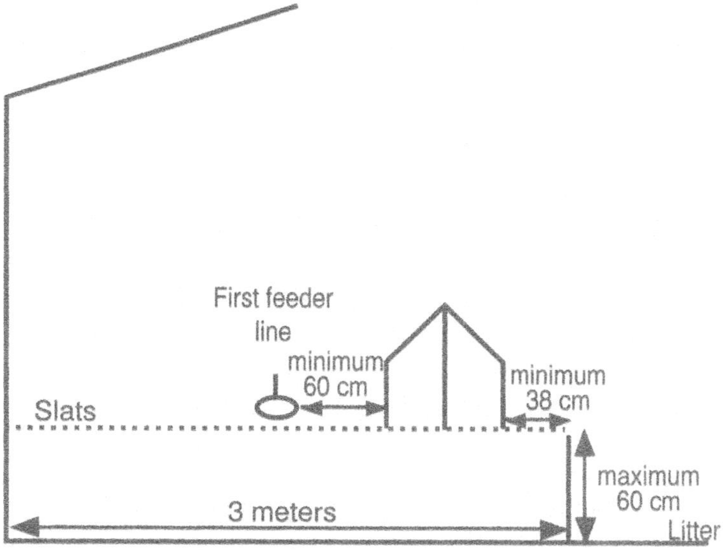

The slats should be no more than 60 cm above the litter, because birds are reluctant to jump up and down when slats are much higher than this. Some managers use ramps,

There should be one nest hole per 4 breeder hens, with one nest per 5 hens regarded as the maximum density. For mechanical nests without individual nest holes, there needs to be at least a 30 cm run of nest space per hen. Traditionally nests have been made of wood, constructed in banks of 20 nests, with 5 top and bottom arranged back-to-back (Fig 8.12). As shown in Fig 8.12, the top of the nest should be fitted with a wire or movable perch such that birds cannot roost on top of the nest. Nest management involves regular cleaning and top dressing with new wood shavings or whatever litter material is used. Depending upon bacterial counts, then nests can be seeded with products such as formaldehyde chips or other antibacterial agents on a biweekly or monthly basis. The slats used in front of both manual and mechanical nests should be hinged, such that they can be used to close off the nest. This prevents immature hens using the nest immediately when they are placed in the breeder house. During the 7-10d prebreeder period, when nests are opened, it may be necessary to close nests at dusk in order to prevent birds roosting here. If this technique is used, the nests obviously have to be opened at dawn. It is very important for the most mature birds to start laying in the nests, since this encourages the remainder of the flock to follow their behavior. The hen is usually attracted to the nest because it is an area of low light intensity. If light enters the nest directly, birds are often reluctant to enter, and this can lead to more floor eggs. This situation can be especially problematic when mechanical nests are used in open-sided buildings that are orientated north-south.

Figure 8.13 shows a situation where sunlight is entering an open-sided breeder house, and illuminating the outside face of the mechanical nests located on the east side of the building. This will happen in the early morning period, which is part of the main period for egg laying. In this example, the eastern face of the mechanical nests are at 500 lux, while the alternate side will be in shadow, and is at 8 lux. The same situation applies to nests on the west side of the building, but because there is no direct sunlight, the effect is much less pronounced. In this example only 13% of eggs were picked up from the nests at 500 lux, compared to 32% of eggs on the alternate side. The same situation is seen on the other slatted area, with 22 vs 33% of eggs being laid in the light exposed vs protected nests. This means overcrowding in certain nests, and unfortunately floor laying is quickly established as a normal habit for the birds. The problem can be solved by having a mesh curtain dropped down on the outside wall, to about 1m from the eaves. The curtain is designed to filter out direct sunlight, but not to unduly restrict air movement.

Fig. 8.12 Traditional wooden nests with (Top) wire or (Middle) wooden tops to prevent roosting. The top photo shows bottom nests closed so as to train young pullets to use the top nests. The bottom photo shows a fully automated nest system. (Campi, Merida, Mexico)

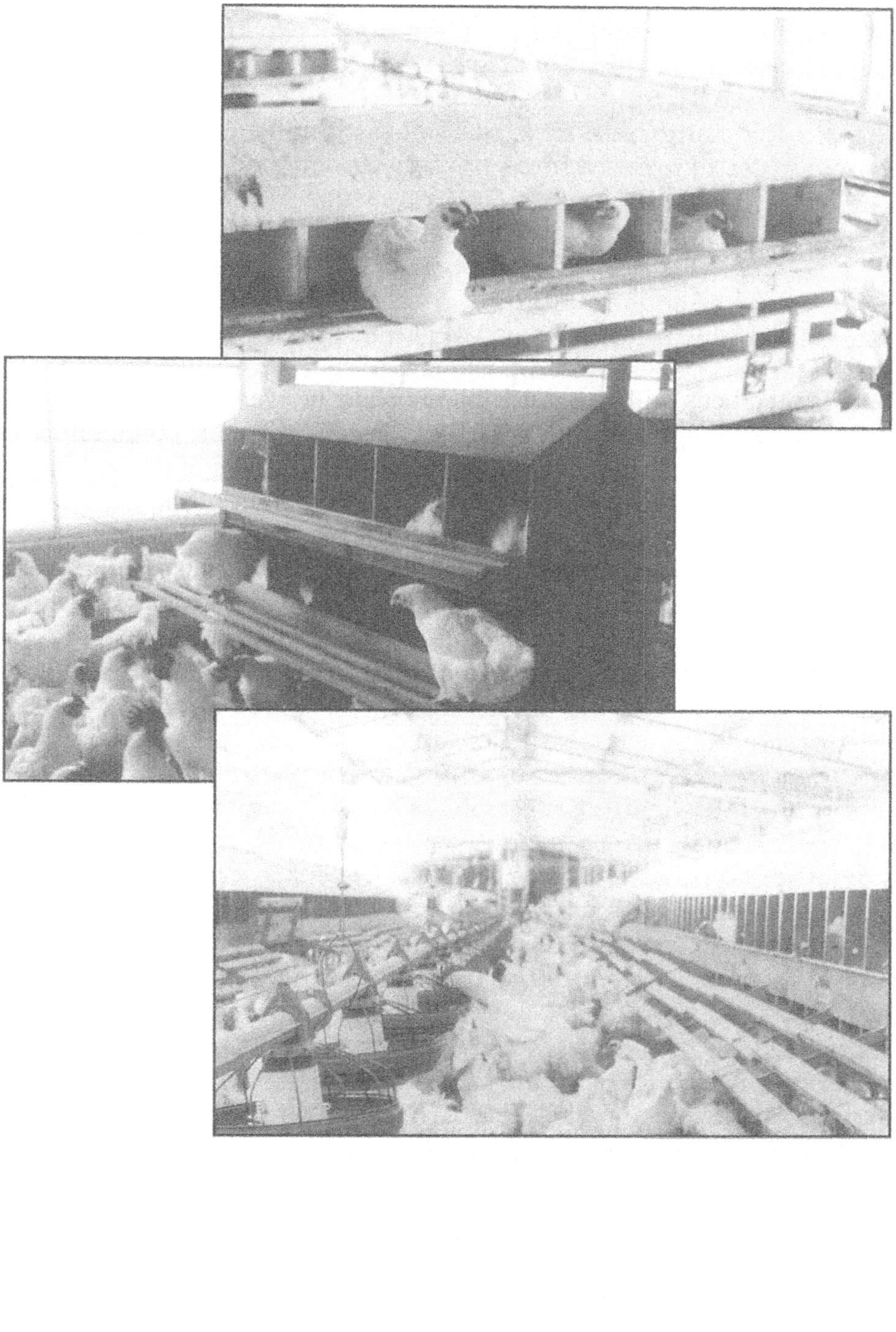

Fig. 8.13 Effect of direct sunlight on light intensity inside breeder house.

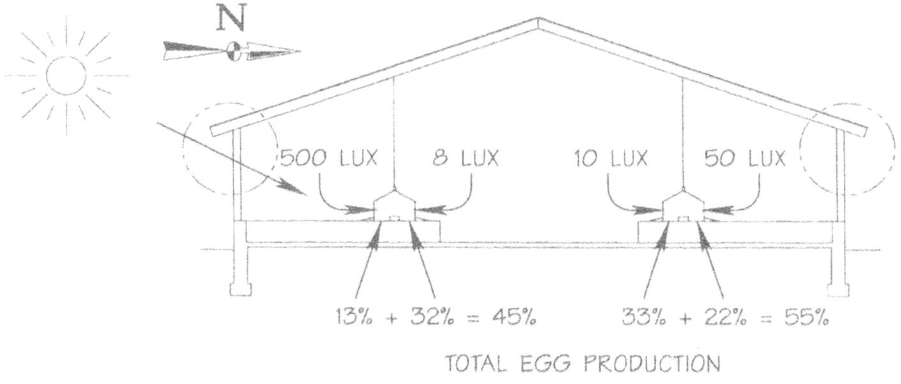

Source: Big Dutchman (1998)

Feeders for the hens will be located on the slats, or evenly spread throughout a litter floored building. Regardless of floor design, it is most common to locate the rooster feeders in a single line running down the middle of the building. The major feature of the rooster feeding system is the height of the pans above the litter, which is usually about 19-21 cm (Fig 8.14). At this height the roosters can adequately feed, while most hens will be excluded because of the excessive height.

Fig 8.14 Male feeder height designed to prevent female access

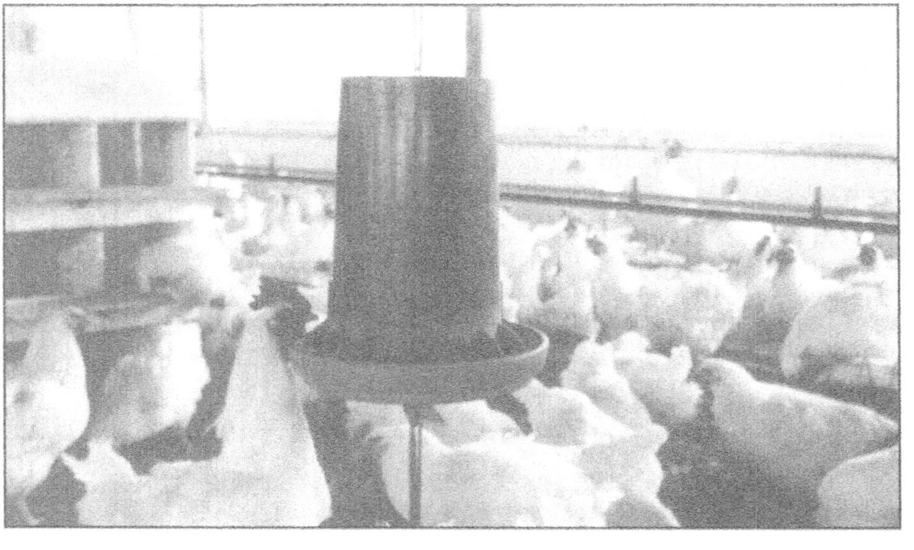

An advantage of moving roosters into the breeder house before moving the hens, is that the roosters can be more easily trained on their feeders. Starting out at a lower height (12-15 cm) the feeders can be gradually raised over 3-4 days, such that they are at full height prior to moving in the hens. Without this prior training, it is more common for roosters to wait around the hen feeder lines. Initially they may be able to gain limited access, because of a smaller head size, but their intake is often inadequate, and these roosters often become caught in the wire grills as their head size increases.

The hens are usually fed from trough or pan type feeders, each being fitted with grills about 43 mm apart that effectively exclude the roosters because of their head width. Fig 8.15 shows these types of feeders in commercial practice.

With continuous trough and chain feeders, the exclusion grills are either high or low profile (Fig 8.16).

The high profile grills are more expensive, but have become popular as managers realize that roosters are sometimes able to bend the low profile grills apart and so gain unlimited access to the hen feed. An alternative approach is to tie a plastic water pipe underneath the apex of the grill, running the length of the trough. This technique prevents most roosters from eating from this feeder. Birds can get their legs caught in the high-profile grills, especially when they are used in grow-out. With high profile grills, it is important to continually adjust the height of the feeder, so that birds can pass beneath, and not necessarily over the top of the feeder, as they move about the house.

If there is no separate male feeder line, then the males can be fed by leaving a proportion (about 10%) of the tube feeders or length of feed trough un-grilled. This is a less satisfactory system of feeding roosters than a dedicated system, but it can be used in older facilities where there is simply no room to install more equipment. A fairly recent innovation has been the so-called nose bars, fitted to roosters before they are transferred to the breeder facilities (Fig 8.17). The plastic bar makes it virtually impossible for the rooster to eat from the grilled hen feeders, regardless of its head size, and so the roosters are truly separate-fed at 21 weeks, or at such time that the two sexes are mixed in the breeder house.

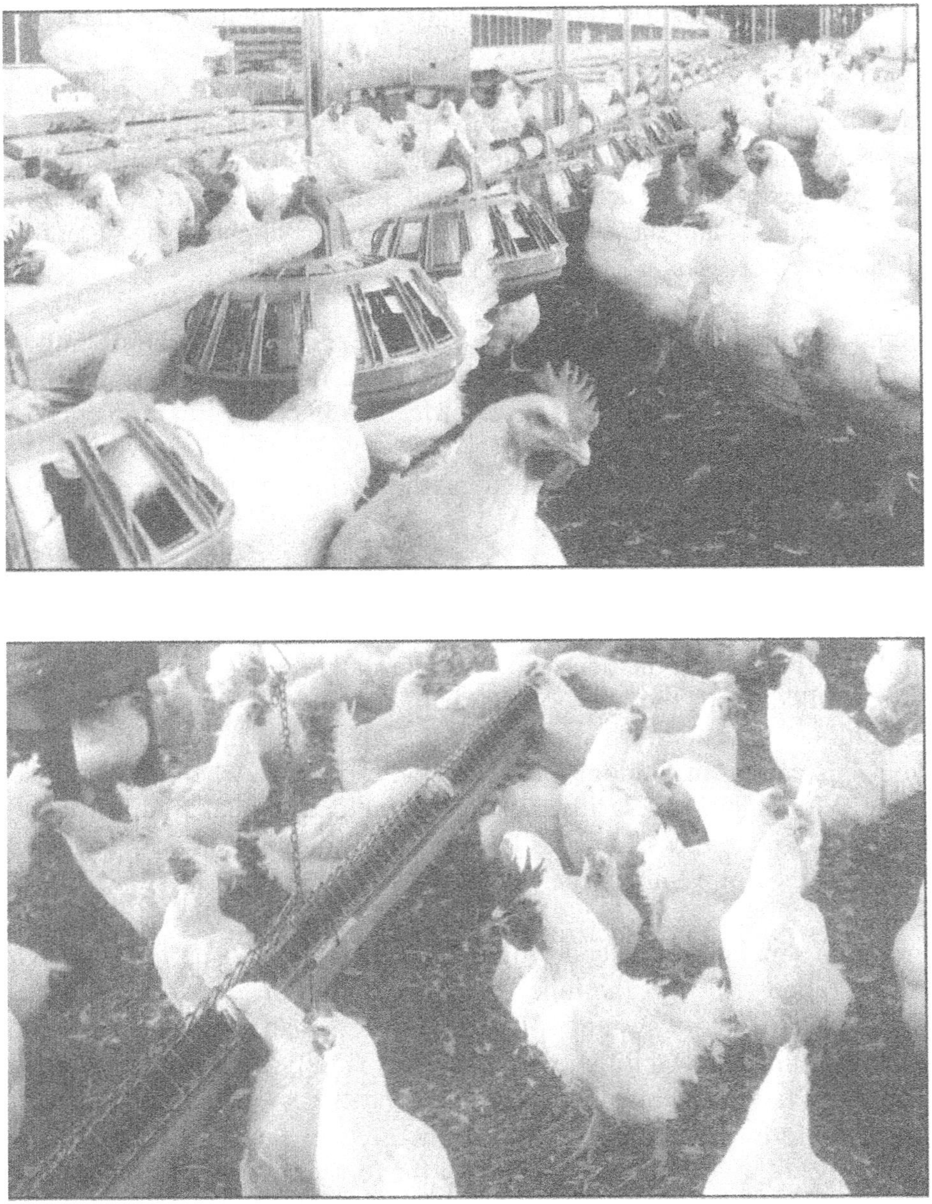

Fig. 8.15 Chain and pan breeder feeders

Fig. 8.16 Feeder grill profiles.

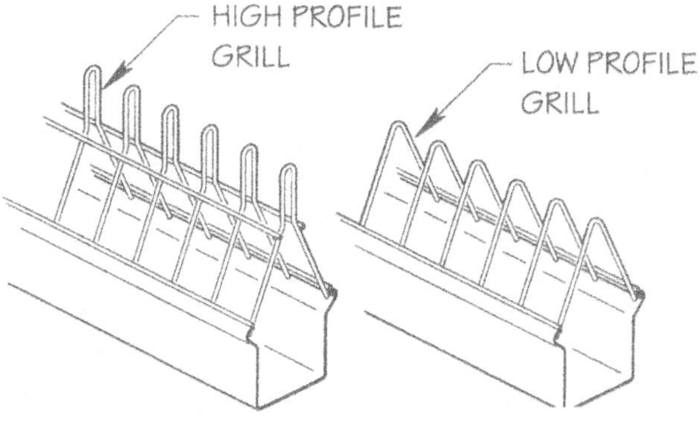

Source: Big Dutchman (1998)

Fig. 8.17 Breeder male fitted with plastic nose bar.

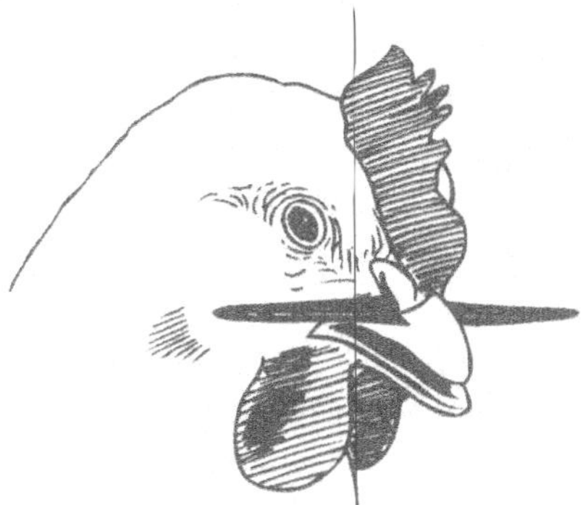

Watering systems are usually bell-type drinkers or nipple drinkers (Fig. 8.18). It seems false economy not to have the recommended number of drinkers, which is usually 1 bell per 60-75 hens, while alternatively there should be at least one nipple per 6-7 birds.

8.4 NEST MANAGEMENT

Eggs laid outside of the nest must be suspect in terms of microbiological content, and so it is essential that young pullets be adequately trained to use the nests. Regardless of design, there needs to be about one nest space for every 4 breeder hens, because the time of egg laying is synchronized by the

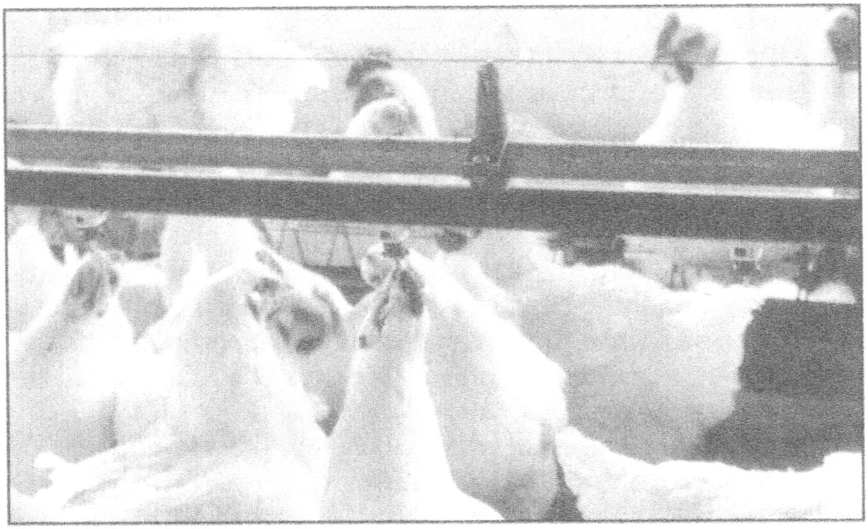

Fig. 8.18 Breeder hens using nipple drinkers

light program, with most eggs appearing during a 3-4 hr period each day. Using a 5 a.m. → 9 p.m. light schedule, then most eggs will be laid between 9 a.m. and 12 noon. If there are a significant number of eggs laid outside of this period, then the lighting system should be re-evaluated.

The desire of a hen to seek out a nest site is a natural behavior, although there also seems to be a learned component that has commercial significance in large flocks. Hens will seek out and use nests of a variety of designs and construction, and there is no single stimulus that is critical to the process. In controlled experiments, hens preferred pre-molded sites to those where the bird had to mold the nest herself. Important features seem to be the need to find a degree of isolation, a site that is darker than the other areas of the house, and is free of drafts, extremes of temperature and unusual noise. The height of the nest above the litter is perhaps one of the most critical features because heavy breeders are sometimes reluctant to use even second tier nests. This latter behavior may be related to the experience of the bird with perching. Studies have shown much greater success with nest use and especially second tier nests, when as pullets, these birds had access to perches.

Floor laying can be virtually eliminated if these hens are continually removed from the floor nests and placed in the nest boxes. Obviously this becomes a tedious task with large commercial flocks, but it does show that hens can be trained to use nest boxes even after establishing a floor laying behavior. It seems as though the nest site used throughout the production cycle is dictated by the site chosen for the first 5-6 eggs. Consequently, it is very difficult to resolve floor laying once the flock is at 28-30 weeks of age. Birds also avoid nest sites where they have experienced a frightening situation, such as unusual noise etc. For this reason, when mechanical nests are first opened, the belt should be run periodically so as to accustom the birds to the noise and vibration associated with belt movement. There is some indication that nest color may have an influence on choice by the hen, where gray is preferred over black or brown nest sites.

Nests should be opened 10-14 d prior to expected first egg. This gives the birds time to inspect the nests and to gain experience in standing on the slatted entry platform. Once production starts, then the slats and litter area should be walked at least 6-8 times each day, picking up floor eggs and moving any nesting birds. If there are obvious floor sites being preferred, then these should be modified by blocking off the area (usually corners etc.) and/or adding extra light to these locations. Leaving 2-3 eggs in a floor nest quickly encourages other hens to use this site. If there is more than 1% of eggs being laid along the feed lines, it is an indication that feed time is occurring too late, and so rather than seek out a nest, the bird's main desire is to feed.

There is a definite trend towards mechanical nests, mainly because of savings in labor. With conventional nests, egg collecting is the major labor input for the breeder farm. Table 8.4 shows time allocation with conventional vs mechanical nests.

TABLE 8.4 Time allocation with conventional vs mechanical egg collection (%)

	Conventional nest	Mechanical nest
Feeding, bird weighing	10%	20%
Egg collection	40%	---
Egg grading, boxing	23%	35%
Floor eggs, walking facility	10%	15%
Culling, ventilation maintenance	15%	20%
Nest maintenance	2%	10%
Hours/10,000 breeders/day	20	14

With conventional nests, there is almost 65% of labor input dedicated to egg handling, and this is reduced to 35% with mechanical nests. This equates to about 14 hours vs 5 hours per day labor for egg handling in a 10,000 bird flock. Mechanical nests are obviously much more expensive to purchase and maintain, and there will be a 1-3% increase in floor eggs with these systems.

Nest pads in mechanical systems need to be cleaned periodically, and it is advisable to inspect and clean 8-10% of the pads daily on a revolving schedule. At the end of the cycle, pads must be thoroughly cleaned and disinfected, which is a somewhat laborious task. Depending upon the size of the operation, concrete mixers are effective in cleaning pre-soaked pads. For large scale operations, concrete trucks, with their revolving tank can be very effective.

With conventional nests, then daily inspection is part of the egg pick up procedure. Nest material should be topped-up as necessary, and totally replaced each 30 days - at this time, 30 g paraformaldehyde flakes can be added to the nest and then covered with new nest material. It may be necessary to close nests at night, especially in the prebreeder period, in order to discourage birds from roosting in the nests. Under these conditions, it is essential to open all nests at first light.

Frequency of manual egg pick up will be discussed more fully in section 8.8. Four to six collections daily are recommended for birds at peak production, with at least three collections before noon each day. Cleanliness of the eggs can be greatly influenced by collection procedures. The operators should wash and disinfect their hands prior to starting a pick up, and egg collection must always be a stand-alone operation - this means that floor eggs, dead birds etc. should be handled at another time. It is tempting for the collector to gather floor eggs at the same time as nest eggs, and this results in the microbial load of the entire collection being only as good as the status of the floor eggs.

There is some controversy about placing floor eggs in the nest during routine operations within the breeder house. Depending upon the level of biosecurity within the organization, this practice is either acceptable or unacceptable in terms of microbial loading of the nest sites.

8.5 EGG STRUCTURE

Figure 8.19 shows the major components of the egg. The cuticle acts as a physical barrier against entry of microbes via the shell pores. Storage of eggs has no effect on the structure of the cuticle, and on many farms the cuticle is removed during the washing process. Loss of the cuticle will increase the rate of water loss, especially for smaller eggs from younger breeders.

Fig. 8.19 Major egg components.

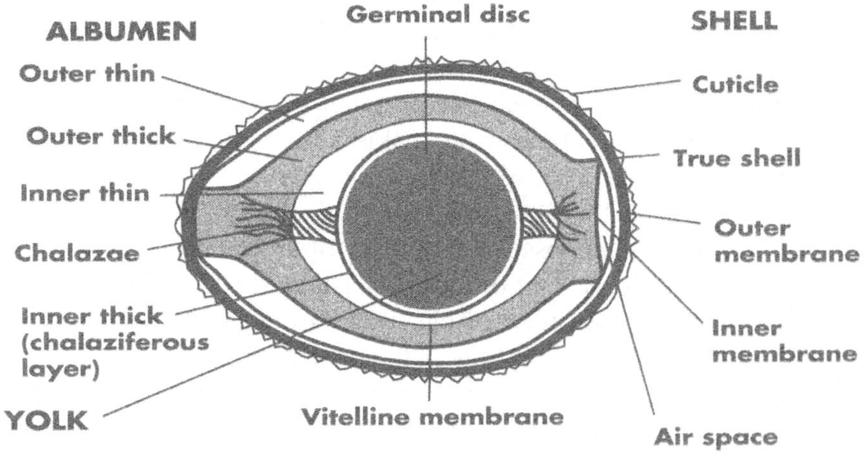

The shell is composed mainly of calcium carbonate, although there are some important quantities of trace minerals such as magnesium. The shape of the egg results in great strength when pressure is applied from the ends, but is very weak when tested around the equator. There is no real difference in resistance of the shell to fracture when pressure is applied from the small or large ends, and so orientation of the egg on trays is not important in this respect. About 90% of hatching eggs should have a characteristic egg shape, and so these eggs are easily placed small end down on setter trays. The remaining 10% of eggs are more difficult to grade, because they have a more rounded shape, and so on average, about 5% of eggs can be incorrectly set small end up.

Shell weight increases at about the same rate as does egg weight, with an increase of about 30% over the 24-64 week period (5→6.5 g shell). However because the volume of the egg is increased over this time, then the shell tends to get thinner with older breeders. This thinner shell may be important to birds on an evolutionary time scale, because as eggs get larger the surface area per unit of egg mass decreases. The larger egg needs to lose more water and CO_2 and take up more O_2 for the larger embryo, and this is more easily accomplished with a thinner shell. A factor influencing moisture and gas exchange is the depth of the pore in addition to the number and diameter of the pores, ie. the deeper the pore, the more resistance to gas exchange and vice versa. Because shell thickness influences moisture and gas exchange, then it becomes a factor in hatchability (see section 8.7). Shell porosity can be measured by placing the shell in concentrated nitric acid for 10 seconds, washing and then drying with a paper towel. Painting or immersing the etched shell in methylene blue then shows up the pores which can be clearly seen under a low power microscope. The pores are the major route of entry for microbes, and when this happens the inner shell membrane is probably the greatest physical barrier to contamination. Should microbes penetrate the membranes, then lysozyme in the albumen is the next line of defense. Another protein in albumen, known as conalbumen tightly binds iron, making this essential nutrient unavailable for microbial multiplication.

The albumen is actually composed of a number of different layers which together make up about 60% of the weight of the egg. The outer thick albumen represents about 57% of the total albumen in a fresh egg, with the outer thin albumen contributing about 23% of the total. The inner thin albumen should be about 17% of albumen mass, while the inner thick which is also called the chalaziferous layer, represents about 3% by weight. These proportions of albumen change with egg storage, and when such changes are extreme, they can adversely influence hatchability. The albumen on average is about 90% water and almost 10% protein. The chalaziferous layer is very important for holding the developing embryo in a central position within the egg, especially when the egg is being turned. It attaches firmly to the outer thick albumen which itself is attached to the shell membranes.

Over time, the structure of the albumen changes as CO_2 diffuses out through the shell pores. Such diffusion continues until the CO_2 concentration of the egg is equivalent to that of the storage environment. Buffer systems within the albumen adjust to this loss of CO_2 and consequently the pH of the albumen increases from around 7.5 in a fresh egg to 8.5 in an egg stored for 48 hrs at 20ºC. The increase in albumen pH causes changes in protein structure, such that there is "thinning" of the albumen over time. Some change in pH of the albumen is thought essential for good hatchability, and lack of thinning is thought responsible for the poorer hatchability seen with eggs set within 24 hr of laying, especially in eggs from young breeders. The rate of change in albumen structure is largely a factor of storage temperature, with changes occurring much more quickly at higher temperatures. For short term storage (<2 days), egg holding temperature is therefore less critical than it is for eggs stored for 5-7d. As the albumen thins, there are characteristic pockets of water that develop in both the albumen and yolk, giving them a mottled appearance.

Albumen quality is best assessed by simply measuring the height of the outer thick albumen or by using this measurement to calculate the Haugh unit. Albumen height is an adequate relative measure of quality as long as eggs are of comparable size. If egg size is variable, or albumen quality is to be tracked over the life of a flock, then Haugh units should be calculated using the following formula:

$$\text{Haugh unit} = 100 \log \left[\frac{H - \sqrt{G}(30W^{.37} - 100)}{100} + 1.9\right]$$

where H = albumen height in millimeters
G = 32.2
W = Egg weight in grams

Alternatively, some tripods used to measure albumen height can be precalibrated for a certain egg weight, and Haugh unit determined directly. A Haugh unit of 90 is regarded as excellent, with 80 being very good, and 70 being good. On the other hand, 65 is poor and anything below 60 is very poor. The decline in Haugh unit with age of the breeder hen is usually predictable with a decrease of about 0.3 units per week.

A number of factors can influence albumen quality, and hence hatchability. During storage, the rate of deterioration in Haugh units is mainly a factor of temperature, with change occurring at double the rate in eggs stored at 20 vs 12°C. Protein and amino acid content of the diet has little effect on albumen composition, although high levels of vanadium (usually as a contaminant of phosphate ingredients) quickly leads to watery albumen. Higher levels than normal of dietary magnesium have been reported to slow the thinning of albumen during storage, although this is usually accompanied by poorer shell quality, and so has little practical application. Challenge with Infectious Bronchitis or Newcastle virus can also lead to thinner albumen.

The yolk is composed of equal quantities of fat and protein that will be used as the major source of nutrients for the developing embryo. The yolk is not depleted 100%, the residual yolk sac is "absorbed" into the body cavity where it may serve as a source of nutrients for the young chick during the first 24-48 hrs. In the fresh egg, the blastoderm is positioned on the yolk as described in section 2.11. The initial pH of the yolk is around 6.0, but this changes over time corresponding to the rate of change in the albumen. There is movement of water from the albumen through the vitelline membrane into the yolk during storage, and this results in the characteristic mottling of the yolk that develops over time. The anticoccidial nicarbazin can also cause yolk mottling and loss of hatchability, but this is usually associated with a characteristic depigmentation of the shell. Cottonseed meal is rarely used in breeder diets, one reason being the potential accumulation of gossypol in the yolk. Cottonseed oils also contain some unusual fatty acids that influence the permeability of the vitelline membrane and subsequent exchange of nutrients between the albumen and yolk.

8.6 EGG SIZE AND APPEARANCE

Egg size is largely a factor of breeder hen body weight, but can also be influenced by nutrition to some extent. As with any bird, egg size increases as the breeder gets older. Depending upon the strain, the first few eggs produced will average around 47g in weight and this will increase quickly to 60 g by 34 weeks and then more slowly increase in size to about 68 g by 62 weeks of age. Table 8.5 shows average egg size of breeders from 24 to 62 weeks of age. Because egg size influences chick size, then there is usually some grading of eggs from young breeder flocks. Traditionally, eggs less than 50 g have not been considered "hatching eggs" and so there is an incentive to maximize early egg size, especially in high-yield strains that tend to lay smaller eggs. Egg size is responsive to protein and especially to the methionine content of the diet. However there is little evidence to suggest that it is economical to use more than the regular level of methionine (around 0.36%) or protein, simply to increase egg size.

TABLE 8.5 Average egg size

Weeks of age	Weight (g)	Weeks of age	Weight (g)
24	47.0	44	65.0
26	50.0	46	65.5
28	56.0	48	66.0
30	58.0	50	66.3
32	59.0	52	66.6
34	60.0	54	66.9
36	61.0	56	67.2
38	62.0	58	67.5
40	63.0	60	67.8
42	64.0	62	68.0

The negative impact of crude protein fortification is reduced fertility, especially in hot weather situations. It is also much more difficult to control body weight of hens fed high vs low protein/amino acid diets. High protein diets at this time are also very detrimental to the fertility of the roosters that are usually eating the same feed. Linoleic acid is another nutrient that can influence egg size, although the effects are more pronounced when deficient dietary levels are used. If corn is used in the breeder diet, there will be no response to linoleic acid. With milo or wheat based diets, linoleic acid could be less than 1% of the diet, and this situation can be corrected by adding 1% supplemental fat to the diet. It seems uneconomical to increase linoleic acid content much beyond 1% of the diet.

Egg size influences chick size, which in turn, affects the final body weight of the broiler chicken. As a generalization each 1g change in egg size, affects the chick size by about 0.5 g, which subsequently results in about a 5 g change in body weight of the broiler at 42 d. Table 8.6 shows the expected relationship between hatching egg size, chick size and live weight of 42 d broilers.

TABLE 8.6 Effect of hatching egg size on broiler performance

Hatching egg weight (g)	Chick weight (g)	Extra liveweight yield per 100,000 broilers (kg)
50	32.5	---
52	33.5	1000
54	34.5	2000
56	35.5	3000
58	36.5	4000
60	37.5	5000
62	38.5	6000
64	39.5	7000
66	40.5	8000
68	41.5	9000

The improved growth rate of birds hatching from larger eggs may in part be due to these chicks hatching with more residual yolk sac, and so they have a greater quantity of potential nutrients prior to placement or initiation of active feeding. Sixty week old breeders produce chicks with about 10% larger residual yolk sacs, and within this yolk there seems to be much more fat. Consequently, these larger chicks have 10-15% increases in levels of blood glucose and triglycerides, suggesting that these chicks are better able to overcome placement delays and/or other management stresses.

Double-yolked eggs, which are usually characterized by being very large and more rounded at the small end should not be sent to the hatchery. Very small and extra large eggs also hatch very poorly, mainly because the average incubation conditions are not suited to these extremes of egg size. Because egg size influences respiratory and water exchange of the developing embryo, it is important to have a consistent size of egg set in any one machine. Small eggs can be made to hatch successfully if they are set as a group, and the resultant small chicks also grow well, if raised as a group without competition from larger chicks. Egg grading by size therefore offers tremendous potential to improve economics within an integrated company. Eggs can also be graded according to their appearance because many deformities are associated with poor hatchability. Table 8.7 gives average loss in hatchability that can be expected with various shell abnormalities.

TABLE 8.7 Hatchability of eggs with various physical characteristics

	% loss of hatchability
Misshapen	12 - 15%
Loss of pigment	20 - 30%
Slightly pimpled	5 - 10%
Heavily pimpled	15 - 20%
Wrinkled	50 - 100%
Belted	80 - 100%
Slab-sided	90 - 100%

Within a flock, eggs with the most pigmentation tend to hatch the best, but there is considerable genetic variance in this trait. Consequently, eggs from strain A that appear depigmented may hatch better than pigmented eggs from strain B.

8.7 EGGSHELL QUALITY

As the number of eggs produced by breeders increases, then eggshell quality becomes more of an issue in breeder management. Both abnormally thick or thin shells are problematic in the hatchery, because moisture and gas exchange are affected, and thin shelled eggs are more likely to break prior to setting.

Shell quality is influenced by breeder age, health status, environmental temperature and the bird's nutrient intake. As detailed in section 5.3, the intake and balance of calcium, phosphorus and vitamin D_3 are critical for maintaining shell quality. As a generalization, shell quality is optimized by a feeding program that increases the bird's intake of calcium and decreases her intake of phosphorus over time. With a two stage breeder feed, this could translate to 3.2% calcium and 0.42% available phosphorus in the first breeder diet, followed by 3.5% calcium and 0.38% available phosphorus in a second diet depending on feed intake. Vitamin D_3 is essential for calcium utilization, and so a common treatment for breeders when shell quality is problematic, is to give extra vitamin D_3 in the drinking water, usually at around 200 IU/breeder/day for three consecutive days per week. As with laying hens, the breeder's need for calcium is greatest starting in the late afternoon, which is the time that shell calcification starts. Because of early morning feeding of restricted quantities of feed, the upper digestive tract is usually empty of feed at this time, and this is not an ideal situation for calcium mobilization. Traditionally, breeders were given oystershell as a scratch feed in the late afternoon (1g per breeder per day) and this had some logic in terms of calcium needs at that time. Broadcasting oystershell (or large particle limestone) onto the litter also has the advantage of attracting birds down from the slatted areas, if used, and this helps to promote mating activity.

Shell quality is best quantitated by simply measuring the thickness of the shell directly, or by an indirect method such as by specific gravity. The shell should be around 0.3 mm in thickness, and with the cuticle and shell membranes the thickness will be 0.4 mm. If shell thickness is routinely used to assess shell quality, then the membranes should be removed. It is also important to assess thickness at 2-3 points around the equator of the egg. The disadvantage of monitoring shell thickness is that the egg is necessarily wasted, although such losses can be minimized if the procedure is combined with checks on fertility etc.

Shell quality can be indirectly measured by assessing the specific gravity of the whole egg. The major variable influencing the buoyancy of the egg is the shell mass. Eggs can therefore be placed in salt solutions of different concentration, and the specific gravity measured as the concentration at which they float. The usual range of specific gravity is from 1.065 to 1.100. Eggs with SG of $\geq$1.088 are acceptable in shell quality. Salt solutions for testing are usually made-up in plastic garbage pails - 3 kg salt added to 38 litres of water gives a SG of around 1.08. Simply by adding extra salt or extra water, SG's of 1.065, 1.070, 1.075, 1.080, 1.085 and 1.090 for example can be prepared. About 50 eggs in a wire basket are then lowered into the solution of lowest SG and any floating eggs removed. The basket is then transferred through the progressively higher SG solutions. The procedure should then be repeated with another 50 egg sample. The SG of eggs laid at various times throughout the day tends to vary, being highest for morning eggs and lowest for eggs laid early in the afternoon. For routine monitoring, therefore, the time of egg collection must be standardized. Specific gravity of the various solutions should be periodically recalibrated with the hydrometer. Table 8.8 shows the relationship between egg specific gravity and shell weight for eggs from 50 to 70 g in weight.

Because shell quality (thickness) affects moisture loss, then hatchability can be affected as shell quality deteriorates over the breeder cycle, or at any one time, due to nutritional or environmental problems. One recent study showed this latter effect to be most pronounced with young breeders where there was a 30% loss in hatch of eggs due to poor shell quality, with most problems relating to early embryonic mortality. With older breeders, the same loss in shell quality caused only a 5-8% loss in hatchability. Specific gravity below 1.080 is negatively correlated with hatchability, although there is no clear relationship between hatch and SG values greater than 1.080. The cause of poor hatchability for eggs of low SG is usually increased moisture loss from the egg. Therefore if eggs are set according to breeder age where shell quality is expected to decline as birds get older, then logically, setter humidity would be increased for eggs from these older flocks.

TABLE 8.8 Prediction of shell weight (g) from estimates of egg specific gravity and egg weight

	Specific gravity						
Egg weight (g)	**1.065**	**1.070**	**1.075**	**1.080**	**1.085**	**1.090**	**1.095**
50	2.96	3.39	3.82	4.25	4.67	5.08	5.50
52	3.08	3.53	3.97	4.42	4.85	5.29	5.71
54	3.20	3.66	4.13	4.59	5.04	5.49	5.94
56	3.31	3.80	4.28	4.76	5.23	5.69	6.16
58	3.43	3.94	4.43	4.93	5.41	5.90	6.38
60	3.55	4.07	4.59	5.10	5.60	6.10	6.60
62	3.67	4.21	4.47	5.27	5.79	6.31	6.82
64	3.79	4.34	4.89	5.43	5.98	6.51	7.04
66	3.91	4.48	5.04	5.61	6.16	6.71	7.26
68	4.02	4.61	5.20	5.78	6.35	6.92	7.48
70	4.14	4.75	5.35	5.95	6.54	7.11	7.70

8.8 EGG HANDLING, CLEANING AND SANITATION

When an egg is laid, the embryo has already been developing for about 24 hrs and is in quite an advanced stage of growth. Consequently the egg must be treated very gently as it is taken from the nest, inspected, stored, and finally transported to the hatchery. Embryo mortality occurs most frequently because of problems with incorrect egg holding temperature and humidity, and because of excessive movement, which can cause shell damage. When laid, the egg is at the hen's body temperature of 41°C, and the main priority in order to prevent pre-incubation, is gradual cooling of the egg down to around 20°C over a 6-9 hr period.

Eggs must be gathered frequently enough such that they can be cooled to the correct temperature, and this usually means 4-6 collections daily. The higher the environmental temperature, the greater the incentive to pick up eggs more quickly. With house temperatures <10°C, the egg may cool down too quickly, and so again more frequent pick-up is desirable. With hand gathering, eggs should be placed directly on plastic egg trays. Cardboard trays do prevent more mechanical damage, but they cannot be re-used since they are virtually impossible to sanitize adequately.

During collection, the egg gatherers should be trained to carry out initial selection of eggs such that obvious defects are not trayed with the regular eggs. Such defects can include double-yolked eggs, eggs that are dirty or cracked or unusually shaped. There is considerable controversy about the use of floor eggs. Some farms do not send floor eggs to the hatchery, while others make a cursory cleaning and mix them with regular eggs. Perhaps the most appropriate compromise is to keep floor eggs separate from the main collection, and to dry clean where appropriate and to discard grossly contaminated eggs. By the time that floor eggs are picked up, they are likely cool, and so bacteria will have already penetrated the shell. Cleaning therefore merely helps reduce contamination of other eggs or chicks at the hatchery. Floor eggs should never be placed in the nest.

An egg that looks perfectly clean is not in fact "sterile" in that it can have up to 500 bacterial cells on its surface when newly laid. Within one hour of laying, the bacterial number can reach 2,000 cells, and while this may sound problematic, it must be compared with a dirty egg that can have in excess of 500,000 bacteria cells on its surface. As the egg cools down in the nest, or on the slats/floor, then some of these bacteria will be drawn into the egg throughout the pores. About 20% of eggs will be contaminated in this way within 1 hour of laying. However most eggs can handle this bacterial invasion, and as previously described, defense mechanisms within the albumen, such as lysozyme, are able to destroy such bacteria. The potential invasion of bacteria through the shell is also affected by shell thickness - with a specific gravity of only 1.070 then there are 2-3 times as many bacteria penetrating the egg compared to eggs with specific gravity at 1.090 *ie.* thinner shells allow more bacterial penetration.

Eggs must be cleaned if they are dirty, although on some farms all eggs are washed. Floor eggs or nest eggs with fecal contamination can best be dry cleaned with fine sandpaper or steel wool. This procedure is very time consuming, and can lead to the removal of the cuticle and the physical clogging of the pores with fecal material and shell dust. If more than 1% of eggs have to be dry cleaned, then nest management should be thoroughly reviewed.

If eggs are to be washed and sanitized, then the procedure should take no longer than 2-3 minutes, because longer washing times usually result in more egg breakage. Washing solutions usually contain a combination of detergent and sanitizers. QUATS are commonly used as a sanitizer, alone or with formalin, using up to 200 ppm. Mechanical washers/disinfectants can remove up to 90% of the shell surface bacteria. After washing, the eggs should be dried quickly, again to prevent any remaining bacteria from being drawn into the egg, as it cools following the 30-35°C washing procedure. Depending upon local disease challenge, many breeder farms also fumigate eggs prior to shipment. Fumigation with formaldehyde gas is the most common procedure, and such treated eggs are virtually sterile on the outside surface. Eggs will ideally be set 3-4 days after being laid - if eggs are much younger or older than this, then some loss in hatchability can be expected. After about 4 days, then the hatchability of eggs declines by about 1% for each day's storage, although this loss can be prevented to some extent by specialized storage conditions. The longer that eggs are held prior to incubation, the longer the hatch time (up to 6 hours), and the greater the loss in broiler market weight. For example, storing eggs for 10 d has been shown to result in a 30 g loss in 42 d broiler weight, while this loss increases to 120 g when eggs are stored for 20 d. However it is usually necessary to store eggs for variable times at the hatchery or farm, and so knowledge of potential changes to egg composition are important in order to prevent these losses in hatch and broiler performance. The most obvious change in the eggs is loss of weight (moisture) over time, which is a factor of temperature and relative humidity (Fig 8.20).

At around 20°C, there is only a small loss in egg weight, even with RH as low as 50%. However as temperature increases to 25°C then weight loss is accentuated, especially at low humidity.

Fig. 8.20 Effects of temperature and humidity on egg weight loss.

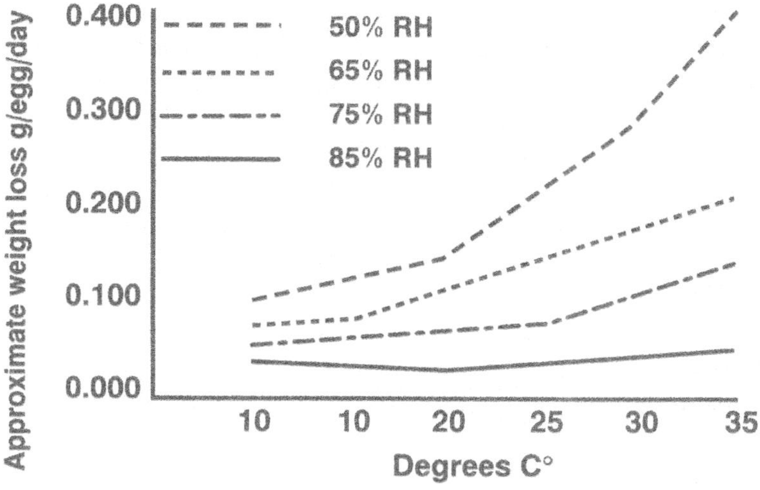

Ideal storage conditions depend upon the expected storage time. In general, the shorter the storage time, the higher the temperature and vice versa. For example, eggs to be stored for just 2-3 d can be held at 19°C while storage for 8-10 d would require a lower temperature closer to 13°C. In all situations, RH should be around 85% in order to control evaporative moisture loss. Higher humidities will prevent more water loss, but can also stimulate mold and fungi growth on the shell. Eggs to be stored for just 3-5 d can be held on open buggies, with adequate air movement around the eggs. If eggs are to be held for longer periods of time, then they can be shrouded with plastic covers. For very prolonged storage, it may also be advisable to flush the eggs with nitrogen gas, and possibly store eggs small end up (Table 8.9).

TABLE 8.9 Conditions for egg storage

	Storage time (days)			
	3-4	**6-7**	**10-14**	**15+**
Temperature (°C)	19	17	15	12
Relative humidity (%)	80	85	85	85
Cardboard boxes	No	No	Yes[1]	Yes[1]
Small end up	No	No	Perhaps	Yes
Plastic shroud	No	No	Perhaps	Yes
Nitrogen gas	No	No	No	Yes

[1]Eggs must be cooled to appropriate storage temperature prior to boxing

Optimum storage conditions and egg handling may in fact be dependant on breeder flock age. Prof. John Brake at North Carolina State Univ., proposes that eggs from young and older breeder flocks should probably be handled differently in order to standardize age related changes that necessarily occur in the egg prior to incubation. Eggs from young breeders are small and have a thicker albumen which is more resistance to change. This thicker albumen must undergo some changes in order to facilitate gas and nutrient exchange for the embryo - without this "thinning" of the albumen, there is more early embryo mortality. With much older breeders, the shell is usually thinner, and so moisture loss can occur more quickly. The albumen is also thinner in eggs from older breeders, and so eggs must not be stored for too long a period because further thinning is detrimental to hatch. These changes in egg structure and composition can be summarized as shown in Table 8.10.

TABLE 8.10 Age related changes in composition of breeder eggs and consequences for egg handling and storage

Breeder age	Egg characteristics	Consequences to egg management
22-35 wks.	Small egg Thick shell Thicker albumen	Longer storage possible Storage at higher temperatures Lower setter humidity Less frequent egg pick up
35-45 wks.	Optimal egg size Optimal shell thickness Optimal albumen thickness	Normal storage for 2-5 days @ 19°C, 80% RH
45-65 wks.	Larger egg Thinner shell Thinner albumen	Maximum 3d storage Lower storage temperature Higher storage humidity More frequent egg collection

8.9 EGG TRANSPORTATION

Hatching eggs will be transported from the farm daily or at least twice weekly depending upon the storage conditions on farm. Where there is no real control over temperature or humidity at the breeder farm, then it is advisable to move the eggs to the hatchery as soon as possible. During transportation, the main concerns are potential physical damage to the egg, control over the environment in the transport vehicle, and prevention of microbial contamination. The latter situation is often most influenced by the flow of egg trolleys, egg flats, etc. from farm to farm via the hatchery. Even with rigorous sanitation, it is preferable to minimize the transfer of egg handling equipment from farm to farm.

The embryo in the 1-2 d old egg is quite sensitive to physical damage. Undoubtedly cardboard or fiber board egg flats offer the egg the most protection, but these have been almost universally replaced by plastic trays because these can be easily disinfected and fumigated. Sudden movement of the egg can increase the chance of early dead embryos, and in this regard, the condition of roads leading up to the farm is often the main culprit. Many companies go to great lengths in designing egg handling facilities and equipment, and at the same time, negate many of these achievements by having poorly maintained access roads to the farm.

If eggs are to be transported for more than 6-8 hrs, then the vehicle should have temperature and humidity control. In very cold environments of 0°C and less, there is always concern about the temperature shock that eggs are exposed to during loading at the farm, and sometimes during unloading at the hatchery. Where effective temperatures (taking into account wind chill) are predictably low in the winter season, then it may be advantageous to shroud egg trolleys with plastic covers. If hatching eggs are shipped by air, then shrouding of eggs with plastic is again useful in winter months since eggs can sit outside the plane for 15-20 minutes in some situations.

8.10 SPIKING

Spiking refers to the practice of introducing new roosters into an established older breeder flock. It is usually practiced in order to try and improve fertility, and to some extent, it is necessary because of other management problems. As roosters get older, their sexual activity declines, and this is especially evident when they are overweight. Spiking was a very common practice before the acceptance of separate male feeding, where it was realized that a proportion of roosters would become overweight and ineffective at mating. The situation should be less severe today, but the concept is still considered when fertility is too low after 45 weeks of age. If spiking is to be considered, then it must be preplanned, because there obviously needs to be a source of new roosters to add to the flock. Young immature (20-28 week old) roosters rarely perform well when mixed with mature birds, and so simply diverting a portion of roosters from a younger flock at this time is rarely successful. On the other hand, it is quite difficult to manage large groups of mature males without there being fighting and generally aggressive behavior.

The major reason for spiking will be low fertility, and the fact that the flock has at least 10 weeks to go before scheduled termination. The costs associated with spiking are the normal rearing costs of the rooster to maturity, and then holding costs prior to introduction to the breeder house. The cost per rooster placed is going to be in the order of $10 per bird, including transportation and culling of inactive roosters from the flock. For break even costs, replacement for each 4% of males in the flock, must result in a 1% increase in fertility of the flock for at least 15 weeks. In order to realize a 7-10% increase in fertility, which is the normal outcome of spiking, then no more than 30-35% of the roosters should be replaced.

The most important management decision to be made regarding spiking, is which roosters to remove from the flock. Simply adding 10-30% extra roosters causes tremendous social problems, and so the original number of roosters must be approximately maintained. Obviously heavy or light weight roosters can be culled, or those with any physical problems such as crooked toes or foot pad lesions. General culling procedures must be applied to the remaining birds, involving such factors as color of comb and wattles, general feather and skin condition, and general alertness when approached for catching. Culling of roosters can be very disruptive to the hens, and is sometimes best be done at dusk with the aid of a flashlight or by using a system of blue lights which has a very calming effect on the flock, while allowing the attendants to easily see and assess the birds.

8.11 COST OF PRODUCING HATCHING EGGS

The major cost of producing hatching eggs is the breeder feed, and so this accounts for regional differences in economics of breeder production management. Table 8.11 provides mean costs for maintaining a breeder female, taking into account an 8% carrying cost of roosters.

TABLE 8.11 Breeder cost of production (assumes 8% roosters, added to costs)

	US$
Cost of hen to 24 weeks	6.25
Breeder feed	7.50
Labor	2.00
Vaccine, medication, equipment depreciation	2.00
TOTAL	17.75
Cost per dozen hatching eggs @ 160 eggs/hen	1.33
Cost per chick @ 82% hatchability	13.5¢

8.12 HATCHABILITY TROUBLESHOOTING

Investigating problems of poor hatchability is often confounded by the fact that contributing events may have occurred weeks or even months previously. Unless the hatchery is undertaking weekly breakout of fresh eggs, then it is often hatch results from eggs laid 3-4 weeks previously that are suspect.

The main question to answer relates to eggs being fertile or not, and while this sounds like a relatively simple question, there is often confusion during diagnosis at the hatchery. Once an egg has been incubated for just a few days, it becomes increasingly more difficult to differentiate between an infertile and an early dead germ. In the warm moist environment of the incubator there is a rapid change in yolk color, consistency and appearance, and so identification becomes more difficult.

As previously described in Section 2.11, fertility is best assessed at the farm by breaking out fresh eggs. In this situation, the fertile egg is characterized by a raised "doughnut" shaped ring of lighter color than the surrounding yolk (Fig 8.21).

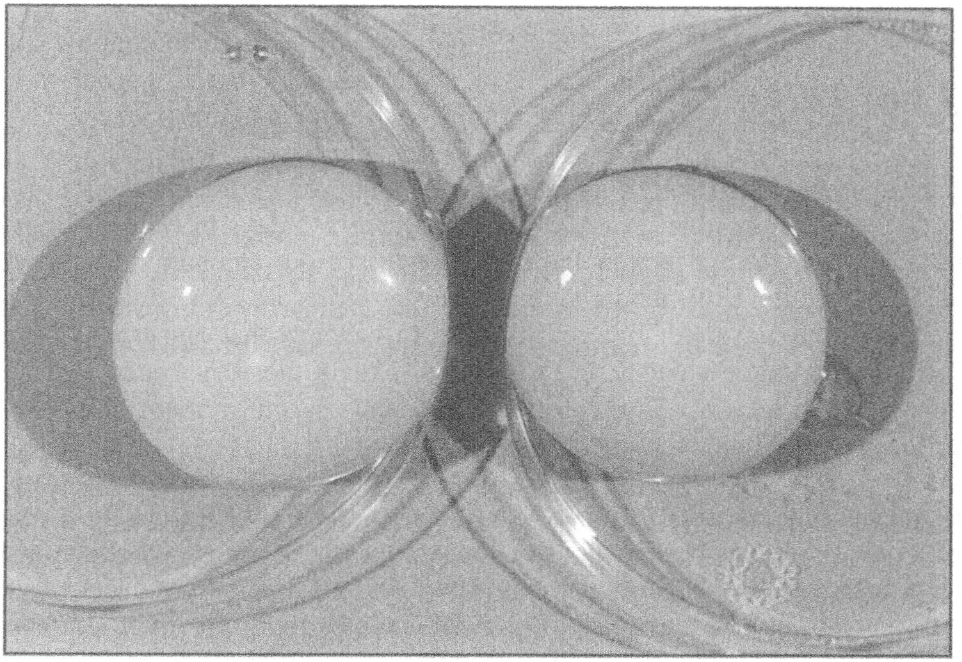

Fig. 8.21 Fertile egg with raised "doughnut" development, and an infertile egg.

If fertility is less than standard, then the check list as shown in Table 8.12 should be followed. Fertility problems usually relate to the male, since if the hen lays an egg then there is little chance of it being infertile if sperm are present in the oviduct. However if the hen is in generally poor condition, the mating activity may be reduced, and patterns of ovulation and fertility may be adversely affected. High temperatures are a fairly common cause of infertility. The male is particularly affected by heat stress and infertility may not occur until 10-14 d following the high temperatures, and low sperm production may continue for 3-4 weeks following the actual stress conditions. Maintaining an effective mating ratio is one of the major factors influencing late cycle fertility. If the number of effective (actively mating) males is much less than 6 per 100 females, then fertility may decline more quickly than expected. This problem, caused by high male mortality, can only practically be resolved by introducing new males into the flock.

If reduced hatchability is due to early dead embryos (less than 5d incubation) then such problems most likely relate to on farm conditions. It is unusual for the very young embryo to die because of improper incubation conditions, unless there are extremes in temperature. The very young embryo is, however, quite sensitive to pre-incubation temperature, humidity and physical handling. Pre-incubation can occur if eggs remain in the nest too long, especially in warmer climates, and this "over-developed" embryo is most likely to die during subsequent cooling and re-heating during actual incubation. Pre-incubation most commonly occurs if eggs are not cooled adequately at the farm or during transport to the hatchery.

Once eggs have been sorted and cleaned they should be ideally cooled to 19-20°C as soon as possible. Such cooling can take 2-3 days to occur if eggs are boxed prior to storage at the farm, and resultant pre-incubation can lead to embryo mortality. Unfortunately, many breeder farms are located some distance from main highways (for biosecurity) and this means that egg trucks have to travel considerable distances on farm roads. Again the very young embryo is susceptible to excessive physical movement, and such movement of eggs does lead to some loss in hatchability.

It is unusual for breeder nutrition to be a factor in early embryo mortality. Unless a breeder diet is grossly deficient in any nutrient (in which case egg production will also be affected) then the embryo can grow for 7-10 d on very meager reserves of most vitamins and minerals. Such deficiencies therefore more commonly result in mid-dead embryo mortality, which occurs characteristically in the 10-14 d period of incubation. During the very early stages of a nutrient deficiency, embryos may in fact develop almost completely, and so the first signs of this are late (18-20 d) morality. As the deficiency proceeds, then mid-dead embryo mortality quickly becomes the characteristic feature (see section 5.6).

Problems with late dead embryo mortality are usually associated with incubator conditions, and are rarely farm related.

TABLE 8.12 Hatchability troubleshooting

Reduced Hatchability

(All flocks?) → **INFERTILE** | (All flocks?) → **FERTILE**

INFERTILE			FERTILE		
Male	**General**	**Female**	**Early Dead**	**Mid Dead**	**Late Dead**
Body weight/ condition	Mating ratio	Body wt/condition	Nest management	Breeder nutrition especially vitamins	Setter/hatcher conditions
Foot pad lesions	Litter condition	ELISA	On-farm egg storage		°C, RH, turning, O_2/ CO_2
ELISA	Environmental temp.	Feather condition	Egg transport		Transfer conditions
Feed intake	Water intake/quality	Feed intake	Hatchery egg holding		Pull-time
	Feed analysis	Feed clean-up time			
	Lighting program	Adequacy of feed grills			

INDEX

Lightning Source UK Ltd.
Milton Keynes UK
UKOW07f0310250717
305955UK00001B/7/P

9 781899 043392